Praise for *Mind Over Mood*

"Only rarely does a book come along that can truly change your life. *Mind Over Mood* is such a book. Dennis Greenberger and Christine A. Padesky have distilled the wisdom and science of psychotherapy and written an easily understandable manual for change."
—*from the Foreword by Aaron T. Beck, MD, developer of cognitive therapy*

"Based on over 40 years of front-line research, this renowned book provides clinically proven strategies to help you manage your mind and the emotions that can so easily destroy your quality of life. Drs. Greenberger and Padesky show how your thoughts affect your feelings and teach step-by-step skills so you can free yourself from painful moods. The first edition of this book was a classic—the second edition is even better, and will be a trusted guide for even more people across the globe."
—*Mark Williams, DPhil, coauthor of* The Mindful Way Workbook

"Over a million people have used *Mind Over Mood* to alleviate—and in many cases eliminate—the suffering caused by depression and other psychological problems. Drs. Greenberger and Padesky are brilliant therapists whose thoroughly updated second edition is informed by the latest research and therapeutic innovations. Science has demonstrated incontrovertibly that changing the way we think about emotional situations is among the most powerful ways to change emotions themselves. Everyone struggling with challenging moods or emotions should read this book."
—*David H. Barlow, PhD, ABPP, coauthor of* 10 Steps to Mastering Stress

"True to its title, this book really can help you transform your thinking so you can make lasting changes."
—*Judith S. Beck, PhD, President, Beck Institute for Cognitive Behavior Therapy*

MIND OVER MOOD

Also Available

For Professionals

Collaborative Case Conceptualization:
Working Effectively with Clients in Cognitive-Behavioral Therapy
Willem Kuyken, Christine A. Padesky, and Robert Dudley

MIND OVER MOOD

SECOND EDITION

Change How You Feel
by Changing the
Way You Think

Dennis Greenberger, PhD
Christine A. Padesky, PhD

Foreword by Aaron T. Beck, MD

**Mishawaka-Penn-Harris
Public Library
Mishawaka, Indiana**

THE GUILFORD PRESS
New York   London

© 2016 Dennis Greenberger and Christine A. Padesky

Published by The Guilford Press
A Division of Guilford Publications, Inc.
370 Seventh Avenue, Suite 1200, New York, NY 10001
www.guilford.com

All rights reserved

The information in this volume is not intended as a substitute for consultation with healthcare professionals. Each individual's health concerns should be evaluated by a qualified professional.

Purchasers of this book have permission to copy worksheets and boxes, where indicated by footnotes, for personal use or use with individual clients. No other part of this book may be reproduced, translated, stored in a retrieval system, or transmitted, in any form or by any means, electronic, mechanical, photocopying, microfilming, recording, or otherwise, without written permission from the publisher.

Printed in the United States of America

Last digit is print number: 9   8   7   6   5   4   3   2   1

Library of Congress Cataloging-in-Publication Data

Greenberger, Dennis.
    Mind over mood : change how you feel by changing the way you think / Dennis Greenberger and Christine A. Padesky. – Second edition.
        pages   cm
    Includes bibliographical references and index.
    ISBN 978-1-4625-2042-8 (pbk. : alk. paper)
    1. Cognitive therapy – Popular works.   2. Affective disorders – Treatment.
 I. Padesky, Christine A.   II. Title.
    RC489.C63G74 2016
    616.89′1425 – dc23
                                                                    2015025241

Contents

	Foreword	*vii*
	Acknowledgments	*xi*
	A Brief Message for Clinicians and Interested Readers	*xv*
	List of Worksheets	*xix*
1	How *Mind Over Mood* Can Help You	*1*
2	Understanding Your Problems	*5*
3	It's the Thought That Counts	*16*
4	Identifying and Rating Moods	*25*
5	Setting Personal Goals and Noticing Improvement	*33*
6	Situations, Moods, and Thoughts	*39*
7	Automatic Thoughts	*50*
8	Where's the Evidence?	*69*
9	Alternative or Balanced Thinking	*95*
10	New Thoughts, Action Plans, and Acceptance	*117*
11	Underlying Assumptions and Behavioral Experiments	*132*
12	Core Beliefs	*152*

13	Understanding Your Depression	188
14	Understanding Your Anxiety	219
15	Understanding Your Anger, Guilt, and Shame	252
16	Maintaining Your Gains and Experiencing More Happiness	280
	Epilogue	292
	Appendix: Duplicate Copies of Selected Worksheets	297
	Index	333
	About the Authors	341

> Purchasers of this book can download and print additional copies of the worksheets from *www.guilford.com/MOM2-materials* for personal use or use with individual clients.

Foreword

Only rarely does a book come along that can truly change your life. *Mind Over Mood* is such a book. Dennis Greenberger and Christine A. Padesky have distilled the wisdom and science of psychotherapy and written an easily understandable manual for change. The first edition of this book has been read, reread, and recommended to others by therapists, patients, and people seeking to improve their lives.

When I first began developing cognitive therapy (CT) in the late 1950s, I had no idea that it would become one of the most effective and widely practiced psychotherapies in the world. Originally, this therapy was designed to help people overcome depression. Our positive results in treating depression were followed by widespread interest in CT. Today CT is the most widely practiced form of psychotherapy in the world, in large part because the treatment has been shown to produce positive, often rapid outcomes with enduring effects.

CT has been successfully used to help patients with depression, panic disorder, phobias, anxiety, anger, stress-related disorders, relationship problems, drug and alcohol abuse, eating disorders, psychosis, and most of the other difficulties that bring people to therapy. This book teaches readers the central principles that have made this therapy successful for all these problems.

Mind Over Mood has proven to be a significant milestone in the evolution of CT. Never before have the nuts and bolts of CT been spelled out so explicitly in a step-by-step fashion for the lay public. Drs. Greenberger and Padesky generously provide the guiding questions, hints and reminders, and worksheets that they have developed in their own clinical practices; these materials can serve as both a vehicle and a road map for people seeking to make fundamental changes in their lives. This is a rare and special book that can easily be used for self-help or as an adjunct to therapy. Not only a self-help book, it has been used to teach graduate students in mental health fields and psychiatric residents how to practice CT effectively. It is unusual for a book to be written so simply that it can be used for self-help and yet teach such important principles that it can guide the highest levels of education. *Mind Over Mood* has proven to be one of the best-selling CT books, with translations in more than 22 languages.

I'm pleased that this second edition of *Mind Over Mood* offers expanded sections on how to use CT for anxiety, which reflect developments in the field since the first edition was published. This new edition also includes sections on mindfulness, acceptance, forgiveness, gratitude, and positive psychology. Readers learn how to incorporate these principles within the CT model to help relieve distress and build happiness.

Drs. Greenberger and Padesky have been students, colleagues, and friends of mine for many years. Together, they have a unique blend of talent, experience, and education that has helped bring this book to fruition. Dennis Greenberger has been an innovator in the application of CT in inpatient and outpatient settings. His work has focused on developing highly effective treatment programs based on psychotherapy research. Dr. Greenberger established and directs the Anxiety and Depression Center, a CT specialty clinic in Newport Beach, California. The Anxiety and Depression Center serves as a model for the provision of warm, compassionate, empirically guided CT for children, adolescents, and adults. In addition to directing this center, Dr. Greenberger teaches and provides supervision to psychiatric residents, graduate students in psychology, and clinicians looking to develop and refine their CT skills. Dr. Greenberger served as the President of the Academy of Cognitive Therapy, an organization that I founded, which certifies the competence of cognitive therapists.

Christine A. Padesky and I have worked together since 1982, teaching CT to thousands of therapists worldwide. After hundreds of hours of conversations together, she understands CT better than almost any other therapist. I have observed and admire the warmth, clarity, and focus she brings to her relationships with clients. Dr. Padesky founded the Center for Cognitive Therapy, now in Huntington Beach, California, in 1983. It has become a major international CT training center for therapists. She personally has taught CT to more than 45,000 therapists in 22 countries. She is well respected by her colleagues and has won statewide, national, and international awards for her many original contributions to the field. Two of her early contributions were the development of the five-part model to understand distress and the seven-column Thought Record. Readers of this book have benefited and will benefit by learning to apply these methods to their own problems. She is a Distinguished Founding Fellow of the Academy of Cognitive Therapy and an international consultant to therapists, clinics, forensic hospitals, and educational programs.

Drs. Greenberger's and Padesky's superb abilities and extensive experience as therapists, innovators, and educators are melded in this exemplary book. In the same way that *Cognitive Therapy of Depression,* which I cowrote with John

Rush, Brian Shaw, and Gary Emery (New York: Guilford Press, 1979), revolutionized how therapy was conducted, *Mind Over Mood* sets the standard for how CT is utilized. Its explicit instructions help therapists and readers adhere more closely to established CT principles and consequently improve the quality of their therapy and their lives. *Mind Over Mood* is an effective tool that puts CT in the hands of the reader.

AARON T. BECK, MD
Professor Emeritus of Psychiatry
University of Pennsylvania

President Emeritus
Beck Institute for Cognitive Behavior Therapy

Acknowledgments

We are indebted to Aaron T. Beck for his pioneering development of cognitive therapy. His work is the foundation and inspiration for *Mind Over Mood*. As mentor, colleague, and friend, he helped both of us define our careers as psychologists. He actively supported this project and generously provided critical feedback to improve the book's value. We hope that this second edition of *Mind Over Mood* is consistent with his vision of cognitive-behavioral therapy (CBT) and provides clear guidance so people can help themselves – a central commitment of his own work, and one that he has passed along to us.

Kathleen A. Mooney critiqued early versions of this book and provided detailed feedback on every chapter. Her gentle honesty, unending enthusiasm, and creativity as a skilled cognitive therapist, as well as her editorial and visual design expertise, substantially enhanced the content and format of the book. For example, she recommended we include Helpful Hints and Reminders and later designed the icons that make these easy to find. Her generous contributions of ideas at every stage made this a better book.

Our editor at The Guilford Press, Kitty Moore, has always been a strong advocate for *Mind Over Mood* and a source of encouragement for us. In fact, everyone with whom we work at Guilford consistently reflects the professionalism, intelligence, and integrity that make Guilford a leader in mental health publishing. We extend special appreciation to Seymour Weingarten, Editor-in-Chief, for sharing our vision.

Rose Mooney's feedback on an early draft of the first edition led to restructuring of several chapters to improve readability. She served as our image of the ideal thoughtful reader as we were writing this book.

The CBT community contributed to this book in innumerable ways. We are grateful to all the researchers around the world who work so hard to learn what people can do to help themselves loosen the grip of troubling moods. We owe a debt of gratitude to the tens of thousands of therapists who embraced the first edition of our book enthusiastically and used it in so many creative ways with their clients. Many of these therapists generously offered their ideas on how we might improve *Mind Over Mood*. We feel privileged to enjoy friendships as well as close working relationships with so many in our field. Our second edition is designed to reflect the art and science of evidence-based therapy, which this dedicated community of therapists and scholars helps shape.

Most importantly, we thank more than a million readers of our first edition of *Mind Over Mood*. Some of you wrote on every page of the book until it was filled with your thoughts and heartfelt emotions. Others copied worksheets over and over again until you mastered the skills. Your efforts, commitment, and thoughtful feedback inspired us as we worked for three years on this second edition. In addition, every one of our clients has asked questions and shared experiences that contributed to our understanding of how people change. Although we are unable to acknowledge you by name, this book is a product of your openness and hard work. You have taught us to be better therapists and writers. Your lessons to us are reflected in this book.

We are also grateful that our own collaborative process in writing this book was such a pleasure; our work was accompanied by laughter and discovery. We literally wrote each page together – a process that was labor-intensive, but led to a book far better than what either of us could have produced alone.

DENNIS GREENBERGER AND CHRISTINE A. PADESKY

On an individual basis:

Thanks to Deidre Greenberger for her warmth and love. Her unwavering faith in me and in this project is a source of continuing strength and inspiration. Her intelligence, humor, spontaneity, curiosity, and wisdom have added to this book and to my life. And thanks also to Elysa and Alanna Greenberger, the two sweetest blessings in my life.

Weekly meetings and informal consultations at the Anxiety and Depression Center with Perry Passaro, Shanna Farmer, David Lindquist, Janine Schroth, Robert Yeilding, Bryan Guthrie, and Jamie Flack Lesser have contributed to this book in significant ways. Our thought-provoking discussions embrace the principles and expand the boundaries of CBT in ways that have influenced this second edition. I always learn from and am impressed by how talented and experienced therapists use the principles and strategies in *Mind Over Mood* to create positive client outcomes. A special acknowledgment to my good friend and trusted colleague Perry Passaro. He has helped sharpen my thinking and added dimension and new meaning to what cognitive therapy can be.

DENNIS GREENBERGER

My entire career is indebted to Aaron T. Beck. His first books set the course for my career, and our nearly 40-year friendship has enriched each year of my life immeasurably. His curiosity, creativity, humor, collaborative spirit, and kindness still inspire me every day.

Kathleen Mooney, my partner for the past 35 years, contributes to all my CBT projects. She has an ability to recognize good ideas and make them better by infusing them with her creative vision, and this book exemplifies her contributions. Kathleen sustains and inspires me with her energetic spirit, honest critique of ideas, unwavering support, and humor. Whether navigating new territory or finding my way home, I rely on her wisdom and guidance. Each day is better because of her.

CHRISTINE A. PADESKY

A Brief Message for Clinicians and Interested Readers

Outcome research demonstrates the effectiveness of cognitive-behavioral therapy (CBT) for a wide variety of psychological problems, including depression, anxiety, anger, eating disorders, substance abuse, and relationship problems. *Mind Over Mood* is a hands-on workbook that teaches CBT skills in a clear, step-by-step format. It is designed to help readers understand their problems better and make fundamental changes in their lives, either with the aid of a therapist or on their own.

Clinicians can use *Mind Over Mood* to structure therapy, to reinforce skills taught to clients, and to help clients continue the therapeutic learning process after formal therapy ends. With extensive worksheets and mood questionnaires, this book actively enlists clients' participation in applying what is learned in therapy to everyday life experiences. CBT skills are taught sequentially, and as readers progress through the book, new skills build upon previously learned skills. The book's structure, along with Helpful Hints and troubleshooting guides on how to navigate common "stuck points," helps readers successfully apply CBT principles so they can resolve their problems and experience greater happiness and life satisfaction.

We are very pleased and humbled by the widespread popularity of the first edition of *Mind Over Mood*. At the time we wrote it, we intended to use empirical findings about what made therapy effective to write a book that therapists could use to improve their own therapy outcomes. One of the exciting features of CBT is that it teaches clients skills to help them become their own therapists. We hoped that a clear manual teaching these skills would resonate both with self-help readers and with therapists as a guide for therapy.

Mind Over Mood was recognized as an inaugural recipient of the Association for Behavioral and Cognitive Therapies Self-Help Book Seal of Merit. This Self-Help Seal of Merit is given only to books that:

- Employ cognitive and/or behavioral principles.
- Have documented empirical support for the methods presented.
- Include no suggestions or methods that are contraindicated by scientific evidence.
- Present treatment methods that have consistent evidence for their effectiveness.
- Are consistent with best psychotherapy practices.

Therapists can feel confident that the skills their clients learn by using *Mind Over Mood* are the skills that have been shown in decades of research to produce the best treatment outcomes for depression, anxiety, and other mood problems. Research demonstrates that clients not only get better but experience longer-lasting improvement (have lower relapse rates) when they learn the skills taught in *Mind Over Mood* and are able to apply these skills on their own, independently of a therapist.

The second edition of *Mind Over Mood* is substantially improved over the first edition, reflecting more than two decades of innovations in research and therapy. This new edition incorporates and integrates additional, empirically supported methods: imagery, acceptance, and mindfulness; fear ladders and exposure for anxiety; tolerating distress and ambiguity; and positive psychology. There is also a fully updated presentation of behavioral activation, relaxation, and cognitive restructuring approaches for mood management. At the same time, this edition retains the core features of the first edition that made it so popular and useful for readers and therapists.

Over the years, we have been surprised and impressed with the creative ways in which *Mind Over Mood* is used by clinicians and readers. Psychology graduate schools and psychiatric residency programs around the world use *Mind Over Mood* as a required text for teaching CBT. *Mind Over Mood* has been translated into more than 22 languages, and the skills taught have proven to be relevant to people in diverse cultures and across the economic spectrum.

A colleague told us that as she was walking into a clinic in Bangladesh, she saw a woman drawing in the dirt with a stick. When she got closer, she realized that the woman was writing out the Thought Record from the first edition of *Mind Over Mood*. Another colleague told us that Aboriginal leaders in Australia found the five-part model from Chapter 2 of *Mind Over Mood* one of the most culturally relevant models for linking CBT ideas with their own long-standing cultural wisdom. The book has been used in well-known addiction treatment centers, psychology clinics, hospitals, and forensic units, as well as with homeless populations. And, of course, the majority of copies have been purchased by individuals who discover it for self-help or have the book recommended to them by mental health professionals. These many uses of *Mind Over Mood* speak to the desires of both clinicians and members of the lay public to learn and use practical, proven strategies for mood management.

The first edition of *Mind Over Mood* was accompanied by a companion book, *Clinician's Guide to Mind Over Mood*, which provided in-depth recommendations for effectively incorporating *Mind Over Mood* into therapy for various client problems and in different clinical settings. A revised edition of this *Clinician's Guide* will be available in 2016.

We hope that this second edition of *Mind Over Mood* will continue to be a useful guide for people who want to positively transform their moods and their lives. Whether *Mind Over Mood* skills are developed by using a stick in the dirt or a digital device, the goal is the same – for people to learn skills that lead to greater happiness and life satisfaction.

We urge clinicians to be curious and take a learning perspective when they use *Mind Over Mood* with clients. Each person's experience of the world is different, and yet common principles can be used to understand how those experiences are formed and can be transformed. Psychological knowledge and the principles of psychotherapy have advanced since *Mind Over Mood*'s first edition. We have done our best to incorporate these new ideas and findings into this second edition, so that it continues to reflect the best of evidence-based therapy practice.

DENNIS GREENBERGER
CHRISTINE A. PADESKY

Sign up at www.guilford.com/MOM2-alerts to receive e-alerts with the latest information from the authors plus special announcements about e-book editions, a Spanish-language edition, the second edition of the *Clinician's Guide to Mind Over Mood* (coming in 2016), and other *Mind Over Mood* news.

List of Worksheets

WORKSHEET 2.1.	Understanding My Problems	14
WORKSHEET 3.1.	The Thought Connections	22
WORKSHEET 4.1.	Identifying Moods	28
WORKSHEET 4.2.	Identifying and Rating Moods	30
WORKSHEET 5.1.	Setting Goals	34
WORKSHEET 5.2.	Advantages and Disadvantages of Reaching and Not Reaching My Goals	35
WORKSHEET 5.3.	What Will Help Me Reach My Goals?	36
WORKSHEET 5.4.	Signs of Improvement	37
WORKSHEET 6.1.	Distinguishing Situations, Moods, and Thoughts	47
WORKSHEET 7.1.	Connecting Thoughts and Moods	57
WORKSHEET 7.2.	Separating Situations, Moods, and Thoughts	58
WORKSHEET 7.3.	Identifying Automatic Thoughts	60
WORKSHEET 7.4.	Identifying Hot Thoughts	64
WORKSHEET 8.1.	Facts versus Interpretations	72
WORKSHEET 8.2.	Where's the Evidence?	88
WORKSHEET 9.1.	Completing Linda's Thought Record	108
WORKSHEET 9.2.	Thought Record	114
WORKSHEET 10.1.	Strengthening New Thoughts	119
WORKSHEET 10.2.	Action Plan	125
WORKSHEET 10.3.	Acceptance	129
WORKSHEET 11.1.	Identifying Underlying Assumptions	140
WORKSHEET 11.2.	Experiments to Test an Underlying Assumption	149
WORKSHEET 12.1.	Identifying Core Beliefs	159
WORKSHEET 12.2.	Downward Arrow Technique: Identifying Core Beliefs about Self	160

WORKSHEET 12.3.	Downward Arrow Technique: Identifying Core Beliefs about Other People	*161*
WORKSHEET 12.4.	Downward Arrow Technique: Identifying Core Beliefs about the World (or My Life)	*162*
WORKSHEET 12.5.	Identifying a New Core Belief	*165*
WORKSHEET 12.6.	Core Belief Record: Recording Evidence That Supports a New Core Belief	*166*
WORKSHEET 12.7.	Rating Confidence in My New Core Belief	*168*
WORKSHEET 12.8.	Rating Behaviors on a Scale	*171*
WORKSHEET 12.9.	Behavioral Experiments to Strengthen New Core Beliefs	*174*
WORKSHEET 12.10.	Gratitude about the World and My Life	*177*
WORKSHEET 12.11.	Gratitude about Others	*178*
WORKSHEET 12.12.	Gratitude about Myself	*179*
WORKSHEET 12.13.	Learning from My Gratitude Journal	*180*
WORKSHEET 12.14.	Expressing Gratitude	*183*
WORKSHEET 12.15.	Acts of Kindness	*185*
WORKSHEET 13.1.	*Mind Over Mood* Depression Inventory	*191*
WORKSHEET 13.2.	*Mind Over Mood* Depression Inventory Scores	*192*
WORKSHEET 13.3.	Identifying Cognitive Aspects of Depression	*197*
WORKSHEET 13.4.	Activity Record	*206*
WORKSHEET 13.5.	Learning from My Activity Record	*208*
WORKSHEET 13.6.	Activity Schedule	*214*
WORKSHEET 14.1.	*Mind Over Mood* Anxiety Inventory	*221*
WORKSHEET 14.2.	*Mind Over Mood* Anxiety Inventory Scores	*222*
WORKSHEET 14.3.	Identifying Thoughts Associated with Anxiety	*232*
WORKSHEET 14.4.	Making a Fear Ladder	*238*
WORKSHEET 14.5.	My Fear Ladder	*239*
WORKSHEET 14.6.	Ratings for My Relaxation Methods	*246*
WORKSHEET 15.1.	Measuring and Tracking My Moods	*253*
WORKSHEET 15.2.	Mood Scores Chart	*254*
WORKSHEET 15.3.	Understanding Anger, Guilt, and Shame	*257*
WORKSHEET 15.4.	Writing a Forgiveness Letter	*265*
WORKSHEET 15.5.	Ratings for My Anger Management Strategies	*266*
WORKSHEET 15.6.	Rating the Seriousness of My Actions	*271*
WORKSHEET 15.7.	Using a Responsibility Pie for Guilt or Shame	*274*
WORKSHEET 15.8.	Making Reparations for Hurting Someone	*275*
WORKSHEET 15.9.	Forgiving Myself	*278*
WORKSHEET 16.1.	*Mind Over Mood* Skills Checklist	*282*
WORKSHEET 16.2.	My Plan to Reduce Relapse Risk	*288*

MIND OVER MOOD

1

How *Mind Over Mood* Can Help You

An oyster creates a pearl out of a grain of sand. The grain of sand irritates the oyster. In response, the oyster creates a smooth, protective coating that covers the sand and provides relief. This protective coating is a beautiful pearl. For an oyster, an irritant becomes the seed for something new and beautiful. Similarly, *Mind Over Mood* will help you develop something new: beneficial skills to lead you out of your current discomfort. The skills you learn by using this book will help you feel better and will continue to have value in your life long after your original problems are gone.

We hope that, like many people who have learned the methods taught in this book, you will look back at the initial discomfort that led you to *Mind Over Mood* as a "blessing in disguise," because it provided you the opportunity and motivation to develop pearls of wisdom and invaluable new perspectives that will help you enjoy the rest of your life more fully.

HOW WILL THIS BOOK HELP YOU?

Mind Over Mood teaches you strategies, methods, and skills that have been shown to be helpful with mood problems such as depression, anxiety, anger, panic, jealousy, guilt, and shame. The skills taught in this book can also help you solve relationship problems, handle stress better, improve your self-esteem, become less fearful, and grow more confident. These strategies also can help you if you are struggling with alcohol or drug use. *Mind Over Mood* is designed to teach you skills in a step-by-step fashion, so you can rapidly make the changes that are important to you.

The ideas in this book come from cognitive-behavioral therapy (CBT), one of today's most effective forms of psychotherapy. "Cognitive" refers to what we think and how we think. Cognitive-behavioral therapists emphasize understanding the thoughts, beliefs, and behaviors connected to our moods, physical experiences, and events in our lives. A central idea in CBT is that our *thoughts* about an event or experience powerfully affects our emotional, behavioral, and physical responses to it.

For example, if we are standing in line at the grocery store and think, "This will take a while. I might as well just relax," we are likely to feel calm. Our bodies stay relaxed, and we may start a conversation with someone standing nearby or pick up a magazine. However, if we think, "They shouldn't have such a long line. They should hire more clerks," we may feel upset and irritated. Our bodies become tense and fidgety, and we may spend our time complaining to other customers and the clerk.

Mind Over Mood teaches you to identify and understand the connections among your thoughts, moods, behaviors, and physical reactions in everyday situations like this one, as well as during major events in your life. You will learn to think about yourself and situations in more helpful ways, and to change the thinking patterns and behaviors that keep you stuck in distressing moods and relationships. You will discover how to make changes in your life when your thoughts alert you to problems that need to be solved. In the end, these changes should help you feel happier, calmer, and more confident. In addition, the skills you learn using *Mind Over Mood* help you create and enjoy more positive relationships.

HOW WILL YOU KNOW IF THIS BOOK IS HELPING?

For any of us, it is much easier to keep trying something when we know we are making progress. For example, when we first learn to read, we often begin by learning the alphabet and recognizing individual letters. Initially, we need to put a lot of effort and practice into recognizing letters. As our skill develops, our recognition of letters becomes easier and more automatic. Over time, we stop paying attention to individual letters, because we have learned to put these letters together and learn simple words. As new readers, we may scan a page looking for words we know. Over time, we develop the skill to read simple sentences, and we know we are making progress when we can read more complicated sentences, paragraphs, and simple books. Soon we are not attending to individual words, but to the meaning of what we are reading. In school, children become better readers year by year, and their reading-level progress can be measured by tests.

Similarly, you will be able to notice and measure the progress you make in using *Mind Over Mood*. In the early weeks, you will learn individual skills. Over time, you will learn to combine these skills in ways that improve your moods and your life. One way to measure your progress is to measure your moods at regular intervals as you develop and practice *Mind Over Mood* skills. Chapter 4 helps you do this and shows you how to graph your scores so you can see your progress over time.

HOW TO USE THIS BOOK

Mind Over Mood is different from other books you may have read. It is designed to help you develop new ways of thinking and behaving that will help you feel better.

These *Mind Over Mood* skills require practice, patience, and perseverance. Therefore, it is important for you to complete the exercises in each chapter. Even some of the skills that look easy can be more complicated than they seem when you actually try to do them. Most people find that the more time they spend practicing each skill, the more benefit they get.

In the beginning, it is helpful to spend some time on these skills every day. You may find it helpful to set aside a regular time each day to read about or practice *Mind Over Mood* skills. If you move too quickly through the book without giving yourself adequate practice time, you will not learn how to apply the skills to your own problems. Thus speed of learning is not the important thing. It is more important to spend enough time with each chapter until you understand the ideas and can use them in your life in a way that is meaningful and helps you feel better. You may find it only takes an hour or so to do this with some chapters of the book. For other chapters, it will take weeks or even months of practice before the skills you learn become automatic and you begin to feel the full benefit.

Mind Over Mood can be customized so that you can read chapters in an order that is likely to be most helpful for you. For example, if you have chosen this book to work on particular moods, at the end of Chapter 4 there is a recommendation that you read the chapters about moods (13, 14, and/or 15) that pertain to you. You can skip any mood chapters that don't apply. After you read those chapters, you can follow the chapter sequence recommended for each particular mood or moods. Alternatively, you may choose to read the book straight through and do the exercises beginning with Chapter 2 and ending with Chapter 16.

If you are using *Mind Over Mood* as part of therapy, your therapist may recommend a different order for reading chapters. There are many ways to customize development of *Mind Over Mood* skills, and your therapist may have their own idea about which sequence will work best for you. If you are bringing this book to the attention of your therapist, you might suggest that he or she read the "A Brief Message for Clinicians and Interested Readers" on pages xv–xvii.

Can You Use *Mind Over Mood* Skills for Issues Other Than Moods?

Yes. The same *Mind Over Mood* skills that help manage moods can also help you with stress; alcohol and drug use; eating issues such as bingeing, purging, or overeating; relationship struggles; low self-esteem; and other issues. It also can be used to develop positive moods, such as happiness and a sense of meaning and purpose in your life.

What If You Want to Use Worksheets More Than Once?

Throughout the book, there are exercises designed to help you learn and apply the important skills introduced in that chapter. The worksheets that accompany these exercises are meant to be practiced over time. Additional copies of many of the exercise worksheets can be found in the Appendix at the end of the book (and all of them are available to download for your personal use at *www.guilford.com/MOM2-materials*), so that you can copy and use them whenever you think they might help.

Mind Over Mood skills and strategies are based on decades of research. These are proven, practical, and powerful methods that, once learned, lead to greater happiness and life satisfaction. By investing time in reading this book and practicing what you learn, you are taking steps to transform your life in a positive way.

Chapter 1 Summary

- Cognitive-behavioral therapy (CBT) is a proven, effective therapy for depression, anxiety, anger, and other moods.

- CBT can also be used to help with eating disorders, alcohol and drug use, stress, low self-esteem, and many other problems.

- *Mind Over Mood* is designed to teach CBT skills in a step-by-step fashion.

- Most people find that the more time they spend practicing each skill, the more benefit they get.

- There are guides throughout the book to help you customize the chapter reading order so you can target the moods that concern you the most.

2
Understanding Your Problems

BEN: *I hate getting old.*

One afternoon a therapist received a telephone call from Sylvie, a 73-year-old woman who was concerned about her husband, Ben. She had read an article about depression, and it seemed to describe him. For the past six months, Ben had complained constantly about feeling tired; yet Sylvie heard him pacing around the living room at three in the morning, unable to sleep. In addition, she said he was not as warm as usual toward her, and he was often irritable and negative. He had stopped visiting his friends and didn't seem interested in doing anything. After his doctor checked him and said he didn't have a medical problem that would explain these symptoms, Ben complained to his wife, "I hate getting old. It feels lousy."

The therapist asked to talk with Ben on the phone, and Ben reluctantly came on the line. He told the therapist not to take it personally, but he didn't think much of "head doctors" and didn't want to see the therapist because he wasn't crazy, just old. "You wouldn't be happy either if you were 78 and ached all over!" He said he would go to one appointment just to satisfy Sylvie, but he was sure it wouldn't help.

How we understand our problems has an effect on how we cope. Ben thought that his sleep problems, tiredness, irritability, and lack of interest in doing things were normal parts of growing older. Growing old was something Ben couldn't change, so he didn't expect that anything could help him feel better.

At their first meeting, the therapist was immediately struck by the difference in Sylvie's and Ben's appearance. In a rose-colored skirt with a coordinating floral blouse, earrings, and shoes, Sylvie had dressed herself carefully for the meeting. She sat upright in her chair and greeted the therapist with an expectant smile and bright, eager eyes. In contrast, Ben sat slumped in his chair, and although he was neatly dressed, he had a slight stubble on the left side of his chin. His eyes were dull and surrounded by the dark circles of fatigue. He stood up stiffly and slowly to greet the therapist, saying grimly, "Well, you got me for an hour."

As the therapist gently questioned Ben over the next 30 minutes, his story slowly unfolded. With each question, Ben sighed deeply and then responded flatly. Ben had been a truck driver for 35 years, making local deliveries for the last 14 of those years. After his retirement, he met regularly with three retired friends to talk, eat a meal, or watch sports. Ben also liked fixing things, working on house projects, and repairing bicycles for his eight young grandchildren and their friends. He regularly saw his three children and the grandchildren, and he felt proud to have a good relationship with each of them.

Eighteen months earlier, Sylvie had been diagnosed with breast cancer. Her cancer had been detected early, and she had recovered well after surgery and radiation treatment, with no further signs of cancer. Ben became teary as he talked about her illness: "I thought I'd lose her, and I didn't know what I'd do." As he said this, Sylvie jumped in quickly, patting Ben on the arm: "But I'm OK, dear. Everything turned out OK." Ben swallowed hard and nodded his head.

While Sylvie was undergoing cancer treatment, one of Ben's best friends, Louie, became suddenly ill and died. Louie had been Ben's friend for 18 years, and Ben felt his loss deeply. He felt angry that Louie had not gone to the hospital sooner, because early treatment might have saved his life. Sylvie said that Ben focused all his attention on tracking her cancer treatment appointments after Louie's death. "I think Ben thought he would be responsible for my death if we missed an appointment," said Sylvie. Ben stopped seeing his friends and devoted himself to Sylvie's care.

"After Sylvie's treatment ended, I knew the relief was only temporary. The rest of my life will be filled with illness and death. I feel half dead already. A young person like yourself can't understand this." Ben sighed. "It's just as well. What use am I, anyway? The grandkids fix their own bikes now. My sons have their own friends, and Sylvie would probably be better off if I wasn't here. I don't know what's worse – to die, or to live and be left all alone because all your friends are dead."

After hearing Ben's story and reviewing his physician's report that there was no physical cause for the way Ben was feeling, it was clear to the therapist that Ben was depressed. He was experiencing physical symptoms (insomnia, appetite loss, fatigue), behavior changes (stopping his usual activities, avoiding friends), mood changes (sadness, irritability, guilt), and a thinking style (negative, self-critical, and pessimistic) consistent with depression. As is often the case with depression, Ben had experienced a number of losses and stresses in the preceding two years (Sylvie's cancer, Louie's death, and the sense that his children and grandchildren didn't need him any more).

Although Ben was skeptical that therapy could help, with Sylvie's encouragement he agreed to go to three more sessions before deciding whether to continue or not.

UNDERSTANDING BEN'S PROBLEMS

During their second meeting, his therapist helped Ben understand the changes he had experienced in the past two years. Using the five-part model in Figure 2.1 on the facing page, Ben noticed that a number of *environmental* changes or major life events (Sylvie's

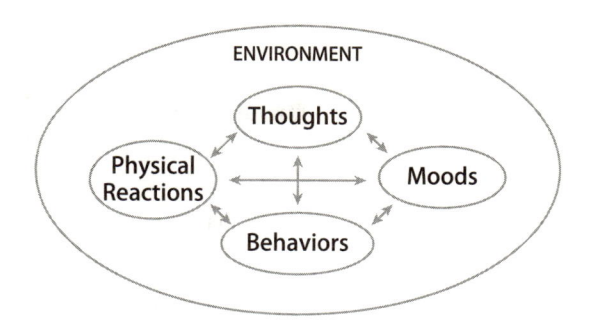

FIGURE 2.1. Five-part model to understand life experiences.
Copyright 1986 by Christine A. Padesky.

cancer, Louie's death) had led to *behavior* changes (the end of regular social time with friends, extra trips to the hospital for Sylvie's cancer treatment). In addition, he began to *think* differently about himself and his life ("Everyone I care about is dying," "My children and grandchildren no longer need me") and to feel worse both *emotionally* (irritable, sad) and *physically* (tired, more trouble sleeping).

Notice that the five areas of Figure 2.1 are interconnected. The connecting arrows show that each different part of our lives influences all the others. For example, changes in our behavior influence how we think and how we feel (both physically and emotionally). Our behavior can also change our environment and life events. Likewise, changes in our thinking affect our behavior, moods, and physical reactions, and can lead to changes in our environment. Understanding how these five parts of our lives interact can help us understand our problems.

Ben could see how each of these five parts of his experience influenced the other four, pulling him deeper into his sad mood. For example, as a result of thinking, "All my friends will die soon because we're getting old" (thought), Ben stopped calling them on the phone (behavior). As Ben became more isolated from his friends, he began to feel lonely and sad (mood), and his inactivity contributed to his sleep problems and tiredness (physical reactions). Since he no longer called his friends or did things with them, many of them stopped calling him (environment). Over time, these interacting forces dragged Ben into a downward spiral of depression.

At first, when Ben and his therapist recognized this pattern, Ben was discouraged: "It's hopeless, then – each of these things will just get worse and worse until I die!" His therapist suggested the possibility that since each of these five areas was connected to the other four, small improvements in any of the areas could contribute to positive change in the others. Ben agreed to experiment to figure out what small changes would make him feel better.

Ben is one of four people described in this chapter whom we follow throughout this book. These four people were experiencing difficulties that are often helped by the strategies and methods described in *Mind Over Mood*. To protect confidentiality, identifying information has been changed, and the descriptive information is a composite of several clients. However, their situations and progress are consistent with our experiences as therapists helping people with these types of problems.

LINDA: *My life would be great if I didn't have panic attacks!*

"One of my friends told me cognitive-behavioral therapy can stop panic attacks. Do you think it would help me?" The phone caller was very direct in her questioning. Her voice was firm and confident as she quizzed the therapist about CBT. She was equally direct in describing her recent experiences that prompted her call. "My name is Linda. I'm 29 years old, and except for a fear of flying in airplanes, I've never had any problems I couldn't handle myself. I'm a marketing supervisor for a company and have always loved my job – until two months ago, that is. Two months ago I was promoted to regional supervisor. Now I need to fly a lot, and I find myself breaking into cold sweats whenever I think about getting on an airplane. I was thinking of going back to my old job when my friend told me to call you first. Can you help me?"

Linda arrived early for her first appointment with her briefcase and a notebook, ready to begin learning what to do. She had been afraid of flying her entire life – a fear she suspected she'd learned from her mother, who always avoided airplanes. Linda's panic attacks had begun eight months ago, before her job promotion.

Linda recalled that her first panic attack happened in a grocery store, when she noticed her heart pounding during her Saturday shopping. She couldn't understand why this was happening and became frightened. This was the first time she broke into a sweat from fear. At the time she thought she was having a heart attack, so she went to the hospital emergency room. After a series of tests, a doctor assured her that she had not had a heart attack and was in good health.

Linda continued to have panic attacks once or twice a month until her recent job promotion. Since her promotion, she had been gripped by fear several times a week. Her heart raced, she broke into a sweat, and she had difficulty breathing. In addition to when she was on an airplane, the panicky feeling sometimes just came "out of the blue – even at home." Her panic would last for a few minutes and then disappear almost as fast as it came. She would feel "on edge" for a few hours afterward.

"I support myself. I have good friends and a supportive family. I don't drink or use drugs. I've always lived a good life. Why is this happening to me?" Linda had in fact led a happy, hard-working, and balanced life. Her only major trauma had been the death of her father a year earlier. She missed him terribly, yet took comfort from her relationship with her mother and two brothers, who lived nearby. Although her job required hard work, Linda seemed to enjoy the pressure, even though she worried a lot about her performance and what others thought of her.

Why was Linda suffering from panic attacks? Throughout this book, we follow Linda's progress in learning to understand her panic attacks. By learning more about the connections among her physical reactions, thoughts, and behaviors, Linda not only learned to overcome her panic and manage her worry, but she also became a relaxed frequent flyer.

UNDERSTANDING LINDA'S PROBLEMS

Linda had panic attacks, worries, and also a fear of flying in airplanes – all anxiety-related problems. Can the model in Figure 2.1 be used to understand anxiety? Notice how the five areas summarize Linda's experiences:

Environment/life changes/situations: My father's death; job promotion.

Physical reactions: Cold sweats; racing heart; difficulty breathing; jumpy.

Moods: Fearful; nervous; panicky.

Behaviors: Avoiding flying; thinking of giving up job promotion.

Thoughts: "I'm having a heart attack," "I'm dying," "What if things go wrong and I can't cope?," "Something bad will happen if I fly."

As you can see, the five-part model describes anxiety as well as it does depression. Notice some of the differences between anxiety and depression. With depression, physical changes often involve a slowing down – trouble sleeping and feeling tired. Anxiety is usually marked by a speeding up of physical reactions – racing heart, increased sweating, feeling jumpy. With depression, the main behavioral change is that people find it difficult to do things, and so they do less and often withdraw from people. Linda described enjoying people and her job, but she avoided specific things that made her anxious. When we are anxious, avoidance is the most common change in our behavior.

Finally, thinking is also quite different in depression and anxiety. Ben's thoughts illustrated depressed thinking, which tends to be negative, hopeless, and self-critical. Linda's thinking was typical of anxiety. It was more catastrophic ("I'm having a heart attack") and involved worry about specific future events (an airplane flight) as well as general worry ("What if things go wrong and I can't cope?"). Depressed thoughts often focus on the past and present, and anxious thoughts focus on the present and future.

Chapters 13, 14, and 15 further summarize the distinguishing characteristics of different moods. Chapter 13 provides a measure of common depression symptoms (see p. 190), and Chapter 14 provides a measure of anxiety symptoms (see p. 220).

MARISSA: *My life isn't worth living.*

Marissa was very depressed. During her first meeting with her therapist, she confided that she was increasingly upset and was beginning to feel out of control. She said that her depression had become worse over the previous six months. This depression frightened her, because she had been seriously depressed twice before – once when she was 18 years old, and again at age 25 – and had made suicide attempts both times. With tears in her eyes, she rolled up her sleeve and showed the scars on her wrist from her first suicide attempt.

Marissa had been sexually molested by her father between the ages of 6 and 14. When she was 14, her parents divorced. By this time, Marissa already thought of herself negatively: "I decided I must be bad for my father to hurt me like he did. I was afraid to get close to other kids, because if they knew what had happened to me, they would think I was a monster. I was also afraid of adults, because I thought they would hurt me too."

Marissa grabbed her first chance to get away from home. She agreed to marry her first boyfriend, Carl. She and Carl were married at age 17 when she became pregnant, and they divorced three years later, shortly after the birth of her second child. Her second marriage, at age 23, lasted only two years. Both of her husbands drank heavily and were physically abusive.

Despite being depressed for 18 months following her second divorce, Marissa emerged from this desperate period in her life feeling stronger. She decided that she could care for her children better on her own, without either of her ex-husbands. She began working and supporting her children by herself. She was a loving mother and was proud of her children. Her older child, now age 19, worked part-time and was a student at a local college; her younger child was doing well in school.

Now, at age 36, Marissa was an administrative assistant for a manufacturing company. Despite her successes as a working mother, Marissa was self-critical. During her first meeting with her therapist, she made minimal eye contact, staring at her hands in her lap. She spoke in a low monotone and did not smile. Her eyes filled with tears on several occasions as she talked about how "worthless" she was and how bleak her future looked to her. "I've been thinking more and more about killing myself. The kids are old enough to take care of themselves. My pain will never end. Death is the only way out."

In response to questions about her life and what made it so painful to her, Marissa described feeling intense sadness all day long. As her depression had become worse over the last six months, Marissa found it increasingly difficult to work and concentrate on her job. She had been given two verbal warnings and a written notice from her supervisor regarding the timeliness, quality, and quantity of her work. She found herself more and more tired, and less and less motivated.

At home, Marissa just wanted to be left alone. She would not answer the phone or talk with family or friends. She prepared minimal meals for her children and then closed herself in her room, watching television until she fell asleep.

At the first meeting, Marissa was not particularly hopeful that CBT would help her, but she had promised her family physician that she would give it a try. She thought that CBT was her last hope, and that if this treatment didn't work, suicide would be her only remaining option. Needless to say, her therapist was very concerned about Marissa and wanted to help her begin to feel better as soon as possible. The therapist referred her to a psychiatrist for a consultation to see if medication might help her, even though she had been helped only a little bit by antidepressants in the past. Marissa and her therapist also agreed that she would track her moods and activities for the upcoming week, so they could see if there was a connection between her mood and what she was doing during each day.

UNDERSTANDING MARISSA'S PROBLEMS

If we use the five-part model in Figure 2.1 to understand Marissa's depression, we can see some similarities between Marissa and Ben in thinking patterns, mood, behavior, and physical experiences. And yet the important life situations contributing to Marissa's depression began back in her early childhood.

Below you see how Marissa and her therapist used the five-part model to understand her depression.

Environment/life changes/situations: My father sexually molested me; both of my husbands were alcoholic and abusive; I'm a single parent of two teenagers; lots of negative feedback from my work supervisor.

Physical reactions: Tired most of the time.

Moods: Depressed.

Behaviors: Difficulty working; I avoid my family and friends; cry easily; cut myself; I tried to kill myself twice.

Thoughts: "I'm no good," "I'm a failure," "I'm never going to get better," "My life is hopeless," "I may as well kill myself."

Some people may think that Marissa was destined to remain depressed because of her harsh life experiences. As you will see, this was not true.

Vic: *Help me be more perfect.*

Vic, a 49-year-old business executive, began therapy three years after he joined Alcoholics Anonymous (AA) to help him stop drinking. Over six feet tall and athletically built, Vic arrived for his first appointment neatly dressed in a gray pin-striped suit and a maroon tie. Every part of Vic's appearance was perfect, from his neatly trimmed hair to his highly polished shoes.

Despite frequent urges to drink, Vic had remained sober most of the past three years. His urge to drink was strongest when he felt sad, nervous, or angry. At these times, he thought, "I can't stand these feelings. I need a drink to feel better." His attendance at AA meetings was irregular, and resisting drinking was still a struggle for him.

Vic was subject to periods of low mood, during which he saw himself as "no good," "worthless," and "a failure." He was often nervous. During these times, Vic worried again and again that he would be fired from his job for poor performance, despite the fact that he consistently received good evaluations. Whenever his phone rang, Vic expected the caller to be his boss, telling him he had been fired. He was surprised and relieved each time this did not happen.

Vic also struggled with periodic outbursts of anger. Although they didn't happen often, these were very destructive, especially in his relationship with his wife, Judy. He quickly became angry when he felt others were disrespecting him, behaving unfairly, mistreating him, or when it seemed as if those close to him didn't care about his feelings. He contained his anger at work, but when these types of situations happened at home, he lost his temper very quickly and exploded in an angry rage. These rages were followed by feelings of intense shame and regret, triggering more thoughts of worthlessness.

Vic described his 25-year battle with alcohol as a result of lifelong feelings of inadequacy, low self-esteem, and a sense that something "awful" was going to happen to him. When he drank he felt better, stronger, and "in control." Becoming sober put the spotlight on his deep feelings of worthlessness, anxiety, and poor self-esteem, which the alcohol had covered up.

Early in therapy, it became clear that Vic was a perfectionist. He had been told by his parents, "If you make a mistake, it's bad," and "If you're going to do something at all, do it right." Vic had concluded, "If I'm not perfect, then I'm a failure."

Vic had grown up with one older brother, Doug, who was a star athlete and straight-A student. As a child, Vic felt that his parents' approval, love, and affection depended on his performance. Although his parents showed their love for Vic in many ways, he never felt that they were as proud of him as they were of Doug. He felt pressured to be the best in school and sports. One year he scored in a big football game, yet Vic was disappointed because a teammate scored twice in the same game. A good performance was not enough for Vic if it was not also the best.

As an adult, Vic found it harder and harder to be the best. He juggled the roles of husband, father, and marketing executive, judging his worth by his performance in each of these areas. He rarely felt perfect in any area of his life and constantly worried about how other people evaluated him. If he worked long hours at the office to please his boss, he worried on the drive home that he was letting down his wife and children.

Vic came to therapy looking for ways to feel better about himself and wanting to feel more confident. He also wanted help staying sober. At the end of the first session, he told the therapist, with a laugh, "Look, all I want is for you to make me perfect, and then I'll be happy." His therapist suggested to Vic that maybe one goal of therapy should be to help him feel happy with himself as he was, imperfections and all. Vic swallowed hard. After a moment, he nodded his head.

UNDERSTANDING VIC'S PROBLEMS

Sometimes we have more than one strong mood. Vic was depressed and anxious, and he also had periodic outbursts of anger. When Vic and his therapist filled out his five-part model, there were some similarities with Ben and Marissa (depression) and also with Linda (anxiety).

Environment/life changes/situations: Mostly sober for three years; lifelong pressure (by parents and myself) to be the best.

Physical reactions: Difficulty sleeping; stomach problems.

Moods: Nervous; depressed; angry; stressed.

Behaviors: Struggling with urges to drink; sometimes I avoid AA meetings; I try to do everything perfectly.

Thoughts: "I'm no good," "I'm worthless," "I'm a failure," "I'll be fired," "I'm inadequate," "Something awful will happen," "If I make a mistake, I'm no good," "If someone criticizes me, they are putting me down."

Vic's thinking was negative and self-critical (typical of depression) and also involved worry, self-doubt, and catastrophic predictions (typical of anxiety). In addition, his thoughts included themes of fairness, disrespect, and being mistreated by others (typical of anger). Difficulty sleeping and stomach problems can be signs of depression, anxiety, or even reactions to anger and stress. Of the three moods, anxiety bothered Vic most often. Like Linda, Vic avoided only particular situations in his life that were connected with his anxiety. As you recall, Ben and Marissa avoided many situations because they were depressed.

In order to better understand how these five areas interact in your life, fill out Worksheet 2.1 on the next page.

EXERCISE: Understanding Your Own Problems

Just as Ben, Marissa, Linda, and Vic used the five-part model to understand their problems, you can begin to understand your own problems by noticing what you are experiencing in these five areas of your life: environment/life changes/situations, physical reactions, moods, behaviors, and thoughts. On Worksheet 2.1, describe any recent changes or long-term problems in each of these areas. If you have difficulty filling out Worksheet 2.1, ask yourself the questions in the Helpful Hints on the facing page.

WORKSHEET 2.1. Understanding My Problems

Environment/life changes/situations: _____

_____

Physical reactions: _____

_____

Moods: _____

_____

Behaviors: _____

_____

Thoughts: _____

_____

From *Mind Over Mood, Second Edition*. Copyright 2016 by Dennis Greenberger and Christine A. Padesky. Purchasers of this book can photocopy and/or download additional copies of this worksheet (see the box at the end of the table of contents).

Can you see some connections among the five parts on Worksheet 2.1? For example, do your thoughts and moods seem connected? Did changes in your environment or life situations lead to any changes in the other four parts? Do your behaviors seem connected to your moods or thoughts? For many people, these five areas are connected. The good news is that because this is so, small positive changes in one area can lead to positive changes in all the other areas as well. In therapy, we look for the smallest changes that can lead to the biggest overall positive improvement. As you use this book, notice what small changes help you feel better. While small changes in several areas may be necessary for you to feel better, changes in your thinking or behavior are often important if you want to create lasting positive improvements in your life. The next few chapters help explain why this is so.

Understanding Your Problems 15

> **HELPFUL HINTS** If you are having trouble filling out Worksheet 2.1, you might find it helpful to look again at the five-part models filled out by Linda, Marissa, and Vic. Then ask yourself the following questions:
>
> *Environment/life changes/situations:* What recent changes have there been in my life (positive as well as negative)? What have been the most stressful events for me in the past year? Three years? Five years? In childhood? Do I experience any long-term or ongoing challenges (e.g., discrimination or harassment by others, physical/health challenges for me or family members, ongoing financial problems)?
>
> *Physical reactions:* What physical symptoms am I having? (Consider general changes in energy level, appetite, pain levels, and sleep, as well as occasional symptoms such as muscle tension, tiredness, rapid heartbeat, stomachaches, sweating, dizziness, and breathing difficulties.)
>
> *Moods:* What single words describe my most frequent or troubling moods (sad, nervous, angry, guilty, ashamed)?
>
> *Behaviors:* What behaviors are connected to my moods? At work? At home? With friends? By myself? (Behaviors are the things we do or avoid doing. For example, Linda avoided airplanes, Vic tried to be perfect, and Ben stopped doing things.)
>
> *Thoughts:* When I have strong moods, what thoughts do I have about myself? Other people? My future? What thoughts interfere with doing the things I would like to do or think I should do? What images or memories come into my mind?

Chapter 2 Summary

▶ There are five parts to any problem: environment/life situations, physical reactions, moods, behaviors, and thoughts.

▶ Each of these five parts interacts with the others.

▶ Small changes in any one area can lead to changes in the other areas.

▶ Identifying these five parts may give you a new way of understanding your own problems and give you some ideas for how to make positive changes in your life (see Worksheet 2.1).

3

It's the Thought That Counts

In Chapter 2, you learned how thinking, mood, behavior, physical reactions, and environment/life situations all affect each other. In this chapter, you learn that when you want to feel better, your thoughts are often the place to start. This chapter describes how learning more about your thoughts can help you in many areas of your life.

WHAT IS THE THOUGHT–MOOD CONNECTION?

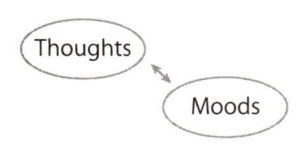

Whenever we experience a mood, there is a thought connected to it that helps define the mood. For example, suppose you are at a party, and a friend introduces you to Alex. As you talk, Alex never looks at you; in fact, throughout your brief conversation, he looks over your shoulder across the room. Following are three different thoughts you might have in this situation. Four moods are listed below each thought. Mark the mood that you believe you would have with each thought:

Thought: Alex is rude. He is insulting me by ignoring me.

    Possible moods (mark one):   Irritated   Sad   Nervous   Caring

Thought: Alex doesn't find me interesting. I bore everybody.

    Possible moods (mark one):   Irritated   Sad   Nervous   Caring

Thought: Alex seems shy. He's probably too uncomfortable to look at me.

    Possible moods (mark one):   Irritated   Sad   Nervous   Caring

This example illustrates that the moods we experience often depend upon our thoughts. Different interpretations of an event can lead to different moods. Since moods are often distressing or may lead to behavior with consequences (such as telling Alex he is rude), it is important to identify what you are thinking and to check out the accuracy of your thoughts before acting. For instance, if Alex is shy, it would be inaccurate to think of him as rude, and you may regret it later if you respond with anger or irritation.

Even situations you might think would create the same mood for everyone – such as losing a job – may, in fact, lead to different moods because of different personal beliefs and meanings. For example, one person facing a job loss might think, "I'm a failure," and feel depressed. Another person might think, "They have no right to fire me; this is discrimination," and feel angry. A third person might think, "I don't like this, but now is my chance to try out a new job," and feel a mixture of nervousness and anticipation.

Thoughts help determine which mood we experience in a given situation. Once a mood is present, we often begin thinking additional thoughts that support and strengthen the mood. For example, angry people think about ways they have been hurt, depressed people think about all the negative aspects of their lives, and anxious people think about danger. This does not mean that our thinking is wrong when we experience an intense mood. But when we feel intense moods, we are more likely to distort, discount, or disregard information that contradicts the validity of our moods and beliefs. In fact, the stronger our moods, the more extreme our thinking is likely to be.

For example, if we are mildly anxious before a party, we might have a thought: "I won't know what to say when I meet new people, and I'll feel really awkward." However, if we are highly anxious, our thought may be "I won't know what to say. I'll blush as red as a beet, and I'll make a complete fool of myself." In addition, we won't remember in this moment that we have been to many parties before, and usually we do think of something to say to new people and generally have a good time. All of us think like this sometimes. This is why it is helpful to be aware of our thoughts when we are most distressed. When we are aware of our thoughts, we more easily see how they are influencing our mood. The following example shows how Marissa's thinking makes her depression worse.

MARISSA: *The thought–mood connection.*

Marissa thought she was unlovable. This belief seemed absolutely true to her. Given her negative experiences with men, she couldn't even imagine that someone could truly love her. This belief, coupled with her desire to be in a relationship, led her to feel depressed. When a colleague, Julio, began to be attracted to her, she had the following experiences:

- A friend teased her about the frequent phone calls she received at work from Julio, saying, "I think you have an admirer, Marissa!" Marissa replied, "What do you mean? He doesn't call that often." (*Not noticing positive information*)

- Julio complimented Marissa, and she thought, "He is just saying this to keep up a good work relationship." (*Discounting positive information*)

- When Julio asked to meet her for lunch, Marissa thought, "I'm probably explaining the work project so poorly that he resents the extra time the project is taking." (*Jumping to a negative conclusion*)

- At lunch, Julio told Marissa he thought that they had both been very creative on the project, and said he had really enjoyed spending the extra time with her. He went on to tell her that he found her attractive. Marissa thought, "Oh, he probably says that to everyone and doesn't really mean it." (*Discounting positive experiences*)

Since Marissa was convinced that she was unlovable, she ignored or distorted information that was not consistent with her belief. Because she was very depressed, she had trouble believing the positive things people said that could help her feel better. Ignoring information that doesn't fit with our beliefs is something we can learn to change. For Marissa, learning to take in positive information about her attractiveness and lovability could be the start of something wonderful.

WHAT IS THE THOUGHT–BEHAVIOR CONNECTION?

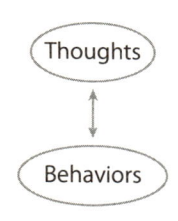

Our thoughts and behaviors are usually closely connected. For example, we are more likely to try to do something if we believe it is possible. For many years, athletes believed it was impossible to run a four-minute mile. In track events around the world, top runners ran a mile in just over four minutes. Then a British miler, Roger Bannister, identified changes he could make in his running style and strategy to break the four-minute barrier. He believed it was possible to run faster and put many months of effort into changing his running technique to reach this goal. In 1954, Roger Bannister became the first man to run a mile in less than four minutes. His belief that he could succeed contributed to behavior change.

Remarkably, once Bannister broke the record, the best milers from around the world also began to run the mile in under four minutes. Unlike Bannister, these runners had not substantially changed their running techniques. What had changed were their beliefs; they now thought it was possible to run this fast, and their behavior followed this thought. Of course, just knowing it is possible to run fast does not mean that everyone can do this. Thinking is not the same as doing. But the more strongly we believe that something is possible, the more likely we are to attempt it and maybe succeed at it.

On a daily basis, we all have "automatic thoughts" that influence our behavior. These are the words and images that pop into our heads throughout the day. For example, imagine that you are at a family reunion. The food has just been laid out, and some family members go over to the buffet tables to fill their plates, while others remain seated and talking. You have been talking with your cousin for 10 minutes. Consider each of the following thoughts and write what behavior you would probably do if you had this thought.

Thought	Behavior
If I don't go now, they'll run out of food.	_____
It's rude to rush to the buffet tables when we're in the middle of a conversation.	_____
My grandfather looks too unsteady to carry a plate.	_____
My cousin and I are having such a wonderful conversation – I've never met anyone so interesting.	_____

Did your behavior change, depending on the thought you had?

Sometimes we are not aware of the thoughts that affect our behavior. Thoughts often occur rapidly, automatically, and just out of our awareness. We sometimes act out of habit, and the original thoughts that led to these habits have been forgotten. For example, perhaps we always give in when someone disagrees with us. This habit may have started with a belief such as "If we disagree, then it is best to just let it go, because otherwise our relationship won't last." We often are not aware of the thoughts guiding our behavior when our actions have become routine. An example from Ben's life illustrates the thought–behavior connection.

BEN: *The thought–behavior connection.*

After his friend Louie died, Ben cut back on meeting his friends for lunch and other activities he used to enjoy. At first, his family thought that avoiding his friends was part of Ben's grief over Louie's death. But as the months passed and Ben still refused to get together with friends, his wife, Sylvie, began to suspect there might be other reasons Ben was staying at home.

One morning, Sylvie sat down with Ben and asked him why he was not returning his friends' telephone calls. Ben shrugged and said, "What's the point? We're at that age where we're all just dying anyhow." Sylvie felt exasperated. "But you're alive now – do the things you enjoy!" Ben shook his head and thought, "Sylvie just doesn't understand."

Sylvie really didn't understand, because Ben was not aware of the thoughts guiding his behavior, and he couldn't fully explain to her why he had stopped doing activities he used to enjoy. As Ben learned to identify his thoughts, he realized that he had a series of thoughts: "Everyone is dying. What's the use in doing things when I'm just going to lose everyone anyhow? If I don't feel like doing something, then I won't enjoy myself."

When Louie died, Ben decided he had reached the age where death was close at hand. This awareness influenced his thoughts and his willingness to do the things he used to enjoy.

By contrast, Sylvie, who was only a little younger than Ben, thought she should do as many enjoyable activities as possible and enjoy life to the fullest. She frequently saw her friends and stayed quite active. As you can see, Sylvie's and Ben's different thoughts about growing older had a big impact on their behavior.

WHAT IS THE THOUGHT–PHYSICAL REACTIONS CONNECTION?

Thoughts also affect our physical reactions. Think about watching a really good movie. When you watch movies, you often anticipate what is coming next. If you think something scary or violent is about to happen, your body reacts as well. Your heart might start to beat more rapidly, and your breathing may actually change as your muscles get tight. If you anticipate a romantic scene, your body may feel warm or even sexually aroused.

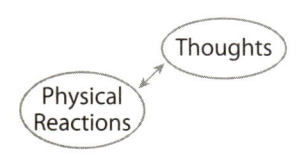

Athletes are trained to use the powerful link between thoughts and physical reactions. Good coaches give their teams inspirational speeches, which they hope will "fire up" the team members, get adrenalin flowing, and lead to top performance. Olympic athletes are often taught to imagine in detail their performance in an event. Research shows that athletes who do this type of vivid imagining actually experience small muscle contractions that reflect the bigger muscle movements they make in their event. This thought–muscle connection improves the athlete's performance.

Research has also discovered that our thoughts, beliefs, and attitudes have an impact on our health. For example, you have probably heard that many medications and health treatments benefit from the "placebo effect." What this means is that our expectation that a medication or treatment will help, increases the likelihood that it does help: Our belief that a pill will help us can itself lead to improvement, even if the pill is just a sugar pill. Modern brain research has found that the placebo effect comes about partly because our beliefs are a type of brain activity and can lead to real changes in physical responses.

LINDA: *The thought–physical reactions connection.*

Just as our thoughts affect our physical reactions, our physical reactions can trigger thoughts. For example, after climbing up a set of stairs, Linda noticed that her heart was beating faster. Because Linda worried about her heart, when her heart rate went up, she had the thought "I'm having a heart attack" (Figure 3.1). This terrifying thought put her whole body on alert, and she experienced a series of physical changes, including quick, shallow breathing and profuse sweating. As Linda's breathing became shallower, she took in less oxygen, which caused her heart to beat even faster. Her brain also temporarily received less oxygen, which caused a sensation of dizziness and light-headedness.

Linda's thought that she was having a heart attack increased her physical reactions

It's the Thought That Counts 21

```
PHYSICAL REACTIONS              THOUGHTS

Increased heart rate  ─────→  "I'm having a heart attack."
        │
More shallow breathing ←┘
        ↓
Less oxygen to heart and brain
        ↓
Increased heart rate  ─────→  "This means I really am having
        │                     a heart attack. I'm going to die."
        ↓                 ┌───┘
Further increase in    ←──┘
physical sensations
        │
        └──→ PANIC
```

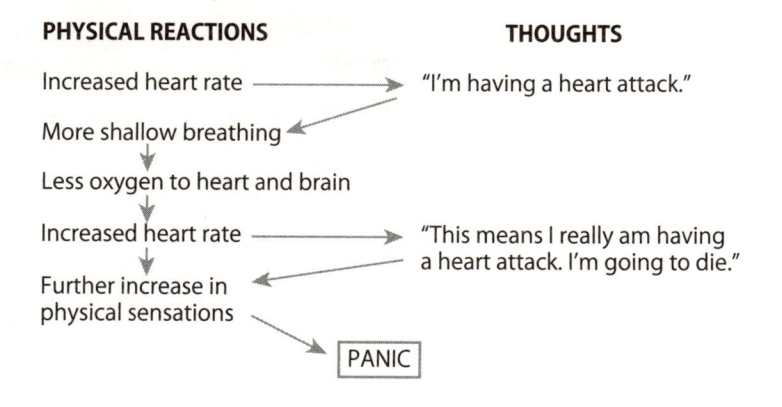

FIGURE 3.1. Linda's panic.

and led her to believe she was in immediate danger of dying. Her physical responses to the idea that she was dying intensified until Linda experienced a full-blown panic attack. After a while, Linda realized that she was not having a heart attack. As she began to think this way, her physical symptoms gradually disappeared.

WHAT IS THE THOUGHT–ENVIRONMENT CONNECTION?

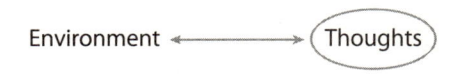

Environment ←────→ (Thoughts)

At the beginning of this chapter, you learned how thoughts influence the moods we experience. You may be wondering why some people are more prone to certain thoughts and moods rather than others. Some portion of these differences may be biological or genetically inherited. But we also know that our environment and life experiences can powerfully shape the beliefs and moods that color our lives. We use the words "environment" and "life experiences" to describe anything outside of us, including our families, our communities, the places we live, interactions with other people, and even our culture. We can be influenced by both present and past experiences that stretch over time from our childhoods to this moment.

Recall that Marissa was sexually and physically abused throughout her childhood and early adult years. These experiences shaped her beliefs that she was worthless, unacceptable, and unlovable, and that men were dangerous, abusive, and uncaring. It is understandable that Marissa's earliest attempts to make sense of her experiences led her to devalue herself and be on the lookout for the negative reactions of others.

It doesn't take traumatic environmental events to influence beliefs. The way we think about ourselves and our lives is influenced by culture, family, neighborhood, gender, religion, and the mass media. As an example of how culture influences beliefs, consider the messages we are given as children. In many cultures, girls are complimented for being pretty, and boys are rewarded for being strong and athletic. A girl might conclude that being pretty is the key to being well liked, and she might value herself for her appearance only. A boy might believe that he should be strong and athletic, and similarly judge himself on his athletic success or failure.

There is nothing inherently more likable about beauty or strength, but some cultures teach us to make these connections. Once these beliefs are formed, they can be difficult to change. Therefore, many girls who are athletic find it difficult to value their skills, and boys with musical or artistic talents but no strong athletic skills may feel cursed rather than blessed.

Vic was raised in a suburban community of educated professionals who valued achievement for themselves and their children. His family and school reflected these community values, emphasizing achievement and excellence. When Vic's performance in school or on the athletic field was not superior, his family, teachers, and friends were disappointed and reacted as if Vic had failed.

From these reactions, Vic concluded that he was inadequate, even though his performance was generally very good. Since Vic believed he was inadequate, it is not surprising that he felt anxious in situations that required him to perform. He dreaded athletic events because there was a risk that he would not win or perform well. To him, those outcomes would mean that he was inadequate.

As you can see, Vic's childhood was not as traumatic as Marissa's. However, the environment he grew up in had a powerful impact on his thoughts that persisted into adulthood.

EXERCISE: The Thought Connections

Worksheet 3.1 provides practice in recognizing the connections between thoughts and mood, behavior, and physical reactions.

WORKSHEET 3.1. The Thought Connections

Sarah, a 34-year-old woman, sat in the back row of the auditorium during a school meeting for parents. She had concerns and questions regarding how her 8-year-old son was being taught, as well as questions about classroom security. As Sarah was about to raise her hand to voice her concerns and questions, she thought, "What if other people think my questions are stupid? Maybe I shouldn't ask these questions in front of the whole group. Someone may disagree with me and this could lead to a public argument. I could be humiliated."

THOUGHT–MOOD CONNECTION

Based on Sarah's thoughts, which of the following moods is she likely to experience? (Mark all that apply.)

- ☐ 1. Anxiety/nervousness
- ☐ 2. Sadness
- ☐ 3. Happiness
- ☐ 4. Anger
- ☐ 5. Enthusiasm

THOUGHT–BEHAVIOR CONNECTION

Based on Sarah's thoughts, how do you predict she will behave?

☐ 1. She will speak loudly and voice her concerns.

☐ 2. She will remain silent.

☐ 3. She will openly disagree with what other people say.

THOUGHT–PHYSICAL REACTIONS CONNECTION

Based on Sarah's thoughts, which of the following physical changes might she notice? (Mark all that apply.)

☐ 1. Rapid heart rate

☐ 2. Sweaty palms

☐ 3. Breathing changes

☐ 4. Dizziness

From *Mind Over Mood, Second Edition*. Copyright 2016 by Dennis Greenberger and Christine A. Padesky. Purchasers of this book can photocopy and/or download additional copies of this worksheet (see the box at the end of the table of contents).

When Sarah had these thoughts, she felt anxious and nervous, remained silent, and experienced a rapid heart rate, sweaty palms, and breathing changes. Were these the reactions you anticipated Sarah would have? Not everyone experiences the same reactions to particular thoughts. However, it is important to recognize that thoughts influence our mood, behavior, and physical reactions.

IS POSITIVE THINKING THE SOLUTION?

Although our thoughts affect our moods, behavior, and physical reactions, positive thinking is not a solution to life's problems. Most people who are anxious, depressed, or angry can tell you that "just thinking positive thoughts" is not that easy. In fact, thinking only positive thoughts is overly simplistic, usually does not lead to lasting change, and can lead us to overlook information that might be important.

Mind Over Mood instead teaches you to consider all information and many different angles on a problem. Looking at a situation from all sides and considering a wide range of information – positive, negative, and neutral – can lead to more helpful ways of understanding things and new solutions to difficulties you face.

If Linda was planning a business trip that required her to fly on an airplane, simply thinking positive thoughts, such as "I won't have a panic attack. Everything will be fine," would not prepare her for the anxiety she might feel. In fact, with positive thinking, Linda might feel like a failure if she felt even a small amount of anxiety. A better solution for Linda would be to anticipate that she might feel anxious and to have a plan for how she will cope with her anxiety in flight. If we only think about the positive, we may not be able to accurately predict and cope with events that are worse than we expect.

IS CHANGING THE WAY YOU THINK THE ONLY WAY TO FEEL BETTER?

Even though the process of identifying, testing, and considering alternative thoughts is a central part of CBT and *Mind Over Mood*, it is often equally important to make changes in your physical reactions and/or your behavior. For example, if you have been anxious for a long time, you probably avoid things that make you anxious. Part of dealing with anxiety may be accepting your anxiety (cognitive shift), learning to relax (physical change), and approaching what frightens you so you can learn to cope with it (behavioral change). People do not usually overcome anxiety until they change their thoughts and overcome avoidance.

Making changes in your environment/life situations can also help you feel better. Reducing stress, learning to say no to unreasonable demands made by others, spending more time with supportive people, working with neighbors to increase neighborhood safety, and taking action to reduce discrimination or harassment on the job are all environmental/life changes that can help you feel better.

Some life situations are so challenging that simply thinking differently about things is not a wise idea. For example, someone who is being abused needs help either to change or to leave the situation. Just changing thoughts is not an adequate solution for abuse: The goal is to stop the abuse. Thought changes might help someone in this situation feel motivated to get help, but simply changing thoughts to permit acceptance of abuse is not a helpful solution.

As you complete the worksheets in this book, you will learn how to identify and change your thoughts, moods, behaviors, physical responses, and environment/life situations.

Chapter 3 Summary

▸ Thoughts help define the moods we experience.

▸ Thoughts influence how we behave and what we choose to do and not to do.

▸ Thoughts and beliefs affect our physical responses.

▸ Life experiences (environment) help determine the attitudes, beliefs, and thoughts that develop in childhood and often persist into adulthood.

▸ *Mind Over Mood* helps you look at all the information available; it is not simply positive thinking.

▸ While changes in thinking are often central, mood improvement may also require changes in behavior, physical reactions, and home or work situations/environments.

4

Identifying and Rating Moods

In order to learn to understand and improve your moods, it is helpful to identify the moods you are experiencing. Moods can be difficult to name. You may feel tired all the time and not recognize that you are depressed. Or you may feel nervous and out of control and not recognize that you are anxious. Along with depression and anxiety, anger, shame, and guilt are very common moods that can be troubling (see Chapters 13–15).

IDENTIFYING MOODS

The list in the box below shows a variety of moods you may experience. This is not a comprehensive list. You can write additional moods on the blank lines. This list helps you name your moods more specifically than simply "bad" or "good." Notice that moods are usually described by one word. When you identify specific moods, you can set goals to improve your moods and track your progress. Learning to distinguish among moods can help you choose actions designed to improve particular moods. For example, certain breathing techniques help nervousness but not depression.

Mood List

Depressed	Anxious	Angry	Guilty	Ashamed
Sad	Embarrassed	Excited	Frightened	Irritated
Insecure	Proud	Mad	Panic	Frustrated
Nervous	Disgusted	Hurt	Cheerful	Disappointed
Enraged	Scared	Happy	Loving	Humiliated
Grief	Eager	Afraid	Content	Grateful

Other moods: _____ _____ _____ _____

If you have trouble identifying your moods, pay attention to your body. Tight shoulders can be a sign that you are afraid or irritated; heaviness throughout your body may mean that you feel depressed or disappointed. Identifying your physical reactions can provide clues to what moods you are feeling.

A second way of getting better at identifying your moods is to pay close attention. See if you can notice three different moods during a day. Or you can choose some of the moods from the list in the box on the previous page and write down situations from your past in which you felt each one. Another strategy is to identify a recent situation in which you had a strong emotional reaction and mark the moods in the list on the previous page that you felt.

When Vic first began therapy, he knew he was feeling anxious and depressed. As he learned to identify moods, he discovered that he was also frequently angry. This was helpful information for Vic, because he was able to learn what was making him angry and set therapy goals to address those issues. Although he had been mostly sober for three years, he reported that he felt the urge to drink whenever he feared he was about to get "out of control." When he and his therapist looked closely at situations when Vic felt "out of control," it became apparent that at these times he was feeling very nervous or angry. When nervous or angry, Vic experienced a rapid heartbeat, sweaty hands, and a sense that something terrible was going to happen. He labeled these sensations as being "out of control," and he would then have the urge to drink because he thought alcohol would help him regain control.

Vic tended not to be very specific about his mood, often saying that he was "uncomfortable" or "numb." When Vic learned that his primary emotional difficulties were with anger and anxiety, he began to focus his attention on the situations in which he felt angry or anxious. He learned to distinguish his irritable anger from the fearful worry of his anxiety. He began to identify these moods, instead of lumping them together as "numbness." As Vic became more specific about what he was feeling, it became apparent to him that when his *mood* was anxious, he was *thinking*, "I'm losing control." When his *mood* was angry, he was *thinking*, "This is not fair – I deserve more respect." Learning which moods he was experiencing was an important step toward a better understanding of his reactions.

It is easy to confuse moods with thoughts. At the beginning of therapy, when Ben's therapist asked him what he was feeling (mood), he would reply, "I feel like I want to be alone." As Ben began to closely analyze the situations in which he wanted to be alone, he discovered that he would often be *thinking* that others (family members or friends) did not need him or want to be with him. He also realized that he was predicting (thinking) that if he got together with other people, he would not have a good time. As he was *thinking*, "They don't want to be with me," and "If I go there, I'm not going to enjoy myself," he recognized that his mood was sad. The thought "I feel like I want to be alone" was connected to Ben's sad mood. Part of developing the ability to identify your moods is learning to distinguish your moods from your thoughts.

It is also important to distinguish moods and thoughts from behaviors and from situational factors (aspects of the environment). Behaviors and situational factors can often be identified by answering the following questions:

1. Who was I with? (situation)

2. What was I doing? (behavior)

3. When did it happen? (situation)

4. Where was I? (situation)

As a general rule, moods can be identified in one word. If you are feeling multiple moods in a situation, you will use one word to describe each mood. For example, you might be "sad, scared, and embarrassed" in one situation. Each of these three moods is described in a single word. If it takes you more than one word to describe a single mood, you may be describing a thought. Thoughts are the words or images, including memories, that go through your mind.

It is helpful to learn to tell the differences among thoughts, moods, behaviors, physical reactions, and situational factors. By doing this, you can begin to figure out which parts of your experience can be changed to help make your life better.

REMINDERS
- Situations and behaviors can be described by asking yourself:

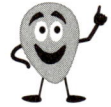

  Who?

  What?

  When?

  Where?

- Moods can be described by one word.
- Thoughts are the words, images, and memories that go through your mind.

To practice linking moods and situations, fill out Worksheet 4.1 on the next page.

> **EXERCISE: Identifying Moods**
>
> One step in learning to feel better is to learn to identify different parts of your experiences – situations, behaviors, moods, physical reactions, and thoughts. Worksheet 4.1 is designed to help you learn to separate your moods from the situations you are in. In order to complete this worksheet, focus on specific situations in which you had a strong mood.

WORKSHEET 4.1. Identifying Moods

Describe a recent situation in which you had a strong mood. Next, identify what moods you had during or immediately after being in that situation. Do this for five different situations.

1. Situation: _____

    Moods: _____

2. Situation: _____

    Moods: _____

3. Situation: _____

    Moods: _____

4. Situation: _____

    Moods _____

5. Situation: _____

    Moods: _____

From *Mind Over Mood, Second Edition*. Copyright 2016 by Dennis Greenberger and Christine A. Padesky. Purchasers of this book can photocopy and/or download additional copies of this worksheet (see the box at the end of the table of contents).

One of Vic's responses on Worksheet 4.1 looked like this:

Situation: *I'm alone, driving in my car, on the way to work at 7:45 A.M.*

Moods: *Frightened, anxious, insecure.*

One of Ben's responses was the following:

Situation: *I received a phone call from Max asking me to lunch.*

Moods: *Sadness, grief.*

As these examples illustrate, knowing the situation does not always help us understand why someone felt a particular emotion. Why would a lunch invitation make Ben feel sad? The presence of strong moods is our first clue that something important is happening. Later chapters teach you why Ben and Vic — and you — experienced the particular moods described on Worksheet 4.1.

RATING MOODS

In addition to identifying moods, it is important to learn to rate the intensity of the moods you experience. Rating the intensity of each mood allows you to observe how your moods fluctuate. Rating your moods also helps alert you to which situations or thoughts are associated with changes in moods. Finally, you can use changes in emotional intensity to evaluate the effectiveness of strategies you are learning.

In order to see how your moods vary, you'll find it convenient to use a rating scale. Ben and his therapist developed the following rating scale for his moods:

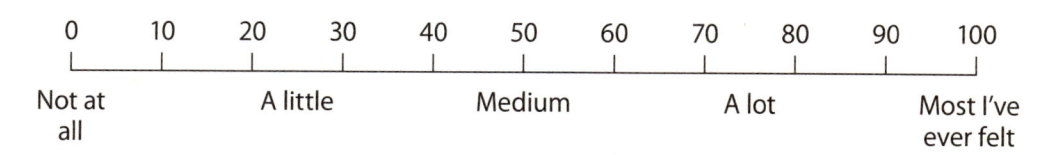

```
0    10   20   30   40   50   60   70   80   90   100
|----|----|----|----|----|----|----|----|----|----|
Not at        A little        Medium         A lot        Most I've
 all                                                      ever felt
```

The therapist then asked Ben to use this scale to rate the moods he listed on Worksheet 4.1. For the lunch invitation, Ben's ratings looked like this:

Situation: *I received a phone call from Max asking me to lunch.*

Moods: *Sadness, grief.*

Sadness 0   10   20   30   40   50 ✗ 60   70   80   90   100

Grief   0   10   20   30   40   50   60   70   80   90 ✗ 100

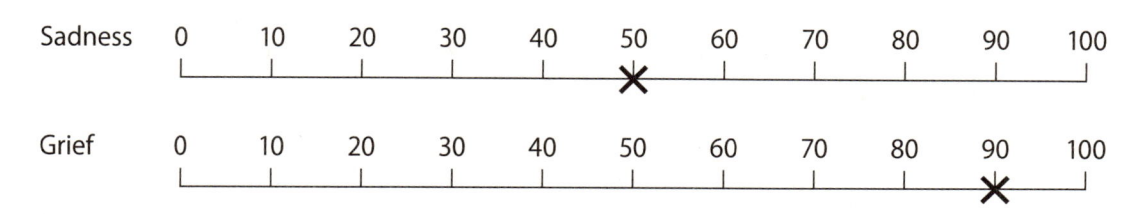

These ratings indicate that Ben experienced a high level of grief (90) and a medium level of sadness (50) while on the phone with Max.

EXERCISE: Rating Moods

On Worksheet 4.2, practice rating the intensity of your moods. On the blank lines, copy the situations and moods you identified on Worksheet 4.1. For each situation, rate one of the moods you identified on the scales provided. Mark the mood you rated.

WORKSHEET 4.2. Identifying and Rating Moods

1. Situation:_____

   Moods: _____

   Not at 0   10   20   30   40   50   60   70   80   90   100   Most I've
   all |⎣___|___|___|___|___|___|___|___|___|___|⎦   ever felt

2. Situation:_____

   Moods: _____

   0   10   20   30   40   50   60   70   80   90   100
   ⎣___|___|___|___|___|___|___|___|___|___|⎦

3. Situation:_____

   Moods: _____

   0   10   20   30   40   50   60   70   80   90   100
   ⎣___|___|___|___|___|___|___|___|___|___|⎦

4. Situation:_____

   Moods: _____

   0   10   20   30   40   50   60   70   80   90   100
   ⎣___|___|___|___|___|___|___|___|___|___|⎦

5. Situation:_____

   Moods: _____

   0   10   20   30   40   50   60   70   80   90   100
   ⎣___|___|___|___|___|___|___|___|___|___|⎦

From *Mind Over Mood, Second Edition*. Copyright 2016 by Dennis Greenberger and Christine A. Padesky. Purchasers of this book can photocopy and/or download additional copies of this worksheet (see the box at the end of the table of contents).

Many people find it helpful to measure their moods weekly or at least twice a month. If you are experiencing depression (unhappiness) and/or anxiety (nervousness), you can use the *Mind Over Mood* Depression Inventory (Worksheet 13.1, p. 191) and the *Mind Over Mood* Anxiety Inventory (Worksheet 14.1, p. 221) to measure these moods. For other moods, you can use Measuring and Tracking My Moods (Worksheet 15.1, p. 253). Once you have measured your moods, mark your score(s) on the relevant worksheet(s). For depression, use Worksheet 13.2 (p. 192); for anxiety, use Worksheet 14.2 (p. 222); and for other moods, use Worksheet 15.2 (p. 254).

Take a few moments right now to fill out the mood measures that apply to the moods you want to improve. It is really helpful to make this first measurement before you begin to read other chapters in this book, so you have a record of where you started.

As you use *Mind Over Mood,* you may also find it helpful to track changes in your positive moods. Use Worksheet 15.1 to rate your happiness over the past week. You can use a copy of Worksheet 15.2 in the Appendix to track your happiness scores if you are already using Worksheet 15.2 on page 254 to track changes in another mood. Alternatively, you can use different colors on the same worksheet to track different moods.

As you use *Mind Over Mood,* rate your happiness on Worksheet 15.1 at least once a month. As you use and practice *Mind Over Mood* skills, you can measure what impact these have on your level of happiness.

Tracking changes in your mood scores is one way to know if *Mind Over Mood* is helping you. If it is, you will feel distressing moods less often and less intensely and your overall level of happiness will increase.

What If You Struggle with Multiple Moods?

It is quite common to struggle with many different moods. Our emotional lives can be complicated. The good news is that *Mind Over Mood* skills are fundamental to helping all mood issues. All the skills you learn can help with a variety of moods. To get the fastest results when you struggle with multiple moods, we recommend you choose the one mood that is most distressing and read that chapter first (see Chapters 13–15). At the end of that chapter, it will recommend which chapters to read next.

For example, if you are both depressed and anxious, decide which mood you most want relief from first. If you want to work on depression first, read Chapter 13 and do the exercises there, and then read the other chapters in this book until your depression improves. When your depression lifts, begin reading Chapter 14 on anxiety, and then follow the recommended chapter sequence to reduce your anxiety. It may surprise you to realize that once you learn skills that help you with depression, these same skills can be helpful for managing anger, guilt, anxiety, and so forth. Skills that help you manage these moods will probably also help boost your happiness at the same time.

If a therapist or other professional has recommended this book to you, he or she may suggest you read the chapters in a different order from the order in the book. There are many different ways to use *Mind Over Mood*. While each chapter adds to your knowledge and abilities, some people will not need to use every chapter to feel better.

Now that you have read and done the exercises in these first four chapters, it is a good time to personalize your use of *Mind Over Mood*. Rather than going immediately to Chapter 5, read the chapter next that teaches you about the mood that is most distressing for you:

- Depression: Chapter 13 (p. 188)
- Anxiety and panic: Chapter 14 (p. 219)
- Anger, guilt, or shame: Chapter 15 (p. 252)

Once you finish that chapter and the exercises in it, there will be directions to which chapter you should read next, so that you can use *Mind Over Mood* most effectively to help you feel better as quickly as possible.

Chapter 4 Summary

▶ Strong moods signal that something important is happening in your life.

▶ Moods can usually be described in one word.

▶ Identifying specific moods helps you set goals and track progress.

▶ It is important to identify the moods you have in particular situations (Worksheet 4.1).

▶ Rating your moods (Worksheet 4.2) allows you to evaluate their strength, track your progress, and evaluate the effectiveness of strategies you are learning.

▶ *Mind Over Mood* can be customized to help with the moods that are most distressing to you. After completing this chapter, go to the recommended mood chapter pertaining to that mood. At the end of that chapter, additional chapters and the order in which you should read them are recommended.

5

Setting Personal Goals and Noticing Improvement

The Lewis Carroll story *Alice in Wonderland* describes a moment when Alice, facing a fork in the road, meets the Cheshire Cat and asks him which road to take. The cat asks Alice where she is going. Alice, who has never been to Wonderland before, says, "I don't much care where –"; the Cheshire Cat happily interrupts, "Then it doesn't matter which way you go." Alice then completes her thought: "– so long as I get *somewhere*."

Just as Alice has never been in Wonderland, you may never have learned skills for managing your moods, and so you don't know what to expect or where you want to be by the end of this book. To make the best use of this book, where you are going does matter. If you know what your goals are, you will have clearer ideas about how to use this book and track your progress. With a goal in mind, it may also be easier to keep practicing what you learn, because you have an end in sight.

Think about the reasons why you picked up this book or why someone recommended it to you. How do you hope you might be different as a result of using *Mind Over Mood*?

Worksheet 5.1 on the next page asks you to write down your goals so you don't forget them and also so you can keep track of your progress as you learn *Mind Over Mood* skills. Would you like to be less depressed? Happier? Have fewer panic attacks? Be less anxious? Improve your relationships? Drink or use drugs less? Go places or do things you are currently avoiding? Have a greater sense of purpose or meaning? Try to make your goals as specific as possible and word them in such a way that you can measure your progress. For example, "improve my relationships" is a good goal, but "having positive and enjoyable conversations with my children more often" is even better because it is easier to tell if you are making progress toward this more specific goal. The mood measures throughout this book help you measure mood changes if these are your goals.

> **EXERCISE: Setting Goals**
>
> Write on the lines in Worksheet 5.1 two changes in your moods or life you hope will result from learning the skills in this book. Each goal you write should be something that you can observe or measure (such as a mood or behavior change). If you have more than two goals, either fit them on the lines below or write them on another piece of paper.

WORKSHEET 5.1. Setting Goals

1. _____
   _____
   _____

2. _____
   _____
   _____

From *Mind Over Mood, Second Edition.* Copyright 2016 by Dennis Greenberger and Christine A. Padesky. Purchasers of this book can photocopy and/or download additional copies of this worksheet (see the box at the end of the table of contents).

    Very often people have mixed feelings about making changes in their lives or spending time learning new skills. For example, Anna often felt anxious and sometimes had panic attacks. She learned that if she stayed home and didn't go out, she would feel less anxious. She grew comfortable staying at home; in fact, she arranged with her employer that she could telecommute most days, so she rarely needed to go out. However, Anna missed the social activities she used to enjoy. The goals she identified on Worksheet 5.1 were to reduce her anxiety and easily leave home whenever she wanted. These goals had both advantages (she would be able to do more activities) and disadvantages (she might have to step outside of her comfort zone).

    With a bit more thought, Anna realized that there would be additional advantages to reducing her anxiety about leaving the house. These included the possibilities that she could see her friends and family more often, she would be able to go on nature walks like she used to enjoy, and she would have more career opportunities. When Anna weighed the advantages and disadvantages of change, she decided that the advantages outweighed the disadvantages. This increased her motivation to change. She reviewed these advantages and disadvantages periodically, especially when the steps she needed to take were more challenging. Worksheet 5.2 asks you to consider the advantages and disadvantages you face if you reach the goals you set above.

> **EXERCISE: Advantages and Disadvantages**
>
> Write the advantages and disadvantages of reaching or not reaching the goals you identified on Worksheet 5.1 in the boxes on Worksheet 5.2. If you have more than two goals, print out extra copies of this worksheet.

WORKSHEET 5.2. Advantages and Disadvantages of Reaching and Not Reaching My Goals

Goal 1: _____

	Reaching This Goal	Not Reaching This Goal
Advantages		
Disadvantages		

Goal 2: _____

	Reaching This Goal	Not Reaching This Goal
Advantages		
Disadvantages		

From Mind Over Mood, Second Edition. Copyright 2016 by Dennis Greenberger and Christine A. Padesky. Purchasers of this book can photocopy and/or download additional copies of this worksheet (see the box at the end of the table of contents).

Did you find that there are both advantages and disadvantages of reaching or not reaching your goals? Are the advantages of reaching your goals and the disadvantages of not reaching your goals big enough that you feel motivated to learn and practice skills to help you reach your goals?

Luckily, most people have knowledge, positive qualities, and skills that offer hope they will be able to reach their goals. For example, when Anna put her mind to something, she generally kept working at it until she succeeded. Her family and friends were loving and supportive. For most of her life, she had been able to leave her home and live a life not affected by anxiety. Each of these qualities and circumstances made it more likely that she would be able to reach her goals of reducing anxiety and panic, as well as living a life with greater freedom of movement.

EXERCISE: What Will Help

On the lines in Worksheet 5.3, write some of your qualities, strengths, experiences, and values that give you hope you can reach your goals. Consider past successes and obstacles you have overcome; any positive qualities you have, such as a sense of humor or other skills that help you through difficult times; spiritual beliefs; a willingness to learn new skills; people who support you; physical health and stamina; or even a single-minded motivation to reach your goals. Write here anything you can think of that will help you reach the goals you have written in Worksheets 5.1 and 5.2.

WORKSHEET 5.3. What Will Help Me Reach My Goals?

_____
_____
_____
_____
_____
_____
_____

From *Mind Over Mood, Second Edition*. Copyright 2016 by Dennis Greenberger and Christine A. Padesky. Purchasers of this book can photocopy and/or download additional copies of this worksheet (see the box at the end of the table of contents).

You may want to mark these pages so that as you work toward your goals; you can refer back to the advantages and disadvantages of reaching them (Worksheet 5.2), as well as the resources you have identified on Worksheet 5.3.

> **EXERCISE: Signs of Improvement**
>
> In addition to rating your mood, it is helpful to actively look for and notice signs of improvement. What do you expect might be different as you begin to improve? Indicate on Worksheet 5.4 what you might notice as you begin to make changes and improve.

WORKSHEET 5.4. Signs of Improvement

Check any of the following that would be early signs of improvement:

- ☐ Sleep better.
- ☐ Talk with people more.
- ☐ Feel more relaxed.
- ☐ Smile more often.
- ☐ Get my work done.
- ☐ Wake up and get out of bed at a regular time.
- ☐ Do activities I currently avoid.
- ☐ Handle disagreements better.
- ☐ Lose my temper less often.
- ☐ Other people tell me I seem better.
- ☐ Feel more confident.
- ☐ Stand up for myself.
- ☐ See hope for the future.
- ☐ Enjoy each day more.
- ☐ Feel appreciation and gratitude.
- ☐ See improvement in relationships.

In addition to what you checked above, write two or three other signs that you could look for to know you are beginning to improve and getting closer to reaching your goals:

_____

_____

_____

From *Mind Over Mood, Second Edition*. Copyright 2016 by Dennis Greenberger and Christine A. Padesky. Purchasers of this book can photocopy and/or download additional copies of this worksheet (see the box at the end of the table of contents).

It's helpful to pay attention and notice small signs of improvement as you use *Mind Over Mood*. Just as problems you experience can gradually get worse over time, positive changes often start small and grow into bigger, more meaningful improvements. If you notice early positive changes, this can encourage you to continue learning and practicing *Mind Over Mood* skills.

Chapter 5 Summary

▶ Setting personal goals for mood or behavior change helps you know where you are headed and can help you track your progress.

▶ People often have mixed feelings about making changes, because there are usually advantages and disadvantages in doing so. Keeping your reasons for change in mind can help you stay motivated.

▶ Supportive people in your life, as well as your personal qualities, past experiences, values, strengths, and motivation to learn new skills, can all offer hope that you will reach your goals.

▶ It is important to pay attention and notice the early signs of improvement you have checked on Worksheet 5.4, because positive changes often start small and grow bigger over time.

6

Situations, Moods, and Thoughts

One warm spring day in central California, a tennis coach was instructing a student on the art of serving the ball. While the student tossed and hit the ball over and over again, the coach focused attention on each part of the student's motion and swing. The coach never criticized the student, but instead gave feedback after each hit about the position of the racquet, the height of the ball toss, the angle of the racquet as it hit the ball, and the student's motion during the racquet follow-through.

In tennis, the ball needs to land in a service square in order to be a successful hit. Yet, remarkably, the coach never once looked to see where the ball landed after the student served it. Instead, the coach focused his feedback exclusively on suggestions for improving each part of the student's service stroke. The coach was confident that once the student learned each of the component skills, the student would be able to combine them so that the ball would consistently land in the proper area.

Just as this coach focused on development of specific skills, music teachers help students become better musicians by teaching notes, rhythms, and performance methods. Skilled laborers instruct their apprentices by showing them how to accomplish individual tasks on a work project. Each of these examples involves teaching *specific skills* and encouraging the learner to *practice* until these skills become familiar and easy to perform. We have all had experience with developing skills through practice (e.g., driving a car, dressing a baby, cooking a meal).

Fortunately, there is a set of specific skills that you can learn to improve your mood and make positive changes in your life. Some of these skills are summarized on a seven-column worksheet called a "Thought Record" (Figure 6.1). Like the student practicing a tennis stroke, you will use parts of Thought Records many times in the weeks ahead to master the skills necessary to complete the whole worksheet.

When Marissa's therapist first showed her a Thought Record, Marissa felt overwhelmed and depressed. The therapist used this reaction to help Marissa complete her first Thought Record (Figure 6.2, pp. 42–43). Notice that the first two columns of Marissa's Thought Record describe the situation she was in and what she was feeling. You learned to identify situations and moods in Chapter 4. As her therapist helped Marissa fill out column 3, labeled "Automatic Thoughts (Images)," they uncovered certain thoughts that accompanied her mood reactions.

Marissa and her therapist next circled the thought ("This is too complicated for me to learn") that was most strongly connected to her feeling overwhelmed. They wrote down evidence in columns 4 and 5 that did and did not support this thought. In column 6, they wrote some alternative ways of looking at the situation, based on the evidence in columns 4 and 5. They rated Marissa's belief in these alternative views 90%, 60%,

THOUGHT

1. Situation Who? What? When? Where?	2. Moods a. What did you feel? b. Rate each mood (0–100%).	3. Automatic Thoughts (Images) a. What was going through your mind just before you started to feel this way? Any other thoughts? Images? b. Circle or mark the hot thought.

FIGURE 6.1. Sample Thought Record. Copyright 1983 by Christine A. Padesky.

and 70%. As you see in column 7, completing this Thought Record lowered Marissa's feeling of being overwhelmed from 95% to 40%, and her depression from 85% to 80%.

The next few chapters teach you how to use the Thought Record as a tool to improve your own moods. You will learn to uncover your automatic thoughts and images in Chapter 7. Chapter 8 shows you how to look for evidence for your automatic thoughts. In Chapter 9, you will learn how to use the evidence you find to construct more adaptive ways of thinking and viewing your life. The rest of this chapter focuses on what you need to know to fill out columns 1–3 of the Thought Record, using skills you have already learned.

RECORD

4. Evidence That Supports the Hot Thought	5. Evidence That Does Not Support the Hot Thought	6. Alternative/ Balanced Thoughts	7. Rate Moods Now
		a. Write an alternative or balanced thought. b. Rate how much you believe each thought (0–100%).	Rerate column 2 moods and any new moods (0–100%).

42   Mind Over Mood

THOUGHT

1. Situation	2. Moods	3. Automatic Thoughts (Images)
Who? What? When? Where?	a. What did you feel? b. Rate each mood (0–100%).	a. What was going through your mind just before you started to feel this way? Any other thoughts? Images? b. Circle or mark the hot thought.
Tuesday 9:30 A.M. In my therapist's office, looking at the Thought Record.	Overwhelmed 95% Depressed 85%	(This is too complicated for me to learn.) I'll never understand this. Image/memory: Taking a report card home with bad grades and being yelled at by my parents. I'll never get better. Nothing can help me. This therapy won't work. I'm doomed to always be depressed.

FIGURE 6.2. Marissa's first Thought Record.

COLUMN 1: SITUATION

In Chapter 4, you learned to describe situations by answering the questions Who? What? When? Where? In filling out column 1 of the Thought Record, be as specific as possible. Limit the "Situation" description to a specific time frame, from as short as a few seconds up to 30 minutes. For example, "all day Tuesday" is not specific enough. Even if you have only one mood "all day Tuesday," there are too many different situations and thoughts that can occur during a day to describe on the Thought Record. Researchers report that we have as many as 50,000 to 70,000 thoughts each day. No one wants to write that many thoughts on a Thought Record! By narrowing the situation down to a

RECORD

4. Evidence That Supports the Hot Thought	5. Evidence That Does Not Support the Hot Thought	6. Alternative/ Balanced Thoughts a. Write an alternative or balanced thought. b. Rate how much you believe each thought (0–100%).	7. Rate Moods Now Rerate column 2 moods and any new moods (0–100%).
I look at this Thought Record and I don't know what to do. I never was very good in school. I don't know what you mean by "evidence."	At work, I learned the computer filing system, which is complicated. Some of the early worksheets seemed hard until my therapist helped me do them a few times — then they seemed easier. My therapist said I need to know how to do only the first two columns now. I can get help from my therapist until I know how to do it on my own.	Even though this seems complicated now, I've learned other complicated things in the past. 90% My therapist will help show me how to do this. 60% With practice, it might make sense and get easier. 70%	Overwhelmed 40% Depressed 80%

specific instance in time when our mood is especially strong, you can focus on the most important thoughts that will help you understand your moods. Marissa's description of her situation as "Tuesday, 9:30 A.M. In my therapist's office, looking at the Thought Record" is a good example of a specific situation.

COLUMN 2: MOODS

In the "Moods" column of a Thought Record, list the moods you experienced in the situation you described. In addition to listing the moods, rate their intensity on a 0–100 scale.

Generally, moods can be described in one word. As you learned in Chapter 4, you can experience more than one mood in any situation. Each mood that you had in the situation you are recording should be listed and rated on the 0–100 scale. If you have trouble identifying the mood you were experiencing, you can refer to the Mood List on page 25 for help. If you describe your mood in an entire sentence, what you wrote may be a thought instead of a mood. If so, write the sentence in the "Automatic Thoughts (Images)" column (column 3) and keep looking for a single word to describe your mood in column 2.

People who experience panic attacks or anxiety may also want to record and rate the physical reactions they experience (see Chapter 14). Since there is not a separate column for these physical responses, they can be recorded in the bottom half of the "Moods" column of the Thought Record. Draw a line below the moods you have listed, and write "Physical reactions" above the line as shown in Figure 6.5 on page 46. Physical reactions can generally be described in one or two words (e.g., "heart racing 85%").

COLUMN 3: AUTOMATIC THOUGHTS (IMAGES)

In the "Automatic Thoughts (Images)" column, identify anything that went through your mind in the situation you have described. Only the thoughts that were actually present in that situation should be recorded. Thoughts can be either verbal or visual. If they are images or memories, describe them in words or draw a picture that shows what went through your mind. Notice that Marissa described one of her thoughts as an image of bringing home a bad report card (Figure 6.2). Chapter 7 provides more detailed information to help you become proficient at identifying your thoughts.

As an example, Marissa brought the Thought Record in Figure 6.3 to her next therapy session, with the first three columns complete.

A second example shows how Vic reacted to an argument with his wife (Figure 6.4).

Linda's Thought Record describing one of her first panic attacks, with the first three columns complete, is shown in Figure 6.5. Notice that she had a number of physical reactions, which she recorded in the bottom half of column 2.

Ben brought the first three columns of the Thought Record in Figure 6.6 to his therapist soon after beginning treatment.

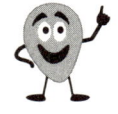

REMINDERS
- In the "Situation" column of the Thought Record (column 1), write down the answers to these questions: Who? What? When? Where?
- Moods are identified in one word and rated for intensity on a 0–100% scale (column 2).
- Physical reactions can be described and rated at the bottom of the "Moods" column (column 2). This is especially helpful for people with anxiety, anger, or health concerns.
- The "Automatic Thoughts (Images)" column (column 3) describes thoughts, beliefs, images, memories, and meanings attached to the situations.

1. Situation Who? What? When? Where?	2. Moods a. What did you feel? b. Rate each mood (0–100%).	3. Automatic Thoughts (Images) a. What was going through your mind just before you started to feel this way? Any other thoughts? Images? b. Circle or mark the hot thought.
Wednesday, 2:45 P.M. My manager is coming to check on the progress I am making on the payroll project.	Depressed 90% Nervous 95% Afraid 97%	The project is not complete. What is complete is not OK. I'm failing. (I'm going to be fired.) I'll feel humiliated to tell my family that I've lost my job.

FIGURE 6.3. The first three columns of Marissa's second Thought Record.

1. Situation Who? What? When? Where?	2. Moods a. What did you feel? b. Rate each mood (0–100%).	3. Automatic Thoughts (Images) a. What was going through your mind just before you started to feel this way? Any other thoughts? Images? b. Circle or mark the hot thought.
Friday, 6:00 P.M. Judy and I were arguing over which movie to go to.	Angry 99% Hurt 95% Sad 70%	She never cares about what I want to do. We always do what she wants to do. (She always has to be in control.) I can't stand feeling this way. I hate being angry all the time. I'm going to explode. This is too much for me. I need a drink.

FIGURE 6.4. The first three columns of Vic's Thought Record.

46 Mind Over Mood

1. Situation Who? What? When? Where?	2. Moods a. What did you feel? b. Rate each mood (0–100%).	3. Automatic Thoughts (Images) a. What was going through your mind just before you started to feel this way? Any other thoughts? Images? b. Circle or mark the hot thought.
It is 2:30 in the afternoon. I'm alone at the mall, where I've been shopping for about 45 minutes.	Fear 100% Panic 100% **Physical Reactions** Racing heart 100% Sweating 80% Dizzy 90% Tight chest 80%	I may stop breathing. I can't get enough air. I'm having a heart attack. I'm losing control. (I'm going to die.) I need to get to a hospital. Image: I see myself lying on the floor, unable to breathe.

FIGURE 6.5. The first three columns of Linda's Thought Record.

1. Situation Who? What? When? Where?	2. Moods a. What did you feel? b. Rate each mood (0–100%).	3. Automatic Thoughts (Images) a. What was going through your mind just before you started to feel this way? Any other thoughts? Images? b. Circle or mark the hot thought.
May 25. I'm preparing to go to a birthday dinner at my daughter's home at 3 P.M.	Sad 85% Remorseful 80%	Birthdays are such a sad time. I have two grown children who live out of town with their families. I don't get to see them nearly as often as I would like. Birthdays are a time when families should be complete and together. We will never be a family like that again. (My life will never be as good as it once was.)

FIGURE 6.6. The first three columns of Ben's Thought Record.

> **EXERCISE:** Distinguishing Situations, Moods, and Thoughts
>
> Worksheet 6.1 is an exercise to help you identify and pull apart the different aspects of your experience. Write on the line at the right whether the item in the left column is a thought, mood, or situation. The first three items have been completed as examples.

WORKSHEET 6.1. Distinguishing Situations, Moods, and Thoughts

	Situation, mood, or thought?
1. Nervous.	Mood
2. At home.	Situation
3. I'm not going to be able to do this.	Thought
4. Sad.	
5. Talking to a friend on the phone.	
6. Irritated.	
7. Driving in my car.	
8. I'm always going to feel this way.	
9. At work.	
10. I'm going crazy.	
11. Angry.	
12. I'm no good.	
13. 4:00 P.M.	
14. Something terrible is going to happen.	
15. Nothing ever goes right.	
16. Discouraged.	
17. I'll never get over this.	
18. Sitting in a restaurant.	
19. I'm out of control.	
20. I'm a failure.	
21. Talking to my mom.	
22. She's being inconsiderate.	
23. Depressed.	
24. I'm a loser.	

(continued on next page)

From *Mind Over Mood, Second Edition.* Copyright 2016 by Dennis Greenberger and Christine A. Padesky. Purchasers of this book can photocopy and/or download additional copies of this worksheet (see the box at the end of the table of contents).

WORKSHEET 6.1 *(continued from previous page)*

	Situation, mood, or thought?
25. Guilty.	
26. At my son's house.	
27. I'm having a heart attack.	
28. I've been taken advantage of.	
29. Lying in bed trying to go to sleep.	
30. This isn't going to work out.	
31. Shame.	
32. I'm going to lose everything I've got.	
33. Panic.	

Following are answers to Worksheet 6.1. Review the pertinent sections of this chapter to clarify any differences between your answers and the ones given.

1. Nervous .... Mood
2. At home .... Situation
3. I'm not going to be able to do this .... Thought
4. Sad .... Mood
5. Talking to a friend on the phone .... Situation
6. Irritated .... Mood
7. Driving in my car .... Situation
8. I'm always going to feel this way .... Thought
9. At work .... Situation
10. I'm going crazy .... Thought
11. Angry .... Mood
12. I'm no good .... Thought
13. 4:00 P.M. .... Situation
14. Something terrible is going to happen ...... Thought
15. Nothing ever goes right .... Thought
16. Discouraged .... Mood
17. I'll never get over this .... Thought

18. Sitting in a restaurant .... Situation

19. I'm out of control .... Thought

20. I'm a failure .... Thought

21. Talking to my mom .... Situation

22. She's being inconsiderate .... Thought

23. Depressed .... Mood

24. I'm a loser .... Thought

25. Guilty .... Mood

26. At my son's house .... Situation

27. I'm having a heart attack .... Thought

28. I've been taken advantage of .... Thought

29. Lying in bed trying to go to sleep .... Situation

30. This isn't going to work out .... Thought

31. Shame .... Mood

32. I'm going to lose everything I've got .... Thought

33. Panic .... Mood

If you had difficulty distinguishing among situations, moods, and thoughts, review Chapters 3 and 4. By separating these components from each other, you will be better able to make changes that are important to you. For example, sometimes it is easier to change a situation or a thought than to change your mood directly.

Chapter 6 Summary

✓ Thought Records help develop a set of skills that can improve your moods and relationships and lead to positive changes in your life.

✓ The first three columns of a Thought Record distinguish a situation from the moods, physical reactions, and thoughts you had in the situation.

✓ The Thought Record is a tool that can help you develop new ways of thinking in order to feel better.

✓ As is true whenever you develop a new skill, you will need to practice using the Thought Record until it becomes a reliable tool to help you feel better.

7
Automatic Thoughts

Marissa was working at her desk when her supervisor came in to say hello. While they were talking, her supervisor said, "By the way, I want to compliment you on the nice report you wrote yesterday." As soon as her supervisor said this, Marissa became nervous and scared. She couldn't shake this mood the rest of the morning.

Vic was putting the dishes on the counter after dinner when his wife said, "I took the car in to get the oil changed today." With irritation, Vic said, "I told you I was going to change the oil on Saturday." His wife replied, "Well, you've been saying you'd take care of it for two weeks, so I just took care of it myself." "Fine!" yelled Vic, throwing a dish towel across the room. "Why don't you just get yourself another husband!" He grabbed his coat and slammed the door as he left the house.

As you begin keeping track of your moods, you will notice times when you, like Marissa, experience a mood that doesn't seem to fit the situation. Most people don't feel anxious after getting a compliment. At other times, you will have a quick, strong reaction like Vic's. An outsider looking on this scene might think that Vic was overreacting in this situation, and yet his reaction might have seemed to be just the right one to him.

How can we make sense of our moods? If we can identify the thoughts we are having, our moods usually make perfect sense. Think of thoughts as clues to understanding moods. For Marissa, we have the following puzzle:

Situation	Clue: Thoughts	Mood
My supervisor compliments me	???	Nervous 80% Scared 90%

How can this make sense? Marissa was confused about why she reacted this way until she talked to her therapist.

THERAPIST: What was scary about this situation?

MARISSA: I don't know – just knowing the supervisor noticed my work, I guess.

THERAPIST: What's scary about that?

MARISSA: Well, I don't always do a good job.

THERAPIST: So what might happen?

MARISSA: Someday the supervisor will notice a mistake.

THERAPIST: And then what might happen?

MARISSA: The supervisor will be mad at me.

THERAPIST: What's the worst that might happen then?

MARISSA: I hadn't thought about it, but I – I guess I could get fired.

THERAPIST: That is a scary thought. And then what might happen?

MARISSA: With a bad recommendation, I'd have trouble getting another job.

THERAPIST: So that helps explain why you felt scared. Can you summarize for me what you've figured out here?

MARISSA: Maybe the compliment made me realize my supervisor is noticing my work. I know I make mistakes, so I worried about what might happen if my supervisor noticed one of these mistakes. I guess I jumped to the conclusion that I'd be fired and not be able to get another job. It sounds a little silly now.

Notice how the thoughts uncovered by Marissa and her therapist provide the necessary clues to understand her emotional reaction.

Situation	Clue: Thoughts	Mood
My supervisor compliments me	My supervisor is noticing my work. When my supervisor finds a mistake, I'll be fired, and won't be able to get another job.	Nervous 80% Scared 90%

Most of us would feel nervous and scared if we thought we were going to be fired and couldn't get another job. Now Marissa's moods make sense. As you can see, an important step in understanding our moods is learning to identify the thoughts that accompany them.

See if you can guess what Vic's automatic thoughts might have been when he got so angry with his wife for changing the oil in the car.

Situation	Clue: Thoughts	Mood
Judy changed oil in car. Judy says, "You've been saying you'd take care of it for two weeks, so I just took care of it myself."		Angry 95%

In the "Clue: Thoughts" column, write any thoughts you can think of that would explain Vic's strong, angry reaction.

After Vic left the house, he realized that he was not upset that his wife had changed the oil in the car. In fact, his week had been very busy, and it was a big help that she had taken care of this chore. His anger was related to the *thoughts* he had about her changing the oil. He thought, "She's mad at me for not doing it. She doesn't appreciate how hard I'm trying to do everything. She is critical of me; she thinks I'm not good enough. No matter how hard I try, she's never happy with me."

These thoughts help us understand Vic's reactions. Thoughts like these are called "automatic thoughts," because they simply pop into our heads automatically throughout the day. We don't plan or intend to think a certain way. In fact, often we are not even aware of our automatic thoughts. One of the purposes of CBT is to bring automatic thoughts into awareness.

Awareness is the first step toward change and better problem solving. Once Vic was aware of his thoughts, a number of possibilities for change became available to him. If he decided that his thoughts were distorted or didn't work for him, he could work to change his understanding of the situation. On the other hand, if Vic concluded that his thoughts were accurate, he could talk directly to his wife to discuss his feelings and ask her to appreciate his efforts more.

HOW DO WE BECOME AWARE OF OUR OWN AUTOMATIC THOUGHTS?

Since we are constantly thinking and imagining, we have automatic thoughts all the time. We daydream about friends or the weekend, or worry about getting errands done. These are all automatic thoughts. When we want to feel better, the automatic thoughts that are most important are the ones that help us understand our strong moods. These thoughts can be *words* ("I'll be fired"), *images* or mental pictures (Marissa might have "seen" herself as a homeless person sitting at a street corner), or *memories* (the memory of being hit on the hand with a ruler by her fifth-grade teacher when she made a mistake might have flashed through Marissa's mind).

> **HELPFUL HINTS** To identify automatic thoughts, notice what goes through your mind when you have a strong feeling or a strong reaction to something.

To practice identifying automatic thoughts, write down what goes through your mind when you imagine yourself in the following situations.

1. **Situation:** You are at a shopping center and are going to buy a very special present for yourself. You saw it there a few weeks ago and have been saving your money to buy it. When you get to the store, the sales clerk tells you that they no longer carry that item.

    Automatic thoughts: _____
    _____
    _____
    _____
    _____
    _____

2. **Situation:** You cooked a dish for a neighborhood party. You are a bit nervous because you tried a new recipe. After 10 minutes, several people come up and say they think the food you made is delicious.

    Automatic thoughts: _____
    _____
    _____
    _____
    _____
    _____

Different people have different automatic thoughts in these situations. For the food situation in example 2, some people think, "Oh, good, the food turned out OK," and they feel relief or pride. Other people think, "These people are just trying not to hurt my feelings; it probably tastes terrible," and they feel ashamed or embarrassed. In any situation, there are many ways to interpret what events mean. The interpretation you make affects your mood.

Actually, we usually have a number of automatic thoughts during situations in our lives. The questions in the following Helpful Hints can help you identify your automatic thoughts. Not every question will help you in every situation, but by asking yourself these questions, you will capture most of your automatic thoughts. There is a hint after each question that suggests which questions might be best to help identify automatic thoughts linked to different moods.

HELPFUL HINTS **Questions to Help Identify Automatic Thoughts**

- What was going through my mind just before I started to feel this way? (General)
- What images or memories do I have in this situation? (General)
- What does this mean about me? My life? My future? (Depression)
- What am I afraid might happen? (Anxiety)
- What is the worst that could happen? (Anxiety)
- What does this mean about how the other person(s) feel(s)/think(s) about me? (Anger, Shame)
- What does this mean about the other person(s) or people in general? (Anger)
- Did I break rules, hurt others, or not do something I should have done? What do I think about myself that I did this or believe I did this? (Guilt, Shame)

From *Mind Over Mood, Second Edition*. Copyright 2016 by Dennis Greenberger and Christine A. Padesky. Purchasers may photocopy this box for personal use or use with individual clients.

To identify automatic thoughts, ask yourself these questions until you have identified the thoughts that help you understand your emotional reactions. You may need to ask yourself some of these questions two or three times to uncover all of the automatic thoughts. To look for images and memories, just let your mind wander and see if any pictures come to mind when you think of the situation in which you had the strong feeling.

You don't need to answer all of these questions. Sometimes the answers to just one or two of these questions are enough to identify the thoughts that are going through your mind when you are having a strong mood. Answer as few, or as many, of the questions in the box as necessary to identify the thoughts associated with your distress.

Begin with General Questions

Usually we start with the first two questions in the Helpful Hints above (the ones labeled "General"). These are questions you can ask yourself with any mood you experience. In the beginning, you may not know what went through your mind just before you started to feel this way. With observation and practice, many people become expert at identifying their key automatic thoughts by just asking the first question in the box.

You might wonder why the second question asks about images and memories. It turns out that most of us do have images when we are experiencing strong moods. These may be visual, or a song or words going through our minds, or a physical feeling. Sometimes these images are completely imaginary (e.g., you see yourself lying on the ground with people staring at you), and sometimes they repeat memories of experiences we have had (e.g., remembering a day when school classmates laughed at you). When you have these images or memories, they tend to evoke very strong moods – stronger than those you experience with word thoughts. So it is very important to notice these images and memories, and to write them down (or draw them) on a Thought Record along with other thoughts.

Next, Ask Specific Mood Questions

After asking and answering the general questions, you may find it helpful to ask yourself the specific mood questions in the Helpful Hints on the facing page. The specific mood questions are labeled "Anxiety," "Depression," "Anger," "Guilt," or "Shame." You are likely to identify the automatic thoughts associated with each of your moods by asking these specific questions. You can answer any of these questions that seem helpful to you, but the specific mood questions are written to help you identify the types of thoughts that tend to go with particular moods.

Depression

For example, when we feel sad or depressed, we tend to be self-critical and have negative thoughts about our lives and futures, as described in Chapter 13. Therefore, if you are experiencing depression or similar moods, like sadness, discouragement, or disappointment, ask yourself, "What does this mean about me?" "What does this mean about my life?" "What does this mean about my future?" These questions help identify the negative automatic thoughts related to those moods.

Anxiety

Chapter 14 describes how, when we are anxious, we tend to imagine a series of "worst-case" events and outcomes: We overestimate danger and underestimate our ability to cope with things that go wrong. Sometimes anxious thoughts begin with "What if . . . ?" and end with a prediction of something terrible happening. When this occurs, in addition to writing down the "What if . . . ?" question, it is helpful to write down the answer you give to that question that makes you feel most anxious. For example, if you think, "What if I have a panic attack at the store?" you might write, "If I have a panic attack at the store, then I will collapse. I see an image of paramedics coming and carrying me away. Everyone is staring, and I'm so embarrassed." Therefore, when you feel anxious, scared, nervous, or similar moods, it is helpful to ask, "What am I afraid might happen? What is the worst that could happen?" When you are asking these questions, it can also be helpful to think about what you imagine your own worst responses might be to the situation (e.g., an image of losing control and running from the room screaming).

Anger

When we feel angry, resentful, or irritated, our thoughts are generally focused on other people and how they have harmed or hurt us. We may think (rightly or wrongly) that others are being unfair, unjust, disrespectful, or are mistreating us in some way. This is why the Helpful Hints on page 54 recommend asking yourself, "What does this mean about how the other person(s) feel(s)/think(s) about me?" and "What does this mean about the other person(s) or people in general?" Chapter 15 teaches more about the thoughts that commonly accompany anger.

Guilt or Shame

Guilt and shame usually are connected to thoughts about having done something wrong. Chapter 15 explains these moods in more detail. A variety of thoughts or behaviors may be associated with feeling guilty or ashamed. For example, you may have let someone down or believe that you have let the person down. You may have broken a rule or moral obligation that is important to you, or you may have had thoughts that violate what you value. Therefore, if your mood is guilt or shame, the Helpful Hints section on page 54 recommends that you ask yourself, "Did I break rules, hurt others, or not do something I should have done? What do I think about myself that I did this or believe I did this?" With shame, it also can be helpful to ask "What does this mean about how the other person(s) feel(s)/think(s) about me?" or "What might they think if they knew this about me?"

Summary of How to Identify Automatic Thoughts

When you are looking for the thoughts linked to a particular mood, be sure to ask yourself the two general questions from the Helpful Hints section on page 54 and the two or three specific questions for the mood you are trying to understand. However, it is also sometimes helpful to ask questions linked to other moods. For example, Aniya, who was socially anxious, answered the question "What is the worst that could happen?" with "I am not going to know what to say, and I'll look stupid." However, by asking the depression question "What does this mean about me?," Aniya uncovered the thought "No one will ever love me." Like Aniya, you can use the mood labels at the end of the questions as guides, but answering some of the questions associated with other moods may help you identify additional important automatic thoughts.

EXERCISE: Connecting Thoughts and Moods

Worksheet 7.1 helps you make the connection between thoughts and specific moods as described on the previous pages. Of the five moods described (depression, anxiety, anger, guilt, shame), write on the line which mood you think is most likely to go with each thought. The first two have been completed as examples.

WORKSHEET 7.1. Connecting Thoughts and Moods

	Depression? Anxiety? Anger? Guilt? Shame?
1. I'm stupid and I'll never understand this.	Depression
2. I'm going to lose my job because I'm so late.	Anxiety
3. She is being so unfair.	
4. I shouldn't have been so hurtful.	
5. If people knew this about me, they wouldn't like me.	
6. When I give my speech, people will laugh at me.	
7. It's wrong for me to think about this.	
8. He's cheating and insulting me.	
9. There's no use in trying any more.	
10. If something goes wrong, I can't cope.	

From *Mind Over Mood, Second Edition.* Copyright 2016 by Dennis Greenberger and Christine A. Padesky. Purchasers of this book can photocopy and/or download additional copies of this worksheet (see the box at the end of the table of contents).

Below are the answers to Worksheet 7.1. Review the relevant paragraphs of this chapter or Chapters 13, 14, and 15 to understand why these specific thoughts might be connected to the moods listed.

1. I'm so stupid that I'll never understand this. .... Depression
2. I'm going to lose my job because I'm so late. .... Anxiety
3. She is being so unfair. .... Anger
4. I shouldn't have been so hurtful. .... Guilt
5. If people knew this about me, they wouldn't like me. .... Shame
6. When I give my speech, people will laugh at me. .... Anxiety
7. It's wrong for me to think about this. .... Guilt
8. He's cheating and insulting me. .... Anger
9. There's no use in trying any more. .... Depression
10. If something goes wrong, I can't cope. .... Anxiety

Now that you understand how thoughts and moods are connected, the following exercise gives you an opportunity to see how this works in your own life.

EXERCISE: Separating Situations, Moods, and Thoughts

Think of a time today or yesterday when you had a particularly strong mood, such as depression, anger, anxiety, guilt, or shame. If there is a particular mood you are working on as you use this book, choose a situation in which you felt that mood. Write about this experience on Worksheet 7.2, describing the situation, your moods, and your thoughts in as much detail as you can remember. This exercise is designed to help you define, separate, and understand the different parts of your experience – an important step in learning to manage your moods.

WORKSHEET 7.2. Separating Situations, Moods, and Thoughts

1. Situation	2. Moods	3. Automatic Thoughts (Images)
Who were you with? What were you doing? When was it? Where were you?	Describe each mood in one word. Rate intensity of mood (0–100%).	**Answer the first two general questions, and then some or all of the questions specific to one of the moods you identified.** What was going through my mind just before I started to feel this way? (General) What images or memories do I have in this situation? (General) What does this mean about me? My life? My future? (Depression) What am I afraid might happen? (Anxiety) What is the worst that could happen? (Anxiety) What does this mean about how the other person(s) feel(s)/think(s) about me? (Anger, Shame) What does this mean about the other person(s) or people in general? (Anger) Did I break rules, hurt others, or not do something I should have done? What do I think about myself that I did this or believe I did this? (Guilt, Shame)

From *Mind Over Mood, Second Edition*. Copyright 2016 by Dennis Greenberger and Christine A. Padesky. Purchasers of this book can photocopy and/or download additional copies of this worksheet (see the box at the end of the table of contents).

Did you find that you experienced more than one mood in the situation you wrote about? Often we have several moods in the same situation. Since there are likely to be different thoughts associated with each mood, it is helpful to circle or mark the one mood in column 2 that is most distressing to you. Then ask yourself the relevant questions to identify thoughts connected to that mood. Learning to identify automatic thoughts can be very interesting, and identifying them will help you understand why you feel the way you feel in different situations. The more you pay attention to your thoughts, the easier it is to identify several thoughts tied to a mood.

The first three columns of the Thought Record take an emotional situation in your life and put it under a psychological microscope. You are learning to take a slice of your personal experience and examine it more closely. This close look at what is going on in the situation and within yourself is necessary before you move on to the second half of the Thought Record, which will help you figure out what changes will help you feel better.

Worksheet 7.3 (on the following page) is designed to give you more practice in identifying your automatic thoughts. Automatic thoughts are the springboard for change throughout the next few chapters of this book. Therefore, it is important for you to become skilled at identifying them. Before reading ahead, complete Worksheet 7.3 for another situation in which you had one or more of the moods you are concerned about.

> **EXERCISE: Identifying Automatic Thoughts**
>
> Remember, if you list more than one mood in column 2, circle or mark the mood you want to put under the microscope. Use the questions at the bottom of column 3 to help you identify the thoughts connected to the mood you circled or marked. Remember, you do not need to answer every question in column 3. Ask yourself the first two general questions, and then some or all of the questions specific to the moods you circled or marked in column 2.

WORKSHEET 7.3. Identifying Automatic Thoughts

1. Situation	2. Moods	3. Automatic Thoughts (Images)
Who were you with? What were you doing? When was it? Where were you?	Describe each mood in one word. Rate intensity of mood (0–100%). Circle or mark the mood you want to examine.	What was going through my mind just before I started to feel this way? (General) What images or memories do I have in this situation? (General) What does this mean about me? My life? My future? (Depression) What am I afraid might happen? (Anxiety) What is the worst that could happen? (Anxiety) What does this mean about how the other person(s) feel(s)/think(s) about me? (Anger, Shame) What does this mean about the other person(s) or people in general? (Anger) Did I break rules, hurt others, or not do something I should have done? What do I think about myself that I did this or believe I did this? (Guilt, Shame)

From *Mind Over Mood, Second Edition.* Copyright 2016 by Dennis Greenberger and Christine A. Padesky. Purchasers of this book can photocopy and/or download additional copies of this worksheet (see the box at the end of the table of contents).

Automatic Thoughts 61

HOT THOUGHTS

Imagine walking into a room, turning on a table lamp, and having no light appear. You may discover that the lamp is unplugged or that the wall switch is turned off. Plugging in the lamp and turning it on causes electricity to flow and the lamp lights up.

Wires that carry electricity are called "hot" wires. Similarly, the automatic thoughts that are most strongly connected to intense moods are called "hot" thoughts. These are the thoughts that conduct the emotional charge, so these are also the thoughts that are most important for us to identify, examine, and consider whether we need to change them to feel better.

To learn about hot automatic thoughts, let's look at one of Vic's Thought Records (Figure 7.1). Vic wanted to identify automatic thoughts and images that would help him

1. Situation Who? What? When? Where?	2. Moods a. What did you feel? b. Rate each mood (0–100%). c. Circle or mark the mood you want to examine.	3. Automatic Thoughts (Images) a. What was going through your mind just before you started to feel this way? Any other thoughts? Images? b. Circle or mark the hot thought.

Handing a monthly report to my supervisor. She reads it while standing in my office. Tuesday, 4:30 P.M.	(Nervous 90%)
	
	Irritated 60%
		(General Question) What was going through my mind just before I got nervous?
		   Why is she reading it here? (Answer that makes me nervous: She's looking for problems and will criticize me.)
		
		(General Question) What images or memories do I have in this situation?
		   A memory of my dad criticizing how I mowed the lawn. His face is red and he looks really upset with me.
		
		(Specific Anxiety Question) What am I afraid might happen?
		   She'll be unhappy with my sales.
		   I bet the other salespeople did better this month.
		
		(Specific Anxiety Question) What is the worst that could happen?
		   I'll get fired or get a pay cut.

FIGURE 7.1. Vic's partial Thought Record.

understand his nervousness, so he circled this mood in Column 2. To help identify his automatic thoughts, Vic asked himself the two general questions in the Helpful Hints "Questions to Help Identify Automatic Thoughts" (p. 54). These questions are underlined in Figure 7.1. In addition, since his feeling of nervousness was most closely related to the mood of anxiety, he asked himself the two anxiety questions from the Helpful Hints, which are also underlined.

Notice that Vic described the situation and then identified and rated his moods. He circled "Nervous" because this was the mood he wanted to learn more about. Because different thoughts are connected to different moods, it is helpful to circle or mark the mood you want to learn about. To figure out the automatic thoughts connected with his nervousness, he asked himself some of the questions listed in the Helpful Hints on page 54. He asked both of the general questions ("What was going through my mind just before I started to feel this way?" and "What images or memories do I have in this situation?"), as well as the specific questions related to anxiety ("What am I afraid might happen?" "What is the worst that could happen?"), because nervousness is similar to anxiety.

To find out which of his thoughts were hottest – most emotionally charged – Vic considered each thought by itself to see how much that thought alone would make him feel nervous. For example, if he thought only the first thought – "Why is she reading it here?" – Vic decided he would have rated his nervousness 10%. However, when he wrote in the answer to this question that made him most nervous, "She's looking for problems and will criticize me," his anxiety rating increased. All of Vic's ratings can be seen here:

Thought	Mood
Why is she reading it here?	Nervous 10%
She's looking for problems and will criticize me.	Nervous 50%
A memory of my dad criticizing how I mowed the lawn. His face is red and he looks really upset with me.	Nervous 40%
She'll be unhappy with my sales.	Nervous 40%
I bet the other salespeople did better this month.	Nervous 80%
I'll get fired or get a pay cut.	Nervous 90%

As you can see, Vic's first thought ("Why is she reading it here?") did not make him very nervous, so it was not particularly hot. His next three thoughts made him more nervous, so these were hotter thoughts. His last two thoughts ("I bet the other salespeople did better this month," and "I'll get fired or get a pay cut") made Vic extremely nervous, and so these were the hottest thoughts. Asking yourself a number of questions, as Vic did, makes it more likely that you will find hot thoughts to help you understand your emotional reactions.

There is one last thing of importance on Vic's Thought Record. Notice that the childhood memory he recalled seemed closely tied to his reaction to the supervisor. Later, Vic learned to look for similarities and differences between the supervisor's reading his report and his dad's criticizing his lawn mowing. Becoming aware of this memory, and learning to see the differences between his childhood experiences and his adult experiences, helped Vic learn to react in more helpful ways with both his supervisor and his wife.

> ### EXERCISE: Identifying Hot Thoughts
>
> Now you are ready to identify your own hot thoughts. For each of the automatic thoughts you listed on Worksheet 7.3 on page 60, rate how much (0–100%) this thought alone led you to feel the emotion you circled. Write the rating next to each thought. These ratings will help you decide which one(s) are the hot thought(s). The hottest thought is the one with the highest rating. Do these thoughts help you understand why you had this particular mood? On Worksheet 7.3, circle or mark the hot thought(s) for the mood you circled or marked in column 2. If none of the thoughts listed are hot, ask yourself the questions in the Helpful Hints on page 54 again, to try to identify additional automatic thoughts.
>
> The skills taught in this chapter are so important that the chapter ends with a special Thought Record. Worksheet 7.4 is similar to Worksheet 7.3, with the addition of a fourth column in which you can rate the hotness of each automatic thought you identify. Notice the helpful hints and questions at the bottom of column 3, which remind you what information to include in the "Automatic Thoughts" column.
>
> Use Worksheet 7.4 until you can successfully identify your automatic thoughts and find the hot thoughts connected to your moods. Before you move on to the next chapter, practice this skill until you are comfortable with it. We recommend that you complete Worksheet 7.4 at least once a day for one week. (We have included four copies of this worksheet here for your convenience. Additional copies can be printed from *www.guilford.com/MOM2-materials*.) It is important to be able to identify your hot thoughts and understand the links between your thoughts and moods before you go on to the next steps. Once you can figure out your hot thoughts, then you are ready to read Chapter 8, which teaches you how to evaluate these thoughts and make changes that can lead to more adaptive ways of thinking.
>
> The more Thought Records you do, the faster you will feel better. Doing a Thought Record is not a test. It is an exercise in identifying your thoughts and the thought patterns that are connected to your moods. With continued practice, you will become more skilled in completing Thought Records. As your skill increases, you are likely to feel better and more in control of your life. Once you are skilled at filling out Worksheet 7.4, you are ready to begin Chapter 8.

WORKSHEET 7.4. Identifying Hot Thoughts

1. Situation	2. Moods	3. Automatic Thoughts (Images)	Rate Hotness of Each Thought
Who were you with? What were you doing? When was it? Where were you?	Describe each mood in one word. Rate intensity of mood (0–100%). Circle or mark the mood you want to examine.	**Answer some or all of the following questions:** What was going through my mind just before I started to feel this way? (General) What images or memories do I have in this situation? (General) What does this mean about me? My life? My future? (Depression) What am I afraid might happen? (Anxiety) What is the worst that could happen? (Anxiety) What does this mean about how the other person(s) feel(s)/think(s) about me? (Anger, Shame) What does this mean about the other person(s) or people in general? (Anger) Did I break rules, hurt others, or not do something I should have done? What do I think about myself that I did this or believe I did this? (Guilt, Shame)	For each thought in column 3, rate (0–100%) how strong your mood would be based on that thought alone.

From *Mind Over Mood, Second Edition.* Copyright 2016 by Dennis Greenberger and Christine A. Padesky. Purchasers of this book can photocopy and/or download additional copies of this worksheet (see the box at the end of the table of contents).

WORKSHEET 7.4. Identifying Hot Thoughts

1. Situation	2. Moods	3. Automatic Thoughts (Images)	Rate Hotness of Each Thought
Who were you with? What were you doing? When was it? Where were you?	Describe each mood in one word. Rate intensity of mood (0–100%). Circle or mark the mood you want to examine.	**Answer some or all of the following questions:** What was going through my mind just before I started to feel this way? (General) What images or memories do I have in this situation? (General) What does this mean about me? My life? My future? (Depression) What am I afraid might happen? (Anxiety) What is the worst that could happen? (Anxiety) What does this mean about how the other person(s) feel(s)/think(s) about me? (Anger, Shame) What does this mean about the other person(s) or people in general? (Anger) Did I break rules, hurt others, or not do something I should have done? What do I think about myself that I did this or believe I did this? (Guilt, Shame)	For each thought in column 3, rate (0–100%) how strong your mood would be based on that thought alone.

From *Mind Over Mood, Second Edition.* Copyright 2016 by Dennis Greenberger and Christine A. Padesky. Purchasers of this book can photocopy and/or download additional copies of this worksheet (see the box at the end of the table of contents).

WORKSHEET 7.4. Identifying Hot Thoughts

1. Situation	2. Moods	3. Automatic Thoughts (Images)	Rate Hotness of Each Thought
Who were you with? What were you doing? When was it? Where were you?	Describe each mood in one word. Rate intensity of mood (0–100%). Circle or mark the mood you want to examine.	**Answer some or all of the following questions:** What was going through my mind just before I started to feel this way? (General) What images or memories do I have in this situation? (General) What does this mean about me? My life? My future? (Depression) What am I afraid might happen? (Anxiety) What is the worst that could happen? (Anxiety) What does this mean about how the other person(s) feel(s)/think(s) about me? (Anger, Shame) What does this mean about the other person(s) or people in general? (Anger) Did I break rules, hurt others, or not do something I should have done? What do I think about myself that I did this or believe I did this? (Guilt, Shame)	For each thought in column 3, rate (0–100%) how strong your mood would be based on that thought alone.

From *Mind Over Mood, Second Edition*. Copyright 2016 by Dennis Greenberger and Christine A. Padesky. Purchasers of this book can photocopy and/or download additional copies of this worksheet (see the box at the end of the table of contents).

WORKSHEET 7.4. Identifying Hot Thoughts

1. Situation	2. Moods	3. Automatic Thoughts (Images)	Rate Hotness of Each Thought
Who were you with? What were you doing? When was it? Where were you?	Describe each mood in one word. Rate intensity of mood (0–100%). Circle or mark the mood you want to examine.	**Answer some or all of the following questions:** What was going through my mind just before I started to feel this way? (General) What images or memories do I have in this situation? (General) What does this mean about me? My life? My future? (Depression) What am I afraid might happen? (Anxiety) What is the worst that could happen? (Anxiety) What does this mean about how the other person(s) feel(s)/think(s) about me? (Anger, Shame) What does this mean about the other person(s) or people in general? (Anger) Did I break rules, hurt others, or not do something I should have done? What do I think about myself that I did this or believe I did this? (Guilt, Shame)	For each thought in column 3, rate (0–100%) how strong your mood would be based on that thought alone.

From *Mind Over Mood, Second Edition*. Copyright 2016 by Dennis Greenberger and Christine A. Padesky. Purchasers of this book can photocopy and/or download additional copies of this worksheet (see the box at the end of the table of contents).

MOOD CHECK-UP

Now that you are beginning to learn how to identify your automatic thoughts, it is a good time to measure your moods again. Remember, you can use the following measures and score sheets:

- Depression/unhappiness: *Mind Over Mood* Depression Inventory
    Worksheet 13.1, page 191, and Worksheet 13.2, page 192

- Anxiety/nervousness: *Mind Over Mood* Anxiety Inventory
    Worksheet 14.1, page 221, and Worksheet 14.2, page 222

- Other moods/happiness: Measuring and Tracking My Moods
    Worksheet 15.1, page 253, and Worksheet 15.2, page 254

Chapter 7 Summary

▶ Automatic thoughts are thoughts that come into our minds spontaneously throughout the day.

▶ Whenever we have strong moods, there are also automatic thoughts present that provide clues to understanding our emotional reactions.

▶ Automatic thoughts can be words, images, or memories.

▶ To identify automatic thoughts, notice what goes through your mind when you have a strong mood.

▶ Specific types of thoughts are linked to each mood. This chapter suggests questions you can ask to identify these mood-specific thoughts.

▶ Hot thoughts are automatic thoughts that carry the strongest emotional charge. These are usually the most valuable thoughts to test on a Thought Record.

8

Where's the Evidence?

VIC: *Stop, look, and relisten.*

One Thursday evening, Vic and his wife, Judy, were standing in the kitchen discussing their plans for the upcoming weekend. Vic told Judy that he had made plans for Saturday morning to meet his friend Jim at an AA meeting. Judy's expression changed as he spoke, and a look of distress came over her face. Vic experienced a surge of anger as he thought, "She's upset that I'm spending time away from her and the kids. It's not fair that she doesn't see my recovery program as important. If she cared about me as much as she cared about the kids, she'd be happy I was going. She doesn't care about me."

Vic exploded at Judy: "If you don't care about my sobriety, then I don't care either!" He slammed his fist on the table and stormed out of the house. As he left, Judy yelled after him, "How can you expect me to care when you act like this? What's wrong with you?"

As Vic drove away from the house, his thoughts were racing: "She's never understood how important AA is to me. She doesn't know how hard it is not to drink. What's the use in trying so hard if she doesn't care if I stay sober? I can't stand being so angry. A drink will make me feel better."

As Vic neared the liquor store, he pulled his car into a parking lot and turned off the ignition. He put his head on the steering wheel to catch his breath. As his anger began to subside, he remembered his therapist telling him that next time he had a strong emotion or urge to drink, he should use that as an opportunity to identify his thoughts and look for evidence on a Thought Record. As much as Vic just wanted to get a drink, he had promised his therapist he would do this at least once. Figure 8.1 shows what Vic wrote on a piece of paper he found in the car.

As you learned to do in Chapter 7, Vic filled out the first three columns of the Thought Record by describing the situation, identifying and rating his mood, and writing down a variety of thoughts connected to his mood. Instead of writing out his ratings of how "hot" each automatic thought was, Vic mentally considered how angry each thought made him feel and circled the hottest thought: "She doesn't care about me." He

70   Mind Over Mood

THOUGHT

1. Situation Who? What? When? Where?	2. Moods a. What did you feel? b. Rate each mood (0–100%). c. Circle or mark the mood you want to examine.	3. Automatic Thoughts (Images) a. What was going through your mind just before you started to feel this way? Any other thoughts? Images? b. Circle or mark the hot thought.
Thursday, 8:30 P.M. Judy gives me an odd look when I tell her I'm going to AA on Saturday.	(Anger 90%)	She's upset that I'm going to AA on Saturday. She doesn't see my recovery program as important. (She doesn't care about me.) She doesn't understand how hard it is not to drink. (I can't stand being so angry. A drink will make me feel better.)

FIGURE 8.1. Vic's Thought Record.

also circled another hot thought – "I can't stand being so angry. A drink will make me feel better." – because Vic realized that these thoughts were pushing him toward drinking, which he knew he would regret later.

Once he identified these two hot thoughts, he remembered his therapist had told him that columns 4 and 5 on the Thought Record ask the most important question in CBT: "Where's the evidence?" Vic began to consider evidence to support his thoughts that Judy didn't care about him and that he needed a drink to cope with his anger.

Vic's anger began when he interpreted the look on his wife's face as irritation with

RECORD

4. Evidence That Supports the Hot Thought	5. Evidence That Does Not Support the Hot Thought	6. Alternative/ Balanced Thoughts a. Write an alternative or balanced thought. b. Rate how much you believe each thought (0–100%).	7. Rate Moods Now Rerate column 2 moods and any new moods (0–100%).
She's not supportive of AA. She nags me to do things. She doesn't seem to appreciate how hard I work. She's always giving me negative looks, like she did tonight. She yelled at me as I was leaving the house.	She stuck with me during all those years of drinking. She attended Al-Anon meetings for a year. She seemed happy to see me when I came home from work tonight. She tells me she loves me and does nice things for me when we're not fighting.		
I hate feeling this way. When I've felt this way in the past, a drink always relaxes me. The alcohol will work quickly.	When the alcohol wears off, I sometimes feel worse. Last month when I got really upset, I didn't drink because I was with Jim, and after an hour I felt better anyway. Although I'm really upset now, I know it won't really last forever. I survived detox, which felt a lot worse than this anger.		

his decision to attend a Saturday AA meeting. He then took that to mean that she didn't care about his recovery program or about him. By looking for evidence that did and did not support his conclusions, Vic put himself in a better position to evaluate and react to his thoughts about what was going on between him and Judy. As shown in the bottom half of columns 4 and 5, Vic also gathered evidence to test out his thought that he couldn't stand feeling angry and needed a drink to help him feel better.

As Vic recalled from his discussion with his therapist, columns 4 and 5 of the Thought Record address the question "Where's the evidence?" (Figure 8.1). These two columns are designed to help you gather information that supports and does not support the hot thoughts you identified in the "Automatic Thoughts" column (column 3). The evidence collected in columns 4 and 5 helps you evaluate your hot thoughts.

When you begin filling out the two evidence columns, it is helpful to think about your hot thoughts as hypotheses, or guesses. If you temporarily suspend your certainty that your hot thoughts are true, you will find it easier to look for evidence that both supports and doesn't support your conclusion.

As Vic sat in his car outside the liquor store considering the evidence for and against his beliefs about Judy and needing a drink, he tried to stick to data, facts, or actual experiences that did or did not support his hot thoughts.

> **EXERCISE: Facts versus Interpretations**
>
> Worksheet 8.1 helps you practice telling the difference between facts and interpretations. "Facts" are generally things that everyone would agree on in a situation – things like "It was Thursday night," or "The expression on Judy's face changed." "Interpretations" are things people looking at the same situation might disagree about. For each of the statements listed in the left column of Worksheet 8.1, write on the line in the right column whether you think this is a fact or an interpretation about what went on between Vic and Judy. The first two have been completed as examples. You may want to refer to the description of Judy and Vic's fight at the beginning of this chapter on page 69 before you decide if a statement is a fact or an interpretation.

WORKSHEET 8.1. Facts versus Interpretations

1. She's always giving me negative looks.	*Interpretation*
2. The expression on Judy's face changed.	*Fact*
3. I'm feeling angry [Vic].	
4. Judy doesn't care if I'm sober or not.	
5. She cares more about the kids than she does about me.	
6. Judy yelled at me as I was leaving the house.	
7. Judy stayed with me through all those years of drinking.	
8. She doesn't support me in AA.	
9. I can't stand being so angry.	
10. You can't expect me to care when you act like this [Judy].	

From *Mind Over Mood, Second Edition*. Copyright 2016 by Dennis Greenberger and Christine A. Padesky. Purchasers of this book can photocopy and/or download additional copies of this worksheet (see the box at the end of the table of contents).

Following are answers to Worksheet 8.1.

1. She's always giving me negative looks. .... Interpretation

2. The expression on Judy's face changed. .... Fact

3. I'm feeling angry [Vic]. .... Fact

4. Judy doesn't care if I'm sober or not. .... Interpretation

5. She cares more about the kids than she does about me. .... Interpretation

6. Judy yelled at me as I was leaving the house. .... Fact

7. Judy stayed with me through all those years of drinking. .... Fact

8. She doesn't support me in AA. .... Interpretation

9. I can't stand being so angry. .... Interpretation

10. You can't expect me to care when you act like this [Judy]. ...... Interpretation

The information in the evidence columns of a Thought Record should consist mostly of objective data or facts. However, when you first begin to fill out these columns, you will probably mix facts with interpretations, as Vic did on his Thought Record. For example, Vic wrote, "She's always giving me negative looks, like she did tonight," which reflected his interpretation that her distressed look was a negative look directed at him. Since Judy didn't really say what she was thinking and feeling when she looked at him, Vic didn't really know for sure that her look was a "negative one" directed at him. Also, "She's always giving me negative looks, like she did tonight" might have been an exaggeration of how often Judy gave him negative looks.

Were you able to tell the difference between facts and interpretations on Worksheet 8.1? The facts are all things described at the beginning of the chapter. Anyone watching Judy and Vic would probably agree that these things occurred: (2) The expression on Judy's face changed, (3) Vic was feeling angry, (6) Judy yelled at Vic as he was leaving the house, and (7) Judy stayed with Vic through many years of drinking.

Interpretations are things we read into situations. These are our thoughts about the situation or another person that may or may not be true. For example, it was possible that (4) Judy didn't care if Vic was sober, or that (5) she cared more about the kids than she did about Vic. But since Judy had not really said these things, we wouldn't know for sure unless we decided to ask her. Similarly, Judy didn't know for sure that (10) Vic couldn't expect her to care when he acted like this. This was her interpretation and might or might not be accurate. Sometimes we need to gather more information before we know if a statement is fact or interpretation. For example, Vic could directly ask Judy if she supported him in AA (8). Also, he could delay his drinking and find out if he could stand being so angry for longer than he imagined (9).

Column 4 ("Evidence That Supports the Hot Thought") and column 5 ("Evidence That Does Not Support the Hot Thought") of the Thought Record are designed to help you test the accuracy of your hot thoughts. As you practice completing the evidence columns for your own automatic thoughts, try to be factual in what you write. However, even if you do include some ideas that are not facts in column 4, the Thought Record will be valuable if you can find evidence to write in column 5. This column is one of the most important on the Thought Record, because it asks you to look for information that doesn't support your conclusions. *Evidence that does not support our beliefs can be hard to uncover when we are experiencing a strong mood. Yet looking at the evidence both for and against our conclusions is one secret to reducing the intensity of our moods.*

If you notice, the first four columns of the Thought Record help us get clear and specific about what is going on when we have strong moods. It isn't until we get to column 5 that we are asked to think about things differently. Perhaps for this reason, column 5 is often the hardest step to master. Some people even draw a blank when they get to column 5. In the Helpful Hints on page 75, we provide some questions you can ask yourself to help complete column 5. It may take a few weeks of practice before you find it easier to find evidence that does not support your hot thought (column 5). As you complete more Thought Records, it will get easier for you to find evidence that doesn't support your hot thoughts.

BEN: *Second thoughts.*

An example from Ben's life further illustrates the importance of using factual evidence to test out our interpretations and conclusions. Approximately three months after his therapy began, Ben felt very sad as he returned home from a day spent visiting his daughter and her family. After he arrived home, Ben decided to fill out a Thought Record in order to understand his sadness better and to try to improve his mood.

After identifying a series of automatic thoughts, Ben decided that they were all "hot." However, the one that seemed most closely connected to his sadness was the idea that he wasn't needed any more by his children and grandchildren. Ben circled this as his hottest thought on the Thought Record in Figure 8.2 on pages 76–77.

When we have negative automatic thoughts, we usually dwell on data that confirm our conclusions. Before Ben filled out his Thought Record, his thoughts were focused on the column 4 events supporting his belief that "The kids and grandkids don't need me any more." Thinking only about the ways in which he was no longer needed by his family led Ben to feel very sad. Thinking about negative experiences is natural when we are depressed.

Column 5 of the Thought Record required Ben to actively search his memory for experiences that did not support his conclusions. When Ben recalled events indicating that he was still needed and loved by his family, his mood lifted. Even though his children were grown up and his grandchildren were doing more things for themselves, Ben was able to remember events suggesting that he was still an important person in their lives.

The realization that he was still important to his family was not available to Ben as long as he focused only on evidence that supported his negative thoughts. Column 5

HELPFUL HINTS — **Questions to Help Find Evidence That Does Not Support Your Hot Thought**

- Have I had any experiences or is there any information that suggests that this thought is not completely true all the time?
- If my best friend or someone I loved had this thought, what would I tell them?
- If my best friend or someone who cares about me knew I was thinking this thought, what would they say to me? What factual evidence (information or experiences) would they point out to me that suggests my hot thought is not 100% true?
- Are there any small pieces of information that contradict my hot thought that I might be ignoring or discounting as not important?
- Are there any strengths or qualities I have that I am ignoring? What are they? How might they help in this situation?
- Are there any positives in this situation that I am ignoring? Is there any information that suggests there might be a positive outcome in this situation?
- Have I been in this type of situation before? What happened? Is there anything different between this situation and previous ones? What have I learned from prior experiences that could help me understand this situation differently?
- When I am not feeling this way, do I think about this type of situation any differently? How? What factual information do I focus on?
- When I have felt this way in the past, what did I think about that helped me feel better?
- Five years from now, if I look back at this situation, will I look at it any differently? Will I focus on any different part of my experience?
- Am I jumping to any conclusions in columns 3 and 4 that are not completely justified by the facts?
- Am I blaming myself for something over which I do not have complete control? What facts can I write down that reflect a more fair, compassionate, or kind view of my responsibility?

From *Mind Over Mood, Second Edition*. Copyright 2016 by Dennis Greenberger and Christine A. Padesky. Purchasers may photocopy this box for personal use or use with individual clients.

encouraged Ben to actively remember and examine information and experiences that did not support his original negative automatic thoughts.

Like Ben, you will probably experience a shift in mood if you can find evidence to write in column 5. However, if you are experiencing a very strong mood or holding a belief that seems absolutely true to you, it can be hard to see the evidence that does not support your beliefs. The questions in the Helpful Hints above, which remind you to

76   Mind Over Mood

THOUGHT

1. Situation Who? What? When? Where?	2. Moods a. What did you feel? b. Rate each mood (0–100%). c. Circle or mark the mood you want to examine.	3. Automatic Thoughts (Images) a. What was going through your mind just before you started to feel this way? Any other thoughts? Images? b. Circle or mark the hot thought.
November 5, 9:00 P.M. Driving home from my daughter's home where I spent the day with my daughter, son-in-law, two of my grandchildren, and my wife.	(Sad 80%)	They all would have had a better time if I hadn't been there today. They didn't pay any attention to me all day. (The kids and grandkids don't need me any more.)

FIGURE 8.2. Ben's Thought Record.

look at a situation from many different perspectives, will help you find evidence that does not support your hot thought.

It is not necessary to answer all the questions in the Helpful Hints on page 75. When you are first learning to complete column 5, it may be helpful to answer a number of the questions. As you gain experience, you will learn which questions are most useful for you and the types of hot thoughts you have.

RECORD

4. Evidence That Supports the Hot Thought	5. Evidence That Does Not Support the Hot Thought	6. Alternative/ Balanced Thoughts a. Write an alternative or balanced thought. b. Rate how much you believe each thought (0–100%).	7. Rate Moods Now Rerate column 2 moods and any new moods (0–100%).
I used to enjoy tying my granddaughter Nicole's shoes, but now she wants to do this on her own. My daughter and son-in-law have their lives together, and they don't need anything from me. Amy, the 15-year-old, left at 7:00 p.m. to be with her friends. Bill, my son-in-law, built new shelves and cabinets in the family room. Three years ago, he would have asked me and needed me to help him with a project that big.	Bill asked for my advice on plans for a room addition to their home. My daughter asked me to take a look at some vegetables in their garden that were dying. I was able to tell her that they weren't getting enough water. I made Nicole laugh often throughout the day. Amy seemed to enjoy my stories about her mom as a teenager. Nicole fell asleep in my lap.		

MARISSA: *Put yourself in someone else's . . . head.*

In the beginning of her therapy, Marissa encountered some difficulty in answering the question "Where's the evidence?" Marissa brought the partially completed Thought Record in Figure 8.3 on pages 78–79 to one of her early therapy sessions.

On her own, Marissa was unable to unearth any evidence that her hot thought was not 100% true. The following exchange with her therapist helped her identify evidence

78 *Mind Over Mood*

to write in column 5. Notice that the questions Marissa's therapist asked are similar to those in the Helpful Hints on page 75.

> THERAPIST: If I understand your Thought Record correctly, your hot thought was "These emotions are so painful that I have to kill myself, because I can't stand them any more."
> You were able to find evidence to support that thought, but you were unable to find any evidence that did not support this thought.
>
> MARISSA: That's right.
>
> THERAPIST: Have you ever felt in the past that your pain was so great that you had to kill yourself?
>
> MARISSA: Dozens of times.
>
> THERAPIST: In the past when you have felt this way, what have you done or thought about that has helped you to feel better?
>
> MARISSA: It's funny, but sometimes talking about my pain helps me feel better.

THOUGHT

1. Situation Who? What? When? Where?	2. Moods a. What did you feel? b. Rate each mood (0–100%). c. Circle or mark the mood you want to examine.	3. Automatic Thoughts (Images) a. What was going through your mind just before you started to feel this way? Any other thoughts? Images? b. Circle or mark the hot thought.
At home alone, Saturday, 9:30 P.M.	Depressed 100% Disappointed 95% Empty 100% Confused 90% Unreal 95%	I want to go numb so I don't have to feel any more. I'm not making any progress. I'm so confused that I can't think clearly. I don't know what's real and what isn't. These emotions are so painful that I have to kill myself, because I can't stand them any more. Nothing helps. Life is not worth living. I'm such a failure.

FIGURE 8.3. Marissa's partially completed Thought Record.

Where's the Evidence?   79

THERAPIST: So talking about it sometimes helps. In addition to talking to someone, have you ever had any thoughts that have helped you feel better?

MARISSA: When I'm feeling the worst, I try to remember that I have felt this way before and have gotten through it every time.

THERAPIST: Well, that is important information. Is there anything about your situation now to suggest that suicide is not the only option?

MARISSA: What do you mean?

THERAPIST: I'm wondering whether or not you have any hope that something other than suicide will lessen your pain.

MARISSA: Well, I guess I'm learning to think differently, but I'm not so sure that's going to help.

THERAPIST: Part of you is doubtful about whether the CBT will help you, and part of you is hopeful.

MARISSA: I am much more doubtful than hopeful.

RECORD

4. Evidence That Supports the Hot Thought	5. Evidence That Does Not Support the Hot Thought	6. Alternative/ Balanced Thoughts a. Write an alternative or balanced thought. b. Rate how much you believe each thought (0–100%).	7. Rate Moods Now Rerate column 2 moods and any new moods (0–100%).
I can't stand this. I want to die. Killing myself is the only way to get rid of the pain. No one has been able to help me.			

THERAPIST: Percent-wise, how much of you is doubtful and how much of you is hopeful that the skills you are learning will help lessen your pain?

MARISSA: I am 90–95% doubtful and 5–10% hopeful.

THERAPIST: We'll keep track of how your levels of doubt and hopefulness fluctuate as you progress in therapy. If you told your best friend, Kate, that "The pain is so great that I have to kill myself," what would she say to you?

MARISSA: I never would tell her, but if I did, she probably would tell me that I have a lot going for me, a lot to look forward to, and a lot to contribute to the world. I wouldn't believe her, though.

THERAPIST: Would she tell you anything else that you might partially believe?

MARISSA: She would probably point out that there are some things in life that give me some enjoyment, and that I have some moments during most days when I feel better and in less pain. She would remind me that some things strike me as funny and I laugh sometimes.

THOUGHT

1. Situation Who? What? When? Where?	2. Moods a. What did you feel? b. Rate each mood (0–100%). c. Circle or mark the mood you want to examine.	3. Automatic Thoughts (Images) a. What was going through your mind just before you started to feel this way? Any other thoughts? Images? b. Circle or mark the hot thought.
At home alone, Saturday, 9:30 P.M.	(Depressed 100%) Disappointed 95% Empty 100% Confused 90% Unreal 95%	I want to go numb so I don't have to feel any more. I'm not making any progress. I'm so confused that I can't think clearly. I don't know what's real and what isn't. (These emotions are so painful that I have to kill myself, because I can't stand them any more.) Nothing helps. Life is not worth living. I'm such a failure.

FIGURE 8.4. Marissa's Thought Record with complete evidence.

THERAPIST: If Kate told you that she was in so much emotional pain that she thought suicide was the only solution, what would you say to her?

MARISSA: I would tell her to keep trying other solutions. There would have to be hope for Kate. But I don't see much hope for me.

THERAPIST: We'll consider how much hope makes sense in a few minutes. First, let's write on the Thought Record the things we just talked about that can go in column 5.

Figure 8.4 reflects the information Marissa gathered with her therapist's help.

It is important to *write down* the evidence you uncover while answering the questions in the Helpful Hints on page 75. Marissa remained quite hopeless while discussing this evidence with her therapist. But when she wrote it down on her Thought Record, she discovered that seeing it all at once did make her feel somewhat more hopeful and less depressed. Similarly, you will benefit more from writing down the evidence you gather rather than simply thinking about it.

RECORD

4. Evidence That Supports the Hot Thought	5. Evidence That Does Not Support the Hot Thought	6. Alternative/ Balanced Thoughts a. Write an alternative or balanced thought. b. Rate how much you believe each thought (0–100%).	7. Rate Moods Now Rerate column 2 moods and any new moods (0–100%).
I can't stand this. I want to die. Whenever I get better it never lasts. Feeling better is always temporary for me. No one has been able to help me.	Sometimes talking to my therapist does help me feel better. This never lasts forever, but it always comes back. This Thought Record is something new that might help, but I'm doubtful. Some days I feel a little better.		

82   Mind Over Mood

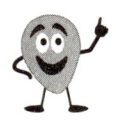

REMINDERS
- To complete column 5 of a Thought Record, ask yourself the questions in the Helpful Hints on page 75.
- *Write down* all the evidence that does not support your hot thought, rather than simply thinking about it.

LINDA: *Heart attack or anxiety?*

As her treatment progressed, Linda became more skilled at asking herself the questions that allowed her to complete column 5 of the Thought Record. This skill helped Linda prevent her anxiety symptoms from escalating into a panic attack. As Linda sat in an airplane waiting for it to take off, she began to feel anxious. She decided to record her

THOUGHT

1. Situation Who? What? When? Where?	2. Moods a. What did you feel? b. Rate each mood (0–100%). c. Circle or mark the mood you want to examine.	3. Automatic Thoughts (Images) a. What was going through your mind just before you started to feel this way? Any other thoughts? Images? b. Circle or mark the hot thought.
Sunday evening, in the airplane, on the runway, waiting for the plane to take off.	(Fear 98%)	I'm feeling sick. My heart is starting to beat harder and faster. I'm starting to sweat. (I'm having a heart attack.) I'll never be able to get off this plane and to a hospital in time. I'm going to die.

FIGURE 8.5. Linda's partially completed Thought Record.

experience on a Thought Record, to see if she could identify and examine the thoughts connected to her anxiety. As shown in Figure 8.5, Linda began by describing the situation, her mood, and automatic thoughts. Once she identified her hot thought – "I'm having a heart attack" – Linda wrote down the evidence that supported this idea in column 4. Then Linda began to gather evidence that did not support her hot thought. As she was sitting on the airplane, Linda thought about what her best friend might tell her if she were sitting next to her. She knew that her friend would tell her that her rapid heartbeat was probably caused by her nervousness and anxiety, and did not necessarily mean that she was having a heart attack. Furthermore, Linda remembered that her physician had told her that her heart was a muscle, and making it beat faster was part of healthy exercise. He told her that a rapid heartbeat is not necessarily dangerous, nor is it a definite sign of a heart attack. He found nothing wrong with her heart after a thorough exam.

Linda also asked herself whether she had had any experiences demonstrating that

RECORD

4. Evidence That Supports the Hot Thought	5. Evidence That Does Not Support the Hot Thought	6. Alternative/ Balanced Thoughts a. Write an alternative or balanced thought. b. Rate how much you believe each thought (0–100%).	7. Rate Moods Now Rerate column 2 moods and any new moods (0–100%).
My heart is racing. I'm sweating. These could be two signs of a heart attack.			

84   *Mind Over Mood*

her hot thought was not true. She realized that, in fact, she had had a rapid heartbeat many times before on airplanes, in airports, and when she was thinking about flying. Even though she had believed that she was having a heart attack in those situations, she understood now that she was having a panic attack, not a heart attack.

Finally, Linda asked herself what she had done or thought about in the past that had helped her feel better. She remembered that in the past it had helped to concentrate on

THOUGHT

1. **Situation** Who? What? When? Where?	2. **Moods** a. What did you feel? b. Rate each mood (0–100%). c. Circle or mark the mood you want to examine.	3. **Automatic Thoughts (Images)** a. What was going through your mind just before you started to feel this way? Any other thoughts? Images? b. Circle or mark the hot thought.
Sunday evening, in the airplane, on the runway, waiting for the plane to take off.	(Fear 98%)	I'm feeling sick. My heart is starting to beat harder and faster. I'm starting to sweat. (I'm having a heart attack.) I'll never be able to get off this plane and to a hospital in time. I'm going to die.

FIGURE 8.6. Linda's Thought Record with complete evidence.

Where's the Evidence? 85

reading a magazine, breathe slowly and deeply, write out a Thought Record, and think about her heart in ways that were not so catastrophic. As she asked herself the questions from the Helpful Hints on page 75, Linda wrote her answers down in column 5, as shown in Figure 8.6. The questions and her answers helped Linda attend to important information that did not fit with her hot thought that she was having a heart attack. As Linda considered this information, her anxiety decreased.

RECORD

4. Evidence That Supports the Hot Thought	5. Evidence That Does Not Support the Hot Thought	6. Alternative/ Balanced Thoughts a. Write an alternative or balanced thought. b. Rate how much you believe each thought (0–100%).	7. Rate Moods Now Rerate column 2 moods and any new moods (0–100%).
My heart is racing. I'm sweating. These could be two signs of a heart attack.	Anxiety can cause a rapid heartbeat. My doctor told me that the heart is a muscle, using a muscle makes it stronger, and a rapid heartbeat is not necessarily dangerous. A rapid heartbeat doesn't mean that I am having a heart attack. I have had this happen to me before in airports, on airplanes, and when thinking about flying. In the past, my heartbeat has returned to normal when I read a magazine, practiced slow breathing, did Thought Records, or thought in less catastrophic ways.		

EXERCISE: Identifying Evidence That Supports and Doesn't Support Hot Thoughts

Just as Linda asked herself the questions from the Helpful Hints on page 75 to help her gather evidence that did not support her hot thought, you can use the same questions to look for evidence that doesn't support the hot thoughts you identified on your copies of Worksheet 7.4 (pp. 64–67). Look back at these copies of Worksheet 7.4 now. Choose two or three of these thoughts to continue working with on Worksheet 8.2 on the following pages. Alternatively, if you do not want to continue working with the thoughts you identified on your copies of Worksheet 7.4, identify two or three situations in which you recently had strong moods, and complete copies of Worksheet 8.2 for them.

On each copy of Worksheet 8.2, circle or mark the hot thought that you will test. In columns 4 and 5, write out information that supports and doesn't support the hot thought you marked.

Try to list in column 4 only factual evidence that supports your hot thought, not your interpretations of the facts. For example, "Peter stared at me" is an example of factual evidence. The statement, "Peter stared at me and thought I was crazy," would not be factual unless Peter had actually said aloud, "I think you are crazy." If Peter had been staring silently, your assumption that you knew what he was thinking is a guess and may or may not be accurate.

Once you have completed column 4, ask yourself the questions in the Helpful Hints on page 75 to look for evidence that does not support your hot thought. Write down in column 5 each piece of evidence you uncover. Completing these two "Evidence" columns of the Thought Record allows you to evaluate your hot thought from different angles, and may provide information that will help you develop an alternative way of seeing things.

> *Before finishing this chapter,
> fill out the first five columns on one or more Thought Records,
> which can be found on the following pages.*

WORKSHEET 8.2. Where's the Evidence?

THOUGHT

1. Situation	2. Moods	3. Automatic Thoughts (Images)
Who were you with? What were you doing? When was it? Where were you?	Describe each mood in one word. Rate intensity of mood (0–100%). Circle or mark the mood you want to examine.	**Answer the first two general questions, and then some or all of the questions specific to the mood you marked in column 2:** What was going through my mind just before I started to feel this way? (General) What images or memories do I have in this situation? (General) What does this mean about me? My life? My future? (Depression) What am I afraid might happen? (Anxiety) What is the worst that could happen? (Anxiety) What does this mean about how the other person(s) feel(s)/think(s) about me? (Anger, Shame) What does this mean about the other person(s) or people in general? (Anger) Did I break rules, hurt others, or not do something I should have done? What do I think about myself that I did this or believe I did it? (Guilt, Shame)

From *Mind Over Mood, Second Edition*. Copyright 2016 by Dennis Greenberger and Christine A. Padesky. Purchasers of this book can photocopy and/or download additional copies of this worksheet (see the box at the end of the table of contents).

RECORD

4. Evidence That Supports the Hot Thought	5. Evidence That Does Not Support the Hot Thought	6. Alternative/Balanced Thoughts	7. Rate Moods Now
Circle hot thought in previous column for which you are looking for evidence. Write factual evidence to support this conclusion. (Try to write facts, not interpretations, as you practiced in Worksheet 8.1 on p. 72.)	Ask yourself the questions in the Helpful Hints (p. 75) to help discover evidence that does not support your hot thought.		

WORKSHEET 8.2. Where's the Evidence?

THOUGHT

1. Situation	2. Moods	3. Automatic Thoughts (Images)
Who were you with? What were you doing? When was it? Where were you?	Describe each mood in one word. Rate intensity of mood (0–100%). Circle or mark the mood you want to examine.	**Answer the first two general questions, and then some or all of the questions specific to the mood you marked in column 2:** What was going through my mind just before I started to feel this way? (General) What images or memories do I have in this situation? (General) What does this mean about me? My life? My future? (Depression) What am I afraid might happen? (Anxiety) What is the worst that could happen? (Anxiety) What does this mean about how the other person(s) feel(s)/think(s) about me? (Anger, Shame) What does this mean about the other person(s) or people in general? (Anger) Did I break rules, hurt others, or not do something I should have done? What do I think about myself that I did this or believe I did it? (Guilt, Shame)

From *Mind Over Mood, Second Edition*. Copyright 2016 by Dennis Greenberger and Christine A. Padesky. Purchasers of this book can photocopy and/or download additional copies of this worksheet (see the box at the end of the table of contents).

RECORD

4. Evidence That Supports the Hot Thought	5. Evidence That Does Not Support the Hot Thought	6. Alternative/Balanced Thoughts	7. Rate Moods Now
Circle hot thought in previous column for which you are looking for evidence. Write factual evidence to support this conclusion. (Try to write facts, not interpretations, as you practiced in Worksheet 8.1 on p. 72.)	Ask yourself the questions in the Helpful Hints (p. 75) to help discover evidence that does not support your hot thought.		

WORKSHEET 8.2. Where's the Evidence?

THOUGHT

1. Situation	2. Moods	3. Automatic Thoughts (Images)
Who were you with? What were you doing? When was it? Where were you?	Describe each mood in one word. Rate intensity of mood (0–100%). Circle or mark the mood you want to examine.	**Answer the first two general questions, and then some or all of the questions specific to the mood you marked in column 2:** What was going through my mind just before I started to feel this way? (General) What images or memories do I have in this situation? (General) What does this mean about me? My life? My future? (Depression) What am I afraid might happen? (Anxiety) What is the worst that could happen? (Anxiety) What does this mean about how the other person(s) feel(s)/think(s) about me? (Anger, Shame) What does this mean about the other person(s) or people in general? (Anger) Did I break rules, hurt others, or not do something I should have done? What do I think about myself that I did this or believe I did it? (Guilt, Shame)

From *Mind Over Mood, Second Edition*. Copyright 2016 by Dennis Greenberger and Christine A. Padesky. Purchasers of this book can photocopy and/or download additional copies of this worksheet (see the box at the end of the table of contents).

RECORD

4. Evidence That Supports the Hot Thought	5. Evidence That Does Not Support the Hot Thought	6. Alternative/Balanced Thoughts	7. Rate Moods Now
Circle hot thought in previous column for which you are looking for evidence. Write factual evidence to support this conclusion. (Try to write facts, not interpretations, as you practiced in Worksheet 8.1 on p. 72.)	Ask yourself the questions in the Helpful Hints (p. 75) to help discover evidence that does not support your hot thought.		

Chapter 9 will teach you what you need to know to complete the last two columns of the Thought Record. Before proceeding to the next chapter, practice identifying evidence for five or six more hot thoughts by completing the first five columns on several more copies of Worksheet 8.2. (Additional copies of this worksheet can be printed from *www.guilford.com/MOM2-materials.*) You can use the thoughts you identified on Worksheet 7.4, or you can use new thoughts. The more you practice looking for evidence for and against hot thoughts, the more quickly you will develop the type of flexible thinking that is linked to feeling better.

Now is a good time to measure your moods again. Remember, you can use the following measures and graphs to record your scores:

- Depression/unhappiness: *Mind Over Mood* Depression Inventory
    Worksheet 13.1, page 191, and Worksheet 13.2, page 192

- Anxiety/nervousness: *Mind Over Mood* Anxiety Inventory
    Worksheet 14.1, page 221; Worksheet 14.2, page 222

- Other moods/happiness: Measuring and Tracking My Moods
    Worksheet 15.1, page 253, and Worksheet 15.2, page 254

Chapter 8 Summary

▶ When we have negative automatic thoughts, we usually think mostly about information and experiences that confirm our conclusions.

▶ It is helpful to think about your hot thoughts as hypotheses or guesses.

▶ Gathering evidence that supports and does not support your hot thoughts can help reduce the intensity of distressing moods.

▶ Evidence consists of factual information, not interpretations.

▶ Column 5 of the Thought Record asks you to actively search for information that doesn't support a hot thought.

▶ It is important to write down all the evidence that does not support your hot thought.

▶ You can ask yourself the specific questions in the Helpful Hints on page 75 to help you complete column 5 of a Thought Record.

9
Alternative or Balanced Thinking

Akiko was at home with the flu and asked her 7-year-old daughter, Yuki, to play quietly while she rested. An hour later, Akiko walked into the kitchen to make some tea and was distressed to see crayons spread all over the floor, shredded colored paper, an open bottle of glue on the table, scissors in the wastebasket, and a half-drunk glass of milk on the counter next to the refrigerator.

Furious about the mess, Akiko went looking for Yuki and found her sleeping soundly in front of the television in the living room. On the cushion near Yuki's head was a large, brightly colored card, covered in hearts that read, "I love you, Mom! Please get well soon!" Akiko shook her head slowly and smiled. She tucked a blanket around Yuki's shoulders and returned to the kitchen to make her tea.

Sometimes a little bit of additional information shifts our interpretation and understanding of a situation 180 degrees. When Akiko first walked into the kitchen, she was not expecting a mess and immediately felt angry that Yuki had made one, especially when Akiko was sick. Akiko's hot thought accompanying her anger was "Yuki is so inconsiderate to make such a mess when she knows I'm sick."

When Akiko discovered the beautiful get-well card, her emotional response shifted immediately. Akiko thought, "Yuki was concerned for me and wanted to help me feel better – how thoughtful!" Feelings of appreciation and tenderness toward Yuki followed this alternative thought. Learning the meaning behind the mess led to a shift in Akiko's attitude and mood.

Vic: *Gathering new evidence.*

Chapter 8 began with a description of Vic's reaction to the change in his wife's facial expression when he told her he had plans to attend a Saturday AA meeting. Vic's interpretation of Judy's facial expression was "She's upset that I'm spending time away from her and the kids." His anger was fueled by further thoughts: "It's not fair that she doesn't see my recovery program as important," "If she cared about me as much as she cares about the kids, she'd be happy I was going to AA," and "She doesn't care about me."

Vic's interpretation of Judy's expression affected his behaviors as well as his emotions. He yelled at Judy, slammed his fist on the table, stormed out of the house, and drove to a nearby liquor store. Fortunately, before going into the liquor store, Vic filled out a Thought Record that looked for evidence both supporting and not supporting the hot thought, "She doesn't care about me" (see Figure 8.1)

As Vic considered all the information on his Thought Record, he realized that Judy did seem to care for him in many important ways. In fact, he began to wonder why she would be upset about his plan to attend an AA meeting. Vic's therapist had pointed out that Vic's distress at work often followed instances where Vic made assumptions about what his supervisor was thinking – assumptions that were often wrong. Vic began to wonder whether he was wrong in his assumption about what Judy was thinking.

THOUGHT

1. Situation Who? What? When? Where?	2. Moods a. What did you feel? b. Rate each mood (0–100%). c. Circle or mark the mood you want to examine.	3. Automatic Thoughts (Images) a. What was going through your mind just before you started to feel this way? Any other thoughts? Images? b. Circle or mark the hot thought.
Thursday, 8:30 P.M. Judy gives me an odd look when I tell her I'm going to AA on Saturday.	Anger 90%	She's upset that I'm going to AA on Saturday. She doesn't see my recovery program as important. She doesn't care about me. She doesn't understand how hard it is not to drink. I can't stand being so angry. A drink will make me feel better.

FIGURE 9.1. Vic's Thought Record.

Instead of buying alcohol at the liquor store, Vic decided to call his AA sponsor. After talking with Vic for a few minutes, his sponsor advised him to go to an AA meeting before heading home. After ending the conversation with his sponsor, Vic decided to telephone Judy. As Vic and Judy began to talk about their argument, Vic decided to test his assumptions by asking Judy about her reaction when he told her he had made plans to go to the AA meeting on Saturday. Judy's response surprised Vic. She said that when he mentioned Saturday, she had remembered that Saturday was her sister's birthday, and she'd forgotten to mail a card. Judy had been concerned that her sister would be upset or hurt if a card didn't arrive on time. Judy had not been aware of a change in her facial expression, but if it had changed, she was certain that these were the thoughts that had caused it – she hadn't been thinking about Vic at all! As shown in Figure 9.1, Vic wrote these alternative explanations in column 6 of his Thought Record.

Vic sheepishly told Judy that he had thought her look meant that she was upset with him for planning to attend an AA meeting on Saturday, and that he had been angry

RECORD

4. Evidence That Supports the Hot Thought	5. Evidence That Does Not Support the Hot Thought	6. Alternative/ Balanced Thoughts a. Write an alternative or balanced thought. b. Rate how much you believe each thought (0–100%).	7. Rate Moods Now Rerate column 2 moods and any new moods (0–100%).
She's not supportive of AA. She nags me to do things. She doesn't seem to appreciate how hard I work. She's always giving me negative looks, like she did tonight. She yelled at me as I was leaving the house.	She stuck with me during all those years of drinking. She attended Al-Anon meetings for a year. She seemed happy to see me when I came home from work tonight. She tells me she loves me and does nice things for me when we're not fighting. Judy explained that her facial expression was due to remembering her sister's birthday. Judy says she is glad I am in AA, and she wants me to go to meetings.	The look on Judy's face was because she remembered her sister's birthday. 100% She is supportive of my AA attendance and wants me to stay sober. 100% She does care about me. 80%	

because he thought this meant that she didn't care about him or his sobriety. Judy voiced her support for Vic's recovery program and told him that she had worried while he was gone that he would drink and be killed driving. She said she loved him very much, although his quick anger was becoming increasingly difficult for her to tolerate. Vic sincerely apologized. He reminded her that he was working on his anger, and he asked her to be patient with him.

Both Akiko's change in mood when she saw the get-well card and Vic's realization that his wife's facial expression had nothing to do with him illustrate how new or additional information can shift one's perspective of a distressing situation. Vic and Akiko each discovered an alternative explanation for an event that was less distressing than their original interpretation. Vic and Akiko each felt better after gathering evidence and understanding their situation in a different way.

In Chapter 8, you learned to ask yourself questions to actively look for evidence that supports and doesn't support your hot thoughts (see the Helpful Hints on p. 75). Sometimes the evidence you find shows that your hot thoughts do not tell the whole story. Akiko discovered that her 7-year-old daughter's mess was the result of her daughter's love and caring. Vic found out that his wife's facial expression was not a negative reaction to him. When the evidence in columns 4 and 5 of the Thought Record does not support your original automatic thought, write an alternative explanation for the situation in column 6, as illustrated in Figure 9.1.

Notice that Vic rated his belief in his alternative thoughts very high. He completely believed that Judy's change in facial expression was due to remembering her sister's birthday, and so he rated his belief in this alternative thought as 100%. He was also completely confident after their discussion that Judy supported his AA attendance and wanted him to stay sober. Vic rated his belief in the last alternative thought – that Judy cared about him – as 80%. He strongly believed that she cared, but he still had a few lingering doubts. The alternative view(s) of a situation you write should take into account all the evidence you have written down in columns 4 and 5.

Vic's perspective changed almost completely. He shifted from a belief that Judy didn't care to one that she did. As it did with Vic, sometimes the evidence leads to a total shift in perspective. At other times, the new view of the situation will be more of a balanced perspective that is based on the evidence supporting and not supporting the hot thought.

To construct a balanced thought, it helps to write one or two sentences that summarize your entries in column 4 of the Thought Record, and another one or two sentences that summarize your entries in column 5. If appropriate, you can connect the two sets of sentences with the word "and." For example, after examining the evidence, someone who originally thinks, "I'm a bad parent," might arrive at this more balanced thought:

"I've made some mistakes as a parent, and yet all parents make mistakes. Making some mistakes doesn't make me a bad parent. I love my children, and I think the good things that I've done outweigh the mistakes that I've made." This statement is probably a more balanced view of all the person's parenting experiences than the original hot thought, "I'm a bad parent," which focuses only on negative parenting experiences.

REMINDERS   Alternative or Balanced Thinking

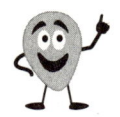

In column 6 of the Thought Record you will want to summarize the important evidence collected and recorded in columns 4 and 5.

1. If the evidence does *not* support your hot thought(s), write an alternative view of the situation that is consistent with the evidence.

2. If the evidence only partially supports your hot thought(s), write a balanced thought that summarizes the evidence supporting and not supporting your original thought.

3. Make sure your alternative thought or your balanced thought is consistent with the evidence summarized in columns 4 and 5.

4. Rate your belief in the new alternative or balanced thought(s) on a 0–100% scale.

Alternative or balanced thinking often results from looking at the evidence you have gathered in columns 4 and 5. Looking at the evidence that both supports and doesn't support your hot thought provides a broader perspective on the situation you are in. Alternative or balanced thinking is often more positive than the initial automatic thought, but it is not merely the substitution of a positive thought for a negative thought. Positive thinking tends to ignore negative information and can be as damaging as negative thinking. For example, you wouldn't want to replace the hot thought "I'm a bad parent" with "I'm a great parent" if you are thinking about a situation in which you made some parenting mistakes. Alternative or balanced thinking takes into account both negative and positive information. It is an attempt to understand the meaning of *all* the available information. With this additional information, your interpretation of an event may change. Questions you can ask yourself to help arrive at a balanced or alternative thought appear in the following Helpful Hints.

> **HELPFUL HINTS**
>
> **Questions to Help Arrive at Alternative or Balanced Thinking**
>
> - Based on the evidence I have listed in columns 4 and 5 of the Thought Record, is there an *alternative* or balanced way of thinking about or understanding this situation?
>
> - If an alternative view of the situation emerges from the evidence in columns 4 and 5, write it in column 6. Otherwise, write a balanced thought.
>
> - To write a *balanced* thought, write one statement summarizing all the evidence that supports my hot thought(s) (column 4), and another statement summarizing all the evidence that does not support my hot thought(s) (column 5). Does combining the two summary statements with the word "and" create a balanced thought that takes into account all the information I have gathered?
>
> - If someone I cared about was in this situation, had these thoughts, and had this information available, what alternative view(s) of the situation would I suggest?
>
> - If someone who cares about me knew I had my hot thought(s), what might this person say is another way of understanding this situation?
>
> - If a hot thought is supported, what is the worst outcome? If a hot thought is supported, what is the best outcome? If a hot thought is supported, what is the most likely outcome?
>
> From *Mind Over Mood, Second Edition*. Copyright 2016 by Dennis Greenberger and Christine A. Padesky. Purchasers may photocopy this box for personal use or use with individual clients.

Column 7 of the Thought Record asks you to rerate the moods you have identified in column 2. If you have constructed a balanced/alternative thought that is believable to you, you will probably notice that the intensity of your negative mood has decreased, and your moods may even change.

The following examples demonstrate how Marissa, Ben, and Linda developed alternative or balanced thoughts and completed columns 6 and 7 of their Thought Records. These examples complete the Thought Records begun in Chapter 8 (Figures 8.2, 8.4, and 8.6).

BEN: *Balanced thinking.*

As described in Chapter 8, Ben completed a Thought Record regarding his experiences after spending the day with his daughter's family (Figure 8.2). Ben identified his hot automatic thought as "The kids and grandkids don't need me any more." Ben then gathered evidence that supported and did not support his hot thought. After writing the evidence in columns 4 and 5 of the Thought Record, Ben reviewed the questions in the Helpful Hints on the facing page, to help construct a balanced thought for column 6.

Ben pondered the questions in the Helpful Hints while he studied the evidence in columns 4 and 5. At first, he struggled to see the situation differently. After looking several times at the evidence in column 5, Ben concluded that the evidence did not consistently support his hot thought, "The kids and grandkids don't need me any more." Ben decided that a more accurate and balanced way of understanding his experiences was: "Even though my children and grandchildren don't need me in the same ways they used to, they still seem to enjoy being with me and asked for my advice a few times. They paid attention to me, although the attention was not the same as it has been in the past." After Ben wrote this balanced thought, he noticed that the intensity rating of his sadness decreased from 80% to 30%. His completed Thought Record is shown in Figure 9.2.

If Ben had simply substituted a positive thought, he might have written, "They need me more than ever." If he had merely attempted to rationalize away his sadness, he might have thought, "They don't need me any more, but what do I care?" Positive thinking and rationalization can both lead to problems. For Ben, positive thinking would have ignored real changes that were taking place in his family (his children and grandchildren were getting older). Rationalization could have led Ben to feel even more isolated and alone. In contrast, Ben's balanced thought emerged from the evidence and allowed Ben to understand his experience in a way that lessened his sadness and increased his connection to his family.

Furthermore, notice that Ben's balanced thoughts were believable to him. He rated his belief in these new thoughts at 85% and 90%. The more an alternative or balanced thought is believable to you, the more it will reduce the intensity of your negative moods or change your mood altogether. If you simply write a rationalization or a positive thought that you do not believe in column 6, it is not likely to have a lasting impact on your mood.

102 Mind Over Mood

THOUGHT

1. Situation Who? What? When? Where?	2. Moods a. What did you feel? b. Rate each mood (0–100%). c. Circle or mark the mood you want to examine.	3. Automatic Thoughts (Images) a. What was going through your mind just before you started to feel this way? Any other thoughts? Images? b. Circle or mark the hot thought.
November 5, 9:00 p.m. Driving home from my daughter's home where I spent the day with my daughter, son-in-law, two of my grandchildren, and my wife.	(Sad 80%)	They all would have had a better time if I hadn't been there today. They didn't pay any attention to me all day. (The kids and grandkids don't need me any more.)

FIGURE 9.2. Ben's Thought Record.

RECORD

4. Evidence That Supports the Hot Thought	5. Evidence That Does Not Support the Hot Thought	6. Alternative/Balanced Thoughts a. Write an alternative or balanced thought. b. Rate how much you believe each thought (0–100%).	7. Rate Moods Now Rerate column 2 moods and any new moods (0–100%).
I used to enjoy tying my granddaughter Nicole's shoes, but now she wants to do this on her own. My daughter and son-in-law have their lives together, and they don't need anything from me. Amy, the 15-year-old, left at 7:00 p.m. to be with her friends. Bill, my son-in-law, built new shelves and cabinets in the family room. Three years ago, he would have asked me and needed me to help him with a project that big.	Bill asked for my advice on plans for a room addition to their home. My daughter asked me to take a look at some vegetables in their garden that were dying. I was able to tell her that they weren't getting enough water. I made Nicole laugh often throughout the day. Amy seemed to enjoy my stories about her mom as a teenager. Nicole fell asleep in my lap.	Even though my children and grandchildren don't need me in the same ways they used to, they still seem to enjoy being with me and asked for my advice a few times. 85% They paid attention to me, although the attention was not the same as it has been in the past. 90%	Sad 30%

MARISSA: *Alternative thinking.*

As described in Chapter 8, Marissa described an experience in which she felt depressed, disappointed, empty, confused, and unreal (Figures 8.3 and 8.4). She identified numerous automatic thoughts and decided that the hot thought was "These emotions are so painful that I have to kill myself, because I can't stand them any more." Marissa completed columns 4 and 5 of the Thought Record with the help of her therapist. To complete column 6, Marissa reviewed the questions in the Helpful Hints (p. 100) with her therapist. The question that was most relevant for Marissa was "If my friend Kate was in this situation, had these thoughts, and had this information available, what alternative view(s) of the situation would I suggest?" Marissa concluded that she would suggest to Kate, "Even though you are in a lot of pain right now, talking to somebody who cares about you has helped you to feel better in the past. You know this feeling won't last forever, and you will feel better at some point. Suicide is not the only solution – you are learning new skills that may help you feel better and stay better longer." Marissa's completed Thought Record is shown in Figure 9.3.

It was easier for Marissa to think of alternatives to suicide when she imagined the

THOUGHT

1. Situation Who? What? When? Where?	2. Moods a. What did you feel? b. Rate each mood (0–100%). c. Circle or mark the mood you want to examine.	3. Automatic Thoughts (Images) a. What was going through your mind just before you started to feel this way? Any other thoughts? Images? b. Circle or mark the hot thought.
At home alone, Saturday, 9:30 p.m.	(Depressed 100%) Disappointed 95% Empty 100% Confused 90% Unreal 95%	I want to go numb so I don't have to feel any more. I'm not making any progress. I'm so confused that I can't think clearly. I don't know what's real and what isn't. (These emotions are so painful that I have to kill myself, because I can't stand them any more.) Nothing helps. Life is not worth living. I'm such a failure.

FIGURE 9.3. Marissa's Thought Record.

advice she would give to Kate. By doing this, she was able to distance herself from her own thoughts and find a different perspective. She was able to see that there was an alternative way of thinking about her emotional pain. Even though her alternative thoughts were only slightly believable to Marissa, they still made a small, positive difference in how she felt. Even this small change had an important effect on Marissa's desire to kill herself. Her therapist reminded her that she had had these automatic thoughts and feelings for a long time, so even small changes could be interpreted as encouraging and hopeful.

The amount of change you notice in your moods when you rerate them in column 7 will depend upon how much you believe your alternative or balanced thoughts. Since Marissa believed her alternative thoughts only slightly (ratings of 10–20%), her mood did not change very much. Over time, if she has experiences that match her alternative views, Marissa's moods will shift more as her hope for improvement becomes more believable to her. It is important that balanced and alternative views are based on evidence gathered in columns 4 and 5. The more your alternative views are linked to real experiences that you have had, the more strongly you are likely to believe these new ideas.

Recall that Ben rated his sadness 80% when he was driving home from his daughter's home thinking, "The kids and grandkids don't need me any more." After con-

RECORD

4. Evidence That Supports the Hot Thought	5. Evidence That Does Not Support the Hot Thought	6. Alternative/ Balanced Thoughts a. Write an alternative or balanced thought. b. Rate how much you believe each thought (0–100%).	7. Rate Moods Now Rerate column 2 moods and any new moods (0–100%).
I can't stand this. I want to die. Killing myself is the only way to get rid of the pain. No one has been able to help me.	Sometimes talking to my therapist does help me feel better. This never lasts forever, but it always comes back. This Thought Record is something new that might help, but I'm doubtful. Some days I feel a little better.	Even though I am in a lot of pain right now, talking to somebody who cares might help me feel better, as it has in the past. 15% This feeling won't last forever, and I will feel better at some point. 10% I am learning new skills that may help me feel better and stay better longer. 15% Suicide is not the only solution. 20%	Depressed 85% Disappointed 90% Empty 95% Confused 85% Unreal 95%

structing the balanced thought "Even though my children and grandchildren don't need me in the same ways they used to, they still seem to enjoy being with me and asked for my advice a few times," Ben's sadness rating dropped to 30%.

Ben's sadness did not disappear completely after he completed a Thought Record, even though his balanced thought was highly believable (85%) to him. Some sadness remained, because some of the evidence reminded Ben of real losses he was experiencing. The goal of a Thought Record is not to eliminate emotions. Instead, the Thought Record is designed to help you gain a broader perspective on a situation, so that your emotional reactions are balanced responses to both the positive and negative aspects of a situation.

WHAT IF YOUR MOOD DID NOT CHANGE?

If your Thought Record was completed properly and your mood did not change, there are two likely possibilities.

1. Sometimes, after you look at all the evidence, it mostly supports your hot thought. The Thought Record is not intended to disprove your hot thought, but to investigate it and find out if you are ignoring important evidence – as we often do when we have strong emotions. If your hot thought is mostly supported by the evidence, then you may need either to complete an Action Plan or to practice acceptance before your mood will improve. Chapter 10 helps you develop Action Plans and/or learn how to develop greater acceptance. An Action Plan outlines steps you can take to make a situation better. Acceptance can be a helpful strategy, especially when you cannot make things better or you are in the midst of a difficult period in your life.

2. Other times, even though all the evidence does not support your hot thought, you have a hard time believing the alternative or balanced thought because your hot thought is a "core belief" – a type of deeply held negative belief that doesn't easily change even in the face of evidence. When you read Chapter 12 you will learn for additional ideas for shifting core beliefs.

What should you think or do if there is no change in your mood ratings after you complete a Thought Record? First, review your Thought Record to make sure you completed it properly. On the following page you will find questions to ask yourself if there has been no change in your moods after you have completed a Thought Record.

Questions to Determine Reason for No Mood Change after Completing a Thought Record

If there is no change in your mood ratings after you complete a Thought Record, ask yourself the following questions:

- Have I described a specific situation?

- Did I accurately identify and rate my moods in column 2?

- Is the thought I am testing a hot thought for the mood I want to change?

- Did I list multiple hot thoughts? If so, I may need to gather data supporting and not supporting each hot thought before my mood shifts.

- Is there an even hotter thought missing from my Thought Record that needs to be tested?

- Did I write down all the evidence that does not support the hot thought(s) I am evaluating? There should have been several pieces of evidence in column 5 before I wrote an alternative or balanced thought.

- Is the alternative or balanced thought I wrote in column 6 believable to me? If not, I will review the evidence again and try to write an alternative or balanced view that seems more believable.

- Does the evidence strongly support my hot thought? Then I may need to do an Action Plan or develop an attitude of acceptance regarding this situation and my reactions to it (see Chapter 10).

- Does the alternative or balanced thought match the evidence but I still don't believe it? Then I may need to gather additional evidence as described in Chapter 11, or work on core beliefs as described in Chapter 12.

From *Mind Over Mood, Second Edition*. Copyright 2016 by Dennis Greenberger and Christine A. Padesky. Purchasers may photocopy this box for personal use or use with individual clients.

LINDA: *Alternative thinking.*

It is sometimes easier to recognize alternative ways of seeing situations for other people than for ourselves. As described in Chapter 8, Linda wrote out a Thought Record that described her fear while sitting in an airplane on a runway awaiting takeoff (see Figures 8.5 and 8.6). Her partially completed Thought Record is duplicated on Worksheet 9.1.

> **EXERCISE: Helping Linda Arrive at an Alternative or Balanced Thought**
>
> In columns 4 and 5, Linda wrote down evidence that supported and did not support her hot thought "I'm having a heart attack." Based on this evidence, write in column 6 of Worksheet 9.1 a believable alternative or balanced thought that would reduce Linda's fear. If you have difficulty completing this exercise, refer to the Helpful Hints on page 100 for suggestions.

WORKSHEET 9.1. Completing Linda's Thought Record

THOUGHT

1. Situation	2. Moods	3. Automatic Thoughts (Images)
Who? What? When? Where?	a. What did you feel? b. Rate each mood (0–100%). c. Circle or mark the mood you want to examine.	a. What was going through your mind just before you started to feel this way? Any other thoughts? Images? b. Circle or mark the hot thought.
Sunday evening, in the airplane, on the runway, waiting for the plane to take off.	(Fear 98%)	I'm feeling sick. My heart is starting to beat harder and faster. I'm starting to sweat. (I'm having a heart attack.) I'll never be able to get off this plane and to a hospital in time. I'm going to die.

From *Mind Over Mood, Second Edition*. Copyright 2016 by Dennis Greenberger and Christine A. Padesky. Purchasers of this book can photocopy and/or download additional copies of this worksheet (see the box at the end of the table of contents).

RECORD

4. Evidence That Supports the Hot Thought	5. Evidence That Does Not Support the Hot Thought	6. Alternative/Balanced Thoughts a. Write an alternative or balanced thought. b. Rate how much you believe each thought (0–100%).	7. Rate Moods Now Rerate column 2 moods and any new moods (0–100%).
My heart is racing. I'm sweating. These could be two signs of a heart attack.	Anxiety can cause a rapid heartbeat. My doctor told me that the heart is a muscle, using a muscle makes it stronger, and a rapid heartbeat is not necessarily dangerous. A rapid heartbeat doesn't mean that I am having a heart attack. I have had this happen to me before in airports, on airplanes, and when thinking about flying. In the past, my heartbeat has returned to normal when I read a magazine, practiced slow breathing, did Thought Records, or thought in less catastrophic ways.		

110 Mind Over Mood

There can be more than one alternative or balanced thought that fits the evidence. When Linda completed column 6, she studied the evidence from columns 4 and 5 and considered alternatives to her hot thought. The evidence suggested that she was not having a heart attack, but that her rapid heartbeat and sweating were caused by her anxiety and were in no way dangerous or harmful. Instead of thinking, "I'm having a heart attack," Linda considered her alternative thoughts: "My heart is racing and I am sweating because I'm anxious/nervous about being on an airplane. My doctor told me that a rapid heartbeat is not necessarily dangerous, and in all likelihood my heartbeat will

THOUGHT

1. Situation	2. Moods	3. Automatic Thoughts (Images)
Who? What? When? Where?	a. What did you feel? b. Rate each mood (0–100%). c. Circle or mark the mood you want to examine.	a. What was going through your mind just before you started to feel this way? Any other thoughts? Images? b. Circle or mark the hot thought.
Sunday evening, in the airplane, on the runway, waiting for the plane to take off.	(Fear 98%)	I'm feeling sick. My heart is starting to beat harder and faster. I'm starting to sweat. (I'm having a heart attack.) I'll never be able to get off this plane and to a hospital in time. I'm going to die.

FIGURE 9.4. Linda's completed Thought Record.

Alternative or Balanced Thinking 111

return to normal in just a few minutes." Linda's completed Thought Record, which she finished while she was still on the runway, is shown in Figure 9.4.

As Linda thought differently about her rapid heartbeat and sweating, her fear dropped considerably. Her fear was connected to her thought "I'm having a heart attack," and not simply to her physical experiences of her heart beating rapidly and of sweating. When she examined the evidence for and against her thought and concluded that she was not having a heart attack, Linda's became less fearful.

RECORD

4. Evidence That Supports the Hot Thought	5. Evidence That Does Not Support the Hot Thought	6. Alternative/ Balanced Thoughts a. Write an alternative or balanced thought. b. Rate how much you believe each thought (0–100%).	7. Rate Moods Now Rerate column 2 moods and any new moods (0–100%).
My heart is racing. I'm sweating. These could be two signs of a heart attack.	Anxiety can cause a rapid heartbeat. My doctor told me that the heart is a muscle, using a muscle makes it stronger, and a rapid heartbeat is not necessarily dangerous. A rapid heartbeat doesn't mean that I am having a heart attack. I have had this happen to me before in airports, on airplanes, and when thinking about flying. In the past, my heartbeat has returned to normal when I read a magazine, practiced slow breathing, did Thought Records, or thought in less catastrophic ways.	My heart is racing and I am sweating because I'm anxious and nervous about being on an airplane. 95% My doctor told me that a rapid heartbeat is not necessarily dangerous, and in all likelihood my heart rate will return to normal in just a few minutes. 85%	Fear 25%

Now you have learned what you need to know to complete all seven columns of a Thought Record. Thought Records help you identify, examine, and perhaps change the thinking and beliefs that contribute to your distress. Constructing alternative or balanced thoughts helps free you from automatic thinking patterns that contribute to the difficulties you are having. If you are able to see yourself and situations from a different perspective, it is likely that you will feel better about yourself and your life.

Complete two or three Thought Records per week to help improve your skills in developing alternative and balanced thinking. (There are additional copies of Worksheet 9.2 in the Appendix of this book.) In the future, whenever you get stuck evaluating a thought, you can write down the evidence and a balanced or alternative thought on a Thought Record.

There are three advantages to completing Thought Records regularly. First, we often respond in emotional ways that can be a bit confusing. For example, at first Linda did not realize why she was panicking on the airplane. Thought Records can help you make sense of your emotional reactions, just as they did for Linda. Second, a Thought Record can help you broaden your perspective on troubling situations, so that you react in ways that are consistent with the "big picture" rather than a narrow and possibly distorted view. Third, repeated practice filling out Thought Records actually helps you learn to think more flexibly. After completing 20–40 Thought Records, many people report that they automatically begin to think alternative or balanced thoughts in distressing situations without writing out a Thought Record. When you reach this point, you will experience fewer and fewer situations as truly distressing, and you can spend your energy on solving what problems remain and on enjoying yourself in more situations.

WHAT IF YOUR HOT THOUGHT IS SUPPORTED BY THE EVIDENCE?

Before we end this chapter, we want to clarify a really important point. Thus far, you might get the impression that Thought Records are designed to show that negative thoughts are always inaccurate or unbalanced. This is not the case.

We usually do a Thought Record when we are experiencing a strong emotion. We know from research that when we have strong emotions, we think mostly about experiences that fit that emotion. When we are sad, for example, we think about sad things;

when we are ashamed, we think about all the bad things we have done. Therefore, most of the time when we decide to fill out a Thought Record, it will help us get a different and more balanced view of things, because it prompts us to think about things that are not consistent with our mood.

However, sometimes our hot thoughts are accurate and good descriptions of difficult situations. For instance, one of our hot thoughts may be "My boss is abusing me," and this may be accurate. Vic might think, "If I keep losing my temper, Judy might get tired of this and leave me." In these instances, the Thought Record does its job in two ways: (1) It helps us test whether our hot thought is accurate, just to make sure we are not jumping to an emotion-driven conclusion; and (2) if we find out that the hot thought is supported by the evidence, it alerts us that this is something we need to manage or change in some way. The next chapter teaches a variety of ways to handle hot thoughts that are supported by the evidence, including problem solving, reexamining the meanings we put on situations, developing acceptance, and learning to be resilient in the face of our difficulties.

MOOD CHECK-UP

As a reminder, as long as you are actively using this book, we recommend you complete mood measures every week or two. At this point in the book, you have learned a lot of *Mind Over Mood* skills. This is a good time to complete mood ratings to see what impact these skills are having on your moods. Be sure to rate and graph all the moods you are tracking, including your happiness. Remember, you can use the following measures and worksheets to record your scores:

- Depression/unhappiness: *Mind Over Mood* Depression Inventory
  Worksheet 13.1, page 191, and Worksheet 13.2, page 192

- Anxiety/nervousness: *Mind Over Mood* Anxiety Inventory
  Worksheet 14.1, page 221; Worksheet 14.2, page 222

- Other moods/happiness: Measuring and Tracking My Moods
  Worksheet 15.1, page 253, and Worksheet 15.2, page 254

EXERCISE: Constructing Your Own Alternative or Balanced Thoughts

On Worksheet 9.2, construct alternative or balanced thoughts for the thoughts you have examined on Worksheet 8.2 in Chapter 8 on pages 88–93. Your alternative or balanced thought(s) will be based on the evidence you gathered in columns 4 and 5 on Worksheet 8.2.

WORKSHEET 9.2. Thought Record

THOUGHT

1. Situation	2. Moods	3. Automatic Thoughts (Images)
Who were you with? What were you doing? When was it? Where were you?	Describe each mood in one word. Rate intensity of mood (0–100%). Circle or mark the mood you want to examine.	**Answer the first two general questions, and then some or all of the questions specific to the mood you circled or marked:** What was going through my mind just before I started to feel this way? (General) What images or memories do I have in this situation? (General) What does this mean about me? My life? My future? (Depression) What am I afraid might happen? (Anxiety) What is the worst that could happen? (Anxiety) What does this mean about how the other person(s) feel(s)/think(s) about me? (Anger, Shame) What does this mean about the other person(s) or people in general? (Anger) Did I break rules, hurt others, or not do something I should have done? What do I think about myself that I did this or believe I did it? (Guilt, Shame)

Copyright 1983 by Christine A. Padesky. Reprinted in *Mind Over Mood, Second Edition*. Copyright 2016 by Dennis Greenberger and Christine A. Padesky. Purchasers of this book can photocopy and/or download additional copies of this worksheet (see the box at the end of the table of contents). All other rights reserved.

Rerate your mood(s) after you have written and rated the alternative or balanced thought. Write the mood(s) and rating(s) in column 7. Is there a relationship between the believability of your alternative or balanced thought and the change in your emotional response?

RECORD

4. Evidence That Supports the Hot Thought	5. Evidence That Does Not Support the Hot Thought	6. Alternative/ Balanced Thoughts	7. Rate Moods Now
Circle hot thought in previous column for which you are looking for evidence. Write factual evidence to support this conclusion. (Try to write facts, not interpretations, as you practiced in Worksheet 8.1 on p. 72.)	Ask yourself the questions in the Helpful Hints (p. 75) to help discover evidence that does not support your hot thought.	Ask yourself the questions in the Helpful Hints in Chapter 9 (p. 100) to generate alternative or balanced thoughts. Write an alternative or balanced thought. Rate how much you believe each alternative or balanced thought (0–100%).	Copy the moods from column 2. Rerate the intensity of each mood (0–100%), as well as any new moods.

Chapter 9 Summary

- Column 6 of the Thought Record, "Alternative/Balanced Thoughts," summarizes the important evidence collected and recorded in columns 4 and 5.

- If the evidence in columns 4 and 5 does not support the original hot thought, write in column 6 an alternative view of the situation that is consistent with the evidence.

- If the evidence in columns 4 and 5 only partially supports your original hot thought, write a balanced thought in column 6 that summarizes the evidence both supporting and not supporting your original thought.

- Ask yourself the questions in the Helpful Hints (p. 100) to help construct an alternative or balanced thought.

- Alternative or balanced thoughts are not merely positive thinking. Instead, they reflect new ways of thinking about the situation based on all the available evidence written in columns 4 and 5.

- In column 7 of the Thought Record, rerate the intensity of the mood(s) you identified in column 2.

- The shift in emotional response to a situation is often related to the believability of your alternative or balanced thoughts. This is why we rate how strongly we believe the alternative or balanced thought.

- If there is no shift in your mood after completing a Thought Record, use the "Questions to Determine Reason for No Mood Change" (p. 107) to discover what else you may need to do to feel better.

- The more Thought Records you complete, the easier it will become to think more flexibly and begin to consider alternative or balanced explanations for events automatically without writing out the evidence.

10
New Thoughts, Action Plans, and Acceptance

Jia enrolled in a Spanish class to prepare for a trip to Mexico. She learned to ask directions, order food, and carry on simple conversations. When Jia arrived in Mexico, her taxi driver spoke English, as did the people working in her hotel. After unpacking, she decided to go to the neighborhood pharmacy to buy some postcards and stamps.

In the pharmacy, everyone was speaking Spanish rapidly. Jia reviewed her digital translator, and then stepped hesitantly up to the counter and spoke the phrases in Spanish she believed would order stamps and postcards. To Jia's surprise, the woman behind the counter smiled and handed her the number of cards and stamps she wanted to purchase.

Why was Jia surprised?

Our first learning of something new tends to be intellectual, or "in our heads." We know that a particular language is supposed to work in another country — but when we actually speak this language, we doubt that it will be understood, because the words and phrases are so different from the language most familiar to us. In the beginning, our native language seems the only true way to speak. A new language begins to feel like true communication only after a lot of practice.

Even though Jia believed that her Spanish phrases were correct, she did not have confidence in the language until she began to receive positive reactions from the people she met in Mexico. As she spoke Spanish more regularly, she gained greater confidence.

Developing new alternative or balanced thoughts may be like writing in a new language for you. Like any new language, new thoughts probably seem awkward and only partly believable. While your automatic thoughts flow easily, like your familiar native language, your alternative thoughts emerge only with great effort. You probably believe the new thoughts "in your head," but they don't feel as if they fit your life experience as well as the old automatic thoughts do.

As Jia did while learning Spanish, the best way to increase the believability of your alternative or balanced thoughts is to try them out in your day-to-day life to gather more evidence. If your life experiences support your alternative and more balanced thoughts, you will begin to believe these new thoughts more, and your improved mood will become more stable. If your experiences do not support your new beliefs, you can use this information to create different alternative thoughts that fit your experiences better.

BEN: *Gathering more evidence and strengthening new thoughts.*

Ben's sad mood on the day he visited his daughter's family improved when he realized that although his children and grandchildren didn't need him in the same ways they used to, they still enjoyed his company and sometimes asked for his advice. Although this alternative thought (see Chapter 9, especially Figure 9.2, pp. 102–103) helped Ben feel better, his new way of thinking was not fully believable to him – even though the evidence seemed to support the new idea. One way for Ben to strengthen his belief in his new conclusion was to gather more information about his alternative thoughts. Ben decided to test his new conclusions ("They still enjoy being with me, even though they don't need me in the same ways they used to"). He called his daughter and son-in-law and offered to help them on a project. His daughter told him that they didn't have any projects that needed help. Rather than concluding that he wasn't needed any more, as he had done in the past, Ben decided to ask her if he could help them in any other way.

After thinking for a moment, his daughter told Ben that his granddaughter Amy's best friend had moved out of town. Amy had been feeling lonely, especially after school when she normally spent time with her friend. She asked if Ben would be able and willing to do something with Amy. Ben eagerly agreed to spend time with Amy two or three times a week after school.

Amy also liked this idea, especially when Ben asked her what she might be interested in doing. She said that she had recently joined a soccer team and would like to practice soccer. Ben agreed to drive her to a field where they would have room to do this. Amy was pleased because the field was too far away to walk or bicycle, and her parents were working and couldn't drive her. Ben was glad to be able to participate in this part of his granddaughter's life.

This experience led to information that strengthened Ben's alternative thought ("They still enjoy being with me, even though they don't need me in the same ways they used to"). His family's reaction increased Ben's belief in his new thought, improved his confidence in acting on this belief, and created enjoyable and positive time with Amy. With his previous style of thinking, Ben would have felt rejected and would have given up when his daughter and son-in-law told him that they didn't have any projects ("What's the use? They don't need me any more"). Ben's alternative thoughts gave him the confidence to find new ways to feel needed, instead of giving up when his initial offer was declined.

> **EXERCISE: Strengthening New Thoughts**
>
> Use Worksheet 10.1 as a guide for testing and strengthening a new alternative thought.

WORKSHEET 10.1. Strengthening New Thoughts

Looking over the Thought Records or other exercises you have completed so far, choose one balanced or alternative thought that you believed less than 50%. Write the thought and your belief rating of it here:

Thought: _____ Rate % belief: _____

Over the next week, look for evidence each day that supports this new thought. Write down whatever evidence you find. If possible, make sure you do things that will provide evidence one way or the other:

_____
_____
_____

At the end of the week, rerate your belief in the new thought: _____ %

Did looking for and recording evidence strengthen your belief in your new alternative or balanced thought?

____ Yes ____ No   Why or why not?

_____
_____
_____

From *Mind Over Mood, Second Edition*. Copyright 2016 by Dennis Greenberger and Christine A. Padesky. Purchasers of this book can photocopy and/or download additional copies of this worksheet (see the box at the end of the table of contents).

MARISSA: *Making an Action Plan to keep a job.*

Sometimes when you gather evidence to test a thought, you find that most of the evidence supports your thought, and so there isn't a very believable alternative thought. When this happens, it usually indicates there is a problem that needs to be solved. Although a change in thinking is often helpful, it is not always the full solution. When most of the evidence supports your thought, you may want to make an Action Plan.

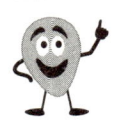

REMINDERS
- If an alternative or balanced thought fits your life experiences but still does not seem believable to you, gather more evidence to test and strengthen the alternative or balanced thought, just as Ben did in his phone conversation with his daughter.
- If the evidence from your life mostly supports your hot thought, then this means you may have a problem to solve, and an Action Plan can help you discover if and how you can solve the problem.

Marissa and her therapist spent several sessions determining the reasons why she had become highly suicidal. One of the main reasons Marissa felt so hopeless was that she was convinced she would be fired from her job and would not be able to support herself and her children. She had a life insurance policy and thought it would provide for her children until they could support themselves.

Marissa tested the automatic thought "I will lose my job" on a Thought Record (see Chapters 6–9). Although this thought could not be considered absolutely true until it happened, Marissa had some pretty convincing evidence that losing her job was a real possibility. In the previous month, she had received three warnings from her supervisor – one for chronically arriving at work late in the morning and after lunch, and two for "poor work product." In her company, three warnings could be followed by termination of employment.

Marissa felt out of control regarding her job. She was so depressed in the mornings that it was hard to get out of bed, even though she knew it would look bad if she was late again. Once she was at work, Marissa had a hard time concentrating, so she made errors – which brought even more negative attention from her supervisor.

Since Marissa's most distressing thought that she would lose her job had a lot of evidence to support it, she and her therapist constructed an Action Plan to help her solve the problem. They discussed and wrote down a variety of actions Marissa could take to improve her performance and make her job more secure. First, she could tell her supervisor that she was trying to do better and ask for help. This supervisor had complimented Marissa on her work only a few months earlier. Marissa acknowledged that her supervisor might be willing to help if he knew she was trying to do better. Second, Marissa decided she could ask Maggie, a friend in the office whom Marissa trusted, to review her work before Marissa handed it to the supervisor. Finally, Marissa considered a variety of strategies to get herself to work on time even when she was depressed.

Marissa's Action Plan led her to become more hopeful about keeping her job. After a few minutes, however, she began to see problems that might interfere. The biggest problem was that she didn't feel comfortable telling her supervisor she was depressed, because she wasn't sure it was safe. She worried that he might tell other people, and then she would feel ashamed. Her therapist suggested to Marissa that she consider what she would be willing to say to her supervisor that might enlist his help.

Marissa decided to tell her supervisor that she was under a lot of stress, but that she was working hard to straighten things out so that her job performance would not be affected. She thought she could remind her supervisor that her work used to be better, let him know that her current problems were temporary, and assure him that she expected her performance to be better soon. Marissa's therapist suggested she also let her supervisor know that she really wanted to keep her job and appreciated his help in letting her know what she needed to do to maintain the company's quality standards. Marissa's completed Action Plan is shown in Figure 10.1 on page 122.

Marissa's hopelessness and thoughts of suicide decreased after she made the Action Plan and began to follow it. Notice that she took several different steps to improve her job performance. Since her depression was making it difficult for her to function well, she enlisted the help of others for a short time. From her boss, she asked for an appropriate level of help and reminded him of her previous good work. She also asked her friend Maggie for help, and she promised to do something for Maggie in return. These steps helped Marissa begin to feel in control again, so she could see light at the end of the tunnel.

Marissa's example shows how to use an Action Plan when the evidence in our lives mostly supports a distressing thought. We can also use Action Plans whenever we identify a problem that needs to be solved.

VIC: *Making an Action Plan to improve his marriage.*

Over time, Vic became more confident that Judy really did care about him and wanted him to stay sober. However, Judy had been complaining for many years that she was frustrated by his frequent angry outbursts. She also told him that she missed the nice things he used to do for her early in their relationship. Vic loved Judy and agreed that his anger was causing real problems in their marriage; he also admitted that he could be kinder to her. He really wanted to improve their marriage, so he decided to make an Action Plan, as shown in Figure 10.2 on pages 123–124.

Vic wrote down two goals that would improve his marriage. First, he would do more positive things for Judy to show that he appreciated her. Second, he wanted to stop his angry outbursts. Working with his therapist, Vic developed the Action Plan in Figure 10.2 to help guide his progress. It is helpful to be specific on an Action Plan, in order to get the most benefit from it. Vic set a time to begin working on his plan, anticipated problems that could interfere with his success, and created strategies for solving the problems in order to keep moving forward on his Action Plan. Finally, the Action Plan provided a place for Vic to record his progress.

Vic's marriage improved once he began to increase his positive interactions with Judy and reduce his angry outbursts. He actually used suggestions from the "Strategies to overcome problems" column on his Action Plan to help him through situations that in previous weeks would have led to explosive anger. The specific coping plans for handling his anger at different intensities, which he developed with his therapist, were successful in reducing his outbursts.

Vic followed his Action Plan for a number of weeks until he learned to handle most situations without losing his temper. When he did become enraged in the following weeks, Vic used these setbacks to better understand his anger and to develop additional, more effective plans for controlling and expressing it.

GOAL: Save my job.

Actions to take	Time to begin	Possible problems	Strategies to overcome problems	Progress
Talk to my supervisor about stress, prior positive work history, problems only temporary, wanting to keep my job, appreciating his help.	Wednesday after staff meeting.	Supervisor might be too busy to meet.	Ask him ahead of time for 15-minute meeting.	Tuesday – Supervisor agreed to Wednesday meeting.
		Supervisor might say it's too late to save my job.	Remind him of my positive work earlier in the year. Ask him to reconsider and give me 30 days to improve.	Wednesday – Meeting went pretty well. I cried, which I didn't want to do, but he seemed glad I talked to him and assured me I could have a few more weeks to improve my work.
Ask Maggie to review my work.	Tuesday at lunch.	It will burden our friendship.	I can promise to help Maggie out next summer when she goes on vacation. I can water her houseplants for her.	Maggie agreed to help.
Get to work on time. Set alarm on other side of room so I have to get out of bed. Lay out clothes night before, so no decisions to make. Leave 10 minutes early and reward myself with time for cup of coffee at office before I begin.	Tuesday A.M.	I'll go back to bed after alarm goes off.	Make a rule that I have to shower and dress before I "rest a few more minutes."	Tuesday – Arrived on time. Wednesday – Arrived 5 minutes early. Thursday – Arrived 8 minutes early and enjoyed my coffee.

FIGURE 10.1. Marissa's Action Plan.

GOAL: _Improve my marriage._

Actions to take	Time to begin	Possible problems	Strategies to overcome problems	Progress
Do five positive things for Judy each day, such as kiss her, give her a compliment, help out, smile at her, massage her neck, ask about her day, call from the office to say, "I love you," bring her coffee.	Today when I get home, and every morning beginning when I wake up.	I could be feeling angry with her.	If I'm angry, I can do easier things (like helping with the dishes, bringing coffee). Use a Thought Record or strategies such as a timeout or imagery (from Chapter 15 of Mind Over Mood) to see if I can reduce my anger.	10/6 – Did 6 positives at night. Felt good. 10/7 – Did 5 positives. Judy hugged me for helping. 10/8 – Felt angry, but did 3 positives anyway. A Thought Record helped.
Reduce angry outbursts (how often and how long it lasts). Reduce to no more than 3 in the first week, 2 in the second week, 1 in the third week, and no more than once a month after that. Try to take a break so I'm not with Judy more than 2 minutes when angry.	Now	A bad day at work, so I arrive home in a bad mood.	Do a Thought Record before leaving the office. Make a plan to handle the work problems before I leave the office. Play good music on the way home. Sit in the car and relax until I feel calm enough to enter the house. Tell Judy that it was a bad day and that I am trying to stay calm. Ask her to help.	10/6 – No problems. 10/7 – Made a plan to handle a work conflict before I left the office. Arrived home pretty relaxed. 10/9 – Played music on the way home. Relaxed for 2 minutes in driveway before going into house. Helped me cope with kids crying without getting angry.

(continued on next page)

FIGURE 10.2. Vic's Action Plan.

Actions to take	Time to begin	Possible problems	Strategies to overcome problems	Progress
Reduce anger outbursts (how often and how long it lasts). Reduce to no more than 3 in the first week, 2 in the second week, 1 in the third week, and no more than once a month after that. Try to take a break so I'm not with Judy more than 2 minutes when angry.	Now	When I feel angry, I explode really quickly.	In conversations with Judy, rate my anger 0–10 every minute when I can see it coming. When my anger gets to a 3, tell Judy I need a break for a few minutes to keep calm. When my anger gets to a 5, take a break and write out a Thought Record. Write out what I hear Judy saying and what I believe to be true. Show Judy this summary to check if we understand each other accurately. If I get above a 5 in my anger ratings, tell Judy I need a longer break. Return to the conversation only when my anger is below 3. Take a walk. Review my Thought Records. Remind myself that Judy loves me, that we have worked out lots of problems in the past, and that we can probably solve this problem too.	10/6 – No anger. 10/7 – Started to get angry, took 3 timeouts, and eventually finished the conversation. Judy seemed impressed that I was sticking to my plan. 10/9 – Lost my temper and shouted at Judy. At least I apologized later.

FIGURE 10.2 (*continued from previous page*)

EXERCISE: Making an Action Plan

Identify a problem in your life that you would like to change, and write your goal on the top line on Worksheet 10.2. Complete the Action Plan, making it as specific as possible. Set a time to begin, identify problems that could interfere with completing your plan, develop strategies for coping with the problems if they should arise, and keep written track of the progress you make. Complete additional Action Plans (more copies of Worksheet 10.2 can be found in the Appendix) for other problem areas of your life that you would like to change.

WORKSHEET 10.2. Action Plan

GOAL: _____

Actions to take	Time to begin	Possible problems	Strategies to overcome problems	Progress

From *Mind Over Mood, Second Edition*. Copyright 2016 by Dennis Greenberger and Christine A. Padesky. Purchasers of this book can photocopy and/or download additional copies of this worksheet (see the box at the end of the table of contents).

ACCEPTANCE

When we can do something to solve a problem, then an Action Plan can help us figure out what to do. Sometimes the problems we have cannot be solved. At other times, we may experience life circumstances that are very difficult to endure, but they are not problems we can work on solving with a Thought Record or an Action Plan. For example, we may become very ill, someone close to us might die, or we might have a task to do that is very unpleasant. In these cases, developing an attitude of acceptance can help us cope and feel better.

Consider Lupe, who was diagnosed with brain cancer six months ago. At first Lupe was in denial about the diagnosis. She frantically sought a second, a third, and even a fourth opinion about her status and prognosis. The physicians she saw were consistent in informing Lupe that there was little they could do, because the cancer was widespread and had progressed beyond the point where treatment could help. Lupe was shocked, then angry that she had cancer. Soon her anger was combined with fear. At 59 years of age, she felt much too young to die, even though her doctors said her cancer was terminal.

It is easy to understand her reactions. Even so, about a month after receiving her diagnosis, Lupe began to feel less angry and scared. She described her change in mood to a friend this way: "I do not want to die. But if I am going to die soon, which seems likely, I want to die with dignity. I am going to make these last few months as good and meaningful as possible for myself, my family, and my friends." Her new attitude helped lift Lupe's spirits and mood. She was still facing death, but acceptance of her illness made it possible for her to focus on what was important to her in her final months. Once she accepted that she had a terminal cancer, Lupe was able to think about how she wanted to spend her remaining days. Lupe's top priority was spending as much time as possible with her family and friends in order to create memorable experiences with them. Acceptance was a turning point for Lupe. Acceptance helped lift her out of despair and focused her attention on how she wanted to live her life.

Acceptance was also very important for Rodney, who visited his elderly father each weekend. Rodney's father had dementia and no longer recognized that Rodney was his son. Each week when he visited, his father would ask, "Who are you? Do I know you?" At first, Rodney would explain, "I'm your son. Don't you recognize me?" His father would become very agitated and upset when Rodney said this. Sometimes his father would cry and say, "I don't know you," or "You are not my son!" It was very sad and painful for Rodney to realize that his father no longer knew who he was. His pain and sadness could have easily filled all his remaining time with his father.

A nurse at the care home helped Rodney develop acceptance. She told him, "Your father does not know who you are. If you understand this and let him experience you as a nice man who comes to visit him, then maybe you can still enjoy his company at times." Rodney considered this and decided to try to accept this new reality in his relationship with his father. When his father asked, "Who are you? Do I know you?," Rodney would reply, "My name is Rodney. I like to come here and talk to people. Would it be OK if I talked to you today?" This satisfied his father and they would sit together, talking and sometimes discussing events long ago in his father's past. These conversations still included pain for Rodney, because he missed having a full relationship with his father. Spending time together reminded him of many things he had lost from his former relationship with his father, such as quick humor and animated sports discussions. But Rodney discovered new pleasure in being able to show his father respect and to lift his spirits through these weekly visits.

As Lupe's and Rodney's experiences demonstrate, acceptance does not mean that we need to think positively about negative events or feel happy about things that we are experiencing. *Mind Over Mood* and CBT do not suggest that it is a good idea simply to substitute a positive thought for a negative thought. It would do Lupe no good to say, "I don't have cancer," or "I don't mind dying." Instead, acceptance of negative circumstances and of painful moods can create a foundation on which to move forward in a way that gives personal meaning to unhappy circumstances. Acceptance means that we acknowledge the difficulties in life, come to our own way of understanding them, and figure out how to live with them in ways consistent with our values and with what is important to us.

These same ideas apply to everyday experiences that are much less dramatic. We do many things that are unpleasant. We may wake up earlier than we would like in order to go to work. If one of our children is sick, we may need to cancel social plans and stay home. We accept these experiences because we have values that are more important to us than our discomfort. We often put our own short-term needs on hold for our family, our work, or other things we value.

The attitudes we hold while we are doing unpleasant activities have a big influence on how we feel. For example, if every day when we wake up early to go to work, we dwell on how tired we are and how we wish we were still in bed, then we are likely to be in a bad mood. However, if we wake up early and say, "Oh, I'm tired and wish I could sleep longer. But I'm so glad to have this job because it helps support my family," our mood is likely to be much better. Keeping in mind our values and what is important to us can be a real help when we face difficult tasks.

Acceptance of thoughts and moods is sometimes a worthwhile alternative to identifying, evaluating, and changing thoughts. Acceptance involves observing your thoughts, moods, and physical reactions without making judgments about them. For example, many people find it helpful to be able simply to observe their thoughts as they appear and as they disappear. Acceptance of your thoughts should not be confused with believing that your thoughts are accurate or adaptive. Acceptance simply means that you recognize these thoughts are present, and that you can observe them without adding any meaning or judgment about them.

For example, Sal understood that an important step in learning to manage anxiety was entering situations that made him anxious, in order to test his fears and practice coping. At first, when he felt anxious in these situations, he negatively judged himself: "What's wrong with me? I'm so weak. I want this anxiety to go away." In fact, such thoughts led to an increase in Sal's anxiety. Ironically, Sal discovered that one step to managing his anxiety was to accept this mood: "I'm feeling anxious now that I'm here. Well, that is to be expected. I'll stay in this situation and notice what happens to my anxiety as I face it. I'll try to understand my reactions, rather than push them away." An accepting, nonjudgmental attitude kept Sal's focus on his thoughts and moods, as well as on his goal to learn to manage anxiety in new and better ways.

As these examples show, there are several pathways to acceptance:

1. We can simply observe our thoughts and feelings without judging them or trying to change them. This was Sal's approach to his anxiety. As one woman said, "I can *see* my thoughts and not *be* my thoughts."

2. We can put our thoughts and feelings in perspective by thinking about the larger picture. For example, Marissa's supervisor had a habit of telling the staff, "Let's be cheerful, ladies," every morning. This annoyed all the staff because it seemed so phony, and it was especially irritating to Marissa when she was depressed. Marissa found it helpful to look at the big picture. When she dwelled on her irritation, her mood really suffered. Marissa considered that this was just one minute out of each day, and thought about how her supervisor was willing to help her keep her job. This big picture thinking helped Marissa accept the irritating comment as a small price to pay for a supervisor who was generally supportive and good to her.

3. Sometimes it is easier to accept internal reactions or external circumstances when we connect our acceptance of thoughts and feelings to values that are important to us. Rodney did this when he put his love and caring for his father above his distress that his father no longer recognized him. Even though Rodney still experienced some distress while sitting with his father, he did not let this stop him from spending time with him. Rodney acknowledged his grief and sadness over his father's declining health, and still spent loving and caring time with him. Grief, love, and caring were each part of Rodney's experience. Over time, the value of these hours spent with his father became more meaningful, as Rodney was able to accept this time as a final phase in his relationship with his father.

EXERCISE: Acceptance

Use Worksheet 10.3 to help you work toward acceptance of situations like the ones discussed above.

WORKSHEET 10.3. Acceptance

Identify one external situation (e.g., family, work, health, relationship) in which you think developing greater acceptance might be helpful. Consider situations that can't be easily changed or solved. Alternatively, write down some internal experiences (thoughts or moods) that recur often and negatively affect your mood.

Situation: _____

_____

Thoughts: _____

_____

Moods: _____

_____

Try out one or more of the following paths to acceptance. It is not necessary to try each path for each situation, thought, or mood. Over time, as you practice acceptance, you might want to try each of these approaches at least once to see if they are helpful.

1. Observe your thoughts and moods (about the situation you have written down above) without judging, criticizing, or trying to change them. Just watch them as they occur. Be curious rather than critical. Try to make these observations for a few minutes each day for a week. This is much more difficult than it may appear. It is OK to notice if you become frustrated, distracted, bored, or judgmental. When you notice these things, just gently turn your attention back to the original thoughts and moods that you are observing.

2. Think about the bigger picture. What are the benefits of accepting this rather than being distressed? Are you focusing on only the negative parts of this experience and not recognizing other dimensions? Are there aspects to the situation that counterbalance the negative parts? If you can accept the parts that distress you, will you be able to enjoy or appreciate the rest of your experience more easily?

3. Sometimes paying too much attention to our distress prevents us from reaching our goals or living according to values that are important to us.

    a. In this situation, is there some value or goal that is more important and meaningful to you than your distress? If so, write that value or goal here: _____
    b. Think about how important that value or goal is for you.
    c. How can you use *Mind Over Mood* skills to help you manage your distressing situation, thought, or mood, so you can approach or reach your values or goals? _____
    d. Can you move in the direction of your values and goals while accepting the distress that you are experiencing?

Whether you followed the first, second, or third path to acceptance, write down what you have learned from this exercise: _____

From *Mind Over Mood, Second Edition.* Copyright 2016 by Dennis Greenberger and Christine A. Padesky. Purchasers of this book can photocopy and/or download additional copies of this worksheet (see the box at the end of the table of contents).

In this chapter, you have learned and practiced three common steps that can be taken after you identify and test thoughts connected to your moods: strengthening new thoughts, using Action Plans, and developing acceptance. Which of these steps you take depends a bit on the thoughts you are working on. Strengthening new thoughts by gathering more evidence is particularly helpful when you have a hard time believing alternative and balanced thoughts, even though these thoughts fit with your life experience. Action Plans are an excellent next step when the evidence from your life experience suggests that you have a real problem that needs to be solved. Acceptance is often the best route if the problems you have cannot be solved, you are in the midst of difficulties that you need to get through, or you want to put your distress in perspective so you can move in the direction of what you value most. Often several of these steps can be used in combination to help you develop a new perspective, so you feel more confident that you can manage troubling situations and moods.

MOOD CHECK-UP

Before going on to the next chapter, measure your moods again and write your scores on the relevant score sheets.

- Depression/unhappiness: *Mind Over Mood* Depression Inventory
    Worksheet 13.1, page 191, and Worksheet 13.2, page 192

- Anxiety/nervousness: *Mind Over Mood* Anxiety Inventory
    Worksheet 14.1, page 221, and Worksheet 14.2, page 222

- Other moods/happiness: Measuring and Tracking My Moods
    Worksheet 15.1, page 253, and Worksheet 15.2, page 254

GOAL CHECK-UP

This is also a good time to review the goals you set on Worksheet 5.1 on page 34. By keeping these goals in mind as you continue to practice *Mind Over Mood* skills, you are likely to make progress toward them. You may also want to review Worksheet 5.4 on page 37, Signs of Improvement, to see what changes you can already notice. You can even make an Action Plan to outline steps you can take to reach your goals more rapidly.

Chapter 10 Summary

▸ Initially, you may not fully believe your balanced or alternative thoughts.

▸ You can strengthen new balanced or alternative thoughts by gathering evidence to support them. This is an ongoing process.

▸ As your belief in your balanced or alternative thoughts increases, your improved mood will stabilize.

▸ Action Plans can help you solve problems that you've identified.

▸ Action Plans are specific and include actions to take, a time to begin, possible problems with strategies to overcome them, and a written record of progress.

▸ Acceptance of thoughts and moods is sometimes a worthwhile alternative to identifying, evaluating, and changing your thoughts.

▸ Developing an attitude of acceptance can help when you are in the midst of life circumstances that can't be changed or are difficult to endure.

▸ Three paths to acceptance are observing your thoughts and moods rather than judging them, keeping the big picture in mind, and acting in accord with your values even when you are distressed.

11

Underlying Assumptions and Behavioral Experiments

Shauntelle and Trey had been married for one year and were deeply in love. But despite their affection for each other, there was a great deal of tension, and they frequently argued when they were getting ready for parties. Trey was always ready 10 minutes before it was time to leave and would stand at the door, tapping his foot. Every few minutes he would text her, asking Shauntelle if she knew what time it was and reminding her that it was time to go. Shauntelle was equally upset and frustrated by Trey's reminders and could not understand why he was always in such a hurry.

In Chapters 6–9, you learned to use a Thought Record to identify and test automatic thoughts – the thoughts that come into your mind automatically in specific situations. In addition to automatic thoughts, we each have beliefs that run quietly beneath the surface. We are often not aware of these thoughts, but they also have a strong influence on our moods, our behavior, and our physical reactions. Because these thoughts usually operate below our awareness, we call them "underlying assumptions." Underlying assumptions are the rules we live by. Each of us has hundreds of underlying assumptions, and each one can be stated as an "If . . . then . . . " statement.

For example, Trey's and Shauntelle's reactions to getting ready for a party seem a bit puzzling at first. Why did Trey continue to stand at the door and text reminders to Shauntelle, when he could clearly see that this upset her? Why did Shauntelle wait so long to get ready, when she knew that this irritated Trey? The underlying assumptions Trey and Shauntelle held can help us make perfect sense of their responses.

Trey grew up in a family that valued punctuality and operated under the rule that an invitation for a party or get-together at 7:00 meant that the guests were expected to arrive at 7:00. In Trey's family, arriving later than 7:00 was a sign of disrespect. Therefore, he held the underlying assumption "If we don't arrive on time, then it will be disrespectful, and others will be upset with us." However, in Shauntelle's family, a party's starting time was viewed as somewhat of a suggestion. No one was expected to be there at the starting time. In fact, in her family, arriving at the stated starting time was unexpected and would put pressure on the hosts, who most likely were still preparing for the party. Shauntelle's underlying assumption was "If we arrive on time, then it will pressure the hosts." It is easy to see how each of their underlying assumptions guided their behavior. However, since Trey and Shauntelle were not yet aware of these assumptions, their conflicting assumptions guaranteed tension in their relationship.

Identifying our underlying assumptions provides a deeper understanding of the roots of our behaviors and our automatic thoughts. Identifying our assumptions allows us the opportunity to evaluate whether they are helpful or unhelpful, and gives us a chance to look at the possibility of constructing new assumptions that may work better in our lives.

Unlike automatic thoughts, our underlying assumptions operate across many situations, guiding our actions and moods. Imagine that you are at a large family reunion. One cousin walks around the room chatting with everyone, and another cousin sits quietly in the corner and only speaks with those who approach and start a conversation. What would lead to such different behaviors? It is easier to wander a crowd and talk freely if you have underlying assumptions such as "If I talk to people, then I will have more fun, because when I meet people they generally like me," or even "If everyone here is family, then we will have a lot to talk about and will enjoy each other's company." On the other hand, the quieter cousin may hold underlying assumptions such as "If I begin a conversation, then I risk saying something wrong, so it is better to wait until someone approaches me for a conversation," or "If someone is elderly like me, then younger family members should come and start a conversation with me to show their respect." Notice that many different underlying assumptions can explain the same behavior. It is impossible to know what people's underlying assumptions are just by looking at their behaviors or knowing their moods.

Luckily, even though they generally operate below the surface, underlying assumptions are easy to identify. Clues that assumptions may be present are situations in which you find you always react with the same mood or do the same behavior. For example, if you always are tidying up your home, then you probably have an underlying assumption that you can figure out by putting your behavior in the "If . . . " part of the sentence: "If I keep the rooms at home tidy, then . . . ". One person might finish this sentence this way: "If I keep the rooms at home tidy, then my home will look nice if friends stop by to chat." Another person might believe: "If I keep the rooms at home tidy, then I will be more relaxed and able to find things when I need them."

Similarly, if you always react to being home alone on Saturday night with sadness, then this is a clue that an underlying assumption is operating in the background. You might be assuming, "If it is Saturday night, then I should be doing something fun. If I am at home and not doing something fun, then this means I am a loser." Someone who holds a different underlying assumption may feel contentment instead of sadness: "If it is Saturday night, then I can do whatever I want to do. Being home alone is a chance to relax and have a nice quiet evening."

Underlying assumptions are sometimes the most important level of thought to identify and test.

- When we are anxious, many of our hottest thoughts are "If . . . then . . ." assumptions, such as these examples: "If I talk, then I'll make a fool of myself," "If my heart beats fast, then it means I am having a heart attack," or "If something bad happens, then I can't cope."

- In our relationships, many misunderstandings come about because each person holds different underlying assumptions. For instance, one partner may assume, "If you care, then you will know what I want without me asking," but the other partner may assume, "If you want something, then you will let me know."

- Behaviors that we do to extremes, such as alcohol or drug misuse, overeating, and even perfectionism, are often driven by underlying assumptions: "If I drink, then I'll be more social," "If I've had a hard day, then I deserve to eat a large dessert," or "If something isn't perfect, then it is worthless."

Underlying assumptions can be identified and tested just like automatic thoughts. However, we don't usually use a Thought Record (Chapters 6–9) for this purpose, because Thought Records are designed to test thoughts in a single situation, and underlying assumptions apply across many situations. The ideal way to test an underlying assumption is to do a series of behavioral experiments. Behavioral experiments are active tests to see if the "If . . . then . . ." rule predicts accurately what happens. There are many types of behavioral experiments, such as doing the "If . . ." part of our belief and seeing whether the "then . . ." part happens or not, trying out a new behavior to find out what happens, or interviewing other people to find out if they hold the same assumptions we do. This chapter teaches you how to identify underlying assumptions and test them with behavioral experiments.

LINDA: *There is nothing to fear but fear itself.*

As you will recall, when Linda's heart began to beat rapidly, she got panicky because she thought she was having a heart attack. When she completed a Thought Record (see Figure 9.4 in Chapter 9, pp. 110–111), Linda's alternative thought, based on the evidence that she gathered, was that her racing heart and sweating were caused by anxiety and not by a heart attack. Although her experiences supported this new idea, Linda did not fully believe the new explanation of her symptoms. While sitting in her therapist's office, Linda was convinced that her bodily changes were merely symptoms of anxiety. But in the middle of a panic attack outside her therapist's office, Linda still believed that she was dying of a heart attack when her heart raced and she began to sweat. Simply using Thought Records was not enough, because Linda only fully believed the alternative thoughts when she was not anxious.

When we have trouble believing an alternative thought even though the evidence supports it, it is likely that our hot thought is fueled by an underlying assumption. In Linda's case, before she began therapy, she had this underlying assumption: "If your heart is racing and you are sweating, then you are having a heart attack." She and her therapist developed an alternative underlying assumption: "If your heart is racing and you are sweating, and your heart is healthy, then a racing heart is not dangerous."

There was a lot of evidence to support this new underlying assumption that her racing heart and sweating were not dangerous. When she went to the emergency room during a panic attack, the doctors checked her heart and said that it was healthy and she was not having a heart attack. She and her therapist discussed how the heart is a muscle, and muscles get stronger when they are exercised. Linda did not think she was in danger when she was exercising and her heart started to beat fast and she started to sweat. But Linda still believed that her racing heart and sweating were signs of a heart attack if they occurred when she was not exercising.

In order to test her new underlying assumption, "Even if my heart beats fast, then I'm not in danger," Linda and her therapist devised a series of behavioral experiments. First, she and the therapist did a variety of experiments in the office in which she increased her heart rate and sweating. By breathing rapidly or remembering a recent panic attack, within a few minutes Linda was able to create all the symptoms that scared her. She and her therapist did this multiple times and discussed her experiences. When she looked at the written summary of these behavioral experiments done in her therapist's office, she saw that even when her heart rate was quite high for several minutes, her heartbeat returned to normal within a brief period of time, she stopped sweating, and she felt calm. This increased her confidence in her new assumption that a rapid heartbeat is not dangerous, but she was not sure how she would think about this outside her therapist's office.

In a second series of experiments, Linda and her therapist decided that she would purposely bring on these symptoms outside the office. On a daily basis, she would raise her heart rate and sweating by breathing fast for a few minutes, and would then rate her confidence that she was not having a heart attack. If she had thoughts like "I'm OK – but if I breathe fast any longer, then I might have a heart attack," she tested this idea by breathing fast for a longer time. (Note: Linda had another physical exam before she began her fast-breathing behavioral experiments, and her physician reconfirmed that she did not have any heart problems and it was medically safe for her to breathe fast and make her heart race, even though she didn't always think she was safe.)

Next, her therapist encouraged Linda to imagine airplane flights from start to finish until she raised her heart rate and began to sweat because of anxiety. These behavioral experiments helped convince Linda that her imagination and anxiety could lead to her increased heart rate and sweating. During these imaginary flights, Linda became more firmly convinced that her physical symptoms were caused by anxiety instead of a heart attack. Finally, she began scheduling the airplane flights she had been avoiding.

On the way to the airport for her flight, Linda hoped that her earlier behavioral experiments would prevent her from feeling anxious. She was surprised to find that her heart began beating wildly from the moment she left home on the morning of the flight. Linda's heart raced and she began to sweat. Linda reminded herself of all the times she had felt this way when breathing fast or feeling anxious and how she had never had a heart attack, even though she thought she would. To test the possibility that the symptoms on the way to the airport were anxiety and not a heart attack, Linda distracted herself from focusing on her body by concentrating on a report she needed to review during the trip. After 10 minutes of concentration on the report, she noticed that her heart rate had slowed. Since distraction can reduce anxiety but not a heart attack, Linda began to breathe easier. She was not dying, just anxious.

Over the following months and after a number of airline trips, Linda found it easier to fly. Occasionally she would still become anxious, especially when the plane encoun-

ASSUMPTION TESTED	If my heart races and I sweat, then it is not dangerous, but instead is probably caused by breathing fast, anxiety, or other factors.				
Experiment	Prediction	Possible problems	Strategies to overcome these problems	Outcome of experiment	What have I learned from this experiment about this assumption?
In my therapist's office, increase my heart rate by breathing fast.	When I stop breathing fast, my heart rate will return to normal.	I may believe that I am having a heart attack and be too scared to go on.	I will tell my therapist that I think I am having a heart attack and am scared; my therapist will help me evaluate how to proceed.	My heartbeat increased soon after I began breathing fast and returned to normal approximately 10 minutes after I stopped.	My heart can beat fast and not be dangerous or cause a heart attack. I don't need to be as afraid of a rapid heartbeat as I thought.
I will imagine myself getting on an airplane, taking off, having a panic attack, and not being able to get off the plane.	My heart rate will increase and I will start to sweat as I am imagining this scene. My heart rate and sweating will return to normal after I stop the imagination exercise.	I might stop this experiment if my heart starts to race too fast. I might start to panic and think I am having a heart attack.	If my heart starts to race really fast, then this is a good chance to test my fears. My therapist will encourage me to stick with the imagination for as long as possible.	My heart rate increased and I started to sweat the more absorbed I became in my imagination. When I stopped imagining, my heart rate returned to normal and I stopped sweating.	A rapid heartbeat can be caused just by thinking about something and feeling scared. When I stop imagining scary thoughts, my heartbeat and sweating go back to normal. It is not dangerous, just uncomfortable.
ALTERNATIVE ASSUMPTION THAT FITS WITH THE OUTCOME(S) OF MY EXPERIMENT(S)	My experiments support the assumption that if my heart races and I sweat, then it is not dangerous, but instead is probably caused by breathing fast, anxiety, or other factors.				

FIGURE 11.1. Linda's Experiments to Test an Underlying Assumption worksheet.

tered turbulence. However, her panic attacks stopped when she gained confidence in her new assumption that her symptoms indicated anxiety, not a heart attack. Figure 11.1 illustrates how Linda planned and charted two of her experiments, using the Experiments to Test an Underlying Assumption worksheet that is provided later in this chapter (Worksheet 11.2).

Even after her anxiety became less frequent, Linda continued doing behavioral experiments to strengthen her belief that her symptoms were not dangerous, just uncomfortable. She occasionally let her racing heart continue for 10 or more minutes, to remind herself that a racing heart was not dangerous. Linda knew she had conquered her anxiety when she earned her first "frequent flyer" free airline ticket and was actually happy to be able to schedule another flight – this time for a vacation!

Linda's experiences provide several good guidelines for planning behavioral experiments:

Guidelines for Planning Behavioral Experiments

1. Write Down the Assumption You Are Testing

In the next part of this chapter, we provide some tips for how to choose an assumption to test. As shown in Figure 11.1, Linda wrote down the new underlying assumption she was testing: "If my heart races and I sweat, then it is not dangerous, but instead is probably caused by breathing fast, anxiety, or other factors."

2. Make Specific Predictions

Make sure the experiments you plan will lead to new information that will help you evaluate your assumption. One way to do this is to **make specific predictions** of what either your old or new assumption tells you will happen. Linda decided to breathe fast to raise her heart rate and cause her to sweat. For a second experiment, she planned an imagination exercise, which she thought would also lead to a racing heart and sweating. For both experiments, she predicted that her heart rate and sweating would return to normal soon after the experiment was over.

3. Break Up Experiments into Small Steps

Small steps are easier to do, and what you learn in each small step can help you take the bigger steps later. Linda began her behavioral experiments in her therapist's office by bringing on her symptoms with fast breathing. Next, she practiced fast breathing at home to experiment without a therapist present. Finally, she began doing experiments in which her symptoms were brought on by anxiety – first in imagination, then in actual airplane flights. Her many experiences with a racing heart brought on by breathing fast (the first small step) helped her cope with a racing heart brought on by anxiety (bigger step).

4. Do a Number of Experiments

We usually need to do a number of experiments before we truly believe a new way of thinking about things. Linda believed that her symptoms were not dangerous when she was not anxious. But it took a number of experiments and plane flights before she believed her new assumption ("A racing heart can be caused by anxiety and is not dangerous") not only when she was calm, but also when she was anxious. Multiple experiments also helped Linda become skilled at handling her anxiety, so that she didn't need to avoid situations in which she anticipated feeling anxious.

5. Problem Solve, Don't Quit

When experiments don't turn out as we hope, it is time to problem-solve, not quit. It's also a good idea to anticipate problems that might occur before you begin doing experiments, so you can plan how to handle these. In Figure 11.1 (on p. 136), Linda wrote these down in the "Possible problems" and "Strategies to overcome these problems" columns. Because Linda had a surprisingly high degree of anxiety on her first plane flight, she made some changes in her coping plan as she planned for her second trip. First, she drank a glass of milk instead of coffee before leaving for the airport. Second, she left a half hour earlier, so that she wouldn't need to rush and would have plenty of time to calm herself if anxious. These two changes reduced two natural causes of increased heart rate (caffeine and rushing). She also took a few minutes for relaxation before leaving the house; this reduced her pre-airport heart rate, which made it easier for her to cope with her anxiety. Even though it was important that she experience a racing heart in order to test her assumptions, Linda found it easier to approach situations that activated her anxiety when she was not rushing and had the time to focus on her experiments.

6. Write Down Your Experiments and Their Outcomes

It is helpful to write down your experiments and their outcomes. Writing down your experiments makes it more likely that you will learn from them. When Linda had taken flights before she began her formal experiments, she had just considered herself "lucky" if the flight went well, and "a mental case" if she had a panic attack. By writing down her experiments, Linda was able to learn from both her good and bad experiences.

From *Mind Over Mood, Second Edition*. Copyright 2016 by Dennis Greenberger and Christine A. Padesky. Purchasers may photocopy this box for personal use or use with individual clients.

Linda's efforts helped prepare her to cope with her first flight successfully. For her, success did not mean having no anxiety; it meant knowing what to do when she felt anxious. She was also successful because she strengthened her assumption that her rapid heartbeat was not dangerous; it was caused by anxiety and not a heart attack.

IDENTIFYING UNDERLYING ASSUMPTIONS

Even though underlying assumptions lie "beneath the surface" they are easy to identify if you know where to look. Since underlying assumptions guide our behaviors and emotional reactions, we know they are active when we want to change a behavior but find it very difficult to do so, when we are avoiding something, and/or when we have strong emotional reactions.

To identify your underlying assumptions in these circumstances, put the behavior or the situation that triggers your reaction (avoidance or strong emotion) into a sentence that begins with "If . . . " and follow that by "then . . . " – and let your mind complete that sentence. It can also be helpful to write a sentence that says the opposite: "If I don't . . . then . . . " Here are a few examples:

RITA: *I can't start my exercise plan.*

Rita wants to exercise so she can lose weight, but she can't figure out why she never begins, even though she has the best intentions. She identifies her underlying assumption by writing:

*If I exercise to lose weight, **then** . . .*

When Rita looks at this sentence, her mind quickly completes it like this:

*If I exercise to lose weight, **then** I will just gain it back, so what's the use?*

She also considers what the "If I don't . . . then . . . " assumption might be:

*If I don't exercise to lose weight, **then** I won't have to get up so early in the morning.*

These two assumptions help Rita understand why she hasn't begun her exercise plan.

DERRICK: *I need it to be perfect.*

Derrick is a perfectionist. He spends hours and hours working on a project at work, but he never hands it in because "it could still be better." What is his underlying assumption? He figures it out by writing:

*If I hand in my project before it is perfect, **then** . . .*

After a few seconds of thought, Derrick completes his assumption this way:

If I hand in my project before it is perfect, **then** *I'll get criticized, and my manager won't ever consider me for a promotion.*

KELLY: *I'm so ashamed.*

Kelly doesn't want people to know what is going on in her personal life, because she is ashamed that she is unemployed and still single at age 35. This is something she accepts about herself, so she is puzzled why she is so ashamed for others to know. Her underlying assumptions help her figure this out:

If others know I am unemployed and single, **then** *they will think I am a loser, gossip about me, and post nasty comments on the internet.*

If I don't let them know I am unemployed and single, **then** *I won't feel anxious, and I'll have a better time.*

You can't really know what people's underlying assumptions are just from looking at their behavior or emotional reactions. For example, Derrick is perfectionistic because he fears criticism. Other people may be perfectionistic because they take pleasure in doing something better than anyone else and they hope for compliments. Only you know what your underlying assumptions are.

> **EXERCISE: Identifying Underlying Assumptions**
>
> Worksheet 11.1 can help you identify some of your assumptions.

WORKSHEET 11.1. Identifying Underlying Assumptions

For items 1 and 2, identify behaviors that you keep doing even when it would be better for you not to do them (e.g., staying up late watching television, drinking too much alcohol, overeating, criticizing someone, dating the wrong types of people, cleaning the house all the time). Write each behavior in the "If . . ." part of the sentence, and then complete the "then . . ." part of the sentence. Do the same for the "If I don't . . ." part.

1. If I _____,

    then _____.

    If I don't _____,

    then _____.

(continued on next page)

From *Mind Over Mood, Second Edition*. Copyright 2016 by Dennis Greenberger and Christine A. Padesky. Purchasers of this book can photocopy and/or download additional copies of this worksheet (see the box at the end of the table of contents).

WORKSHEET 11.1 *(continued from previous page)*

2. If I _____,

   then _____.

   If I don't _____,

   then _____.

For items 3 and 4, identify things you typically avoid, and see what underlying assumptions can help explain your avoidance:

3. If I avoid _____,

   then _____.

   If I don't avoid _____,

   then _____.

4. If I avoid _____,

   then _____.

   If I don't avoid _____,

   then _____.

For items 5 and 6, identify some specific times when you have especially strong emotions (e.g., someone criticizes you, you make a mistake, people are late, you get interrupted, someone tries to take advantage of you, a telemarketer calls you). What underlying assumptions might explain your reaction? Write the situation that triggers your emotion in the "If . . . " section, and then complete the other sections.

5. If _____,

   then it means _____.

   If this does not happen,

   then it means _____.

6. If _____,

   then it means _____.

   If this does not happen,

   then it means _____.

From *Mind Over Mood, Second Edition.* Copyright 2016 by Dennis Greenberger and Christine A. Padesky. Purchasers of this book can photocopy and/or download additional copies of this worksheet (see the box at the end of the table of contents).

Were you able to identify at least several assumptions in this exercise? If so, do your assumptions help you better understand your behavior and your emotional reactions? Underlying assumptions, just like automatic thoughts, can be tested and even changed. Because underlying assumptions consist of "If . . . then . . . " predictions, the best way to test them is by doing behavioral experiments. One type of experiment is to do the "If . . . " part and see if the "then . . . " part always follows. Another type of experiment is to observe other people and see if your "If . . . then . . . " rule applies to them. Sometimes we do the opposite of our underlying assumption to learn what happens when we change our behavior. The following examples illustrate these three types of experiments.

EXPERIMENT 1: DOES "THEN . . ." ALWAYS FOLLOW "IF . . ."?

Mike experienced a lot of anxiety in social situations. When he was in work meetings, he avoided eye contact, hoping that his supervisor wouldn't call on him to speak. At parties, he wanted to meet other people, but felt very shy and stayed on the edges of the crowd, because he was afraid of looking or sounding foolish. He identified his underlying assumptions as these:

If I say something, then I will sound stupid, and people will laugh at me.

If I talk to someone new, then they will think I am boring.

Mike decided to do some experiments to test his assumption about sounding stupid and people laughing at him. As shown in Figure 11.2, Mike decided to do one experiment three times. He wanted to start with a relatively easy experiment, so he planned to talk about his weekend plans with store clerks when he did his shopping. Rather than avoiding eye contact, he decided to look directly at each clerk to gather evidence of whether the clerk was laughing at him or in any way negatively judging him. Mike predicted that at least two of the clerks would make fun of him or say something negative.

As shown in Figure 11.2, even though he was nervous, none of the clerks laughed at Mike or said anything negative. In fact, two of them seemed to genuinely enjoy talking about the weekend with him. Mike was pleasantly surprised by these outcomes. His prediction, " . . . then I will sound stupid, and people will laugh at me or say something negative," did not come true. Instead, his experiments supported an alternative assumption: "If I talk to people, some of the time they seem genuinely interested, and they don't look like they are criticizing me." Based on these results, he planned additional experiments at work and in other social situations to see if this new assumption predicted what would occur most of the time.

ASSUMPTION TESTED	If I say something, then I will sound stupid, and people will make fun of me or say something negative.				
Experiment	Prediction	Possible problems	Strategies to overcome these problems	Outcome of experiment	What have I learned from this experiment about this assumption?
Talk about my weekend plans with three store clerks.	I will sound stupid, and at least two of the clerks will make fun of me or say something negative.	I will feel too nervous and avoid doing it. I may avoid eye contact and not get the evidence I need.	Remind myself that it is important to test my assumption. It is OK to be nervous, and this will be over in a few minutes. My therapist told me that being nervous means I am on the right track. Make sure I look at the clerk while I'm talking.	First clerk: Smiled and told me her plans for the weekend. Second clerk: Seemed to listen but did not say much back. Third clerk: Joked with me, but it did not seem like he was making fun of me. He was just being friendly.	Even though I was nervous, nothing happened that supported my prediction that I would sound stupid. None of the clerks laughed at me or said anything negative. Two clerks seemed to enjoy talking with me.
ALTERNATIVE ASSUMPTION THAT FITS WITH THE OUTCOME(S) OF MY EXPERIMENT(S)	If I talk to people, some of the time they seem genuinely interested, and they don't look like they are criticizing me.				

FIGURE 11.2. Mike's Experiments to Test an Underlying Assumption worksheet.

EXPERIMENT 2: OBSERVE OTHERS AND SEE IF YOUR "IF . . . THEN . . ." RULE APPLIES TO THEM

Claudia was a single mother and worked as a waitress to support her daughter. She held herself and her daughter to perfectionistic standards. She demanded that her daughter get the best grades in school; Claudia cleaned their home every day to keep it spotless; she made sure she and her daughter were always perfectly groomed; and she raced around during the work day to make sure that all her orders were delivered quickly and without any mistakes. Although she always felt compelled to try to do her best, Claudia was often very tired, and her relationship with her daughter was becoming strained. With her therapist's prompting, Claudia identified the following underlying assumptions:

If what I do is not perfect, then I'm a failure.

If something is not perfect, then it's worthless.

Her therapist encouraged Claudia to consider an experiment to test these assumptions and see if imperfection always led to failure or a sense of worthlessness. Claudia couldn't imagine attempting to do things less than perfectly. Her therapist suggested that as a first step, Claudia could observe others doing things less than perfectly and see if her rules applied to them. Claudia had no trouble spotting mistakes other people made, so she thought this experiment would be easier.

In the beginning, Claudia found herself being critical of the other waitresses' mistakes. But when she wrote down the outcomes of their mistakes on her Experiments to Test an Underlying Assumption worksheet, Claudia noticed that her predictions did not come true. The other waitresses did not seem to feel they were worthless; in fact, customers still gave good tips even after their mistakes. So evidently the customers thought the waitresses' service had worth, even if it was not perfect. None of the other waitresses seemed to feel like failures after making errors; in fact, one of them just laughed about it, as shown in Figure 11.3. This suggested that not everyone held the same assumptions about being perfect. Even though she was not completely convinced, Claudia had to admit that it was possible for people or activities to have some worth even when they were less than perfect. This idea made Claudia more willing to do some experiments where she did things less than perfectly.

EXPERIMENT 3: DO THE OPPOSITE AND SEE WHAT HAPPENS

Gabriela constantly worried about her children. Whenever her oldest daughter, Angelina, went out with her teenage friends, Gabriela sat home worrying until her daughter returned. She imagined her daughter getting into a car accident, being abducted, making poor choices, talking to strangers, or being the victim of a violent crime. Her constant worry kept Gabriela awake at night and distressed throughout the day.

When she put her worry into the "If . . . then . . . " sentence, Gabriela identified several assumptions she held:

If I worry, then I can anticipate bad things and protect my children.

If I don't worry, then my children will be more vulnerable.

If I don't worry, then I'm not being a good mother.

Although her assumptions made Gabriela's worry look like a good thing, Gabriela was anxious all the time. She wondered if she could protect her children and be a good mother without paying such a high price in distress and tension. For example, she noticed that her sister seemed to be a very good mother without being nearly as anxious

ASSUMPTION TESTED	If something is not perfect, then it is worthless, and the person doing it is a failure.				
Experiment	Prediction	Possible problems	Strategies to overcome these problems	Outcome of experiment	What have I learned from this experiment about this assumption?
Observe other waitresses at the restaurant making mistakes or errors.	When waitresses make a mistake, their work is worthless, and they are failures.	I might be too busy myself to notice their mistakes.	I can ask them at break if they had any problems with their orders or customers.	One waitress delivered food to the wrong table. Customer pointed out it was wrong. The waitress apologized and brought the correct meal. The customer was understanding and even gave a good tip.	It is possible for something to be less than perfect and still have worth (she still got a good tip). Making a mistake does not mean you are a failure. That waitress laughed about her mistake, and the customer didn't seem to mind. I guess not everyone has the same rules about perfection that I do.
ALTERNATIVE ASSUMPTION THAT FITS WITH THE OUTCOME(S) OF MY EXPERIMENT(S)	It is possible for something to be less than perfect and still have worth. If I make a mistake, then it doesn't mean I'm a failure.				

FIGURE 11.3. Claudia's Experiments to Test an Underlying Assumption worksheet.

or worried. When she talked to her sister about this, her sister said, "I try not to worry too much. Things I worried about in the past didn't happen, and the bad things that happened, I never thought to worry about! But I was able to handle them when they happened. So I just try to take things as they come."

After this discussion with her sister, Gabriela decided to do an experiment in which she would do the opposite of worry, to see if worry was necessary to protect her children or to be a good mother. She decided that the opposite of worry would be something that helped her mind relax. Even better, she thought it would help to do something enjoyable and meaningful to her. When her daughter went out the next weekend, she decided she would plan fun activities at home that would keep her mind engaged so she was less likely to worry. She talked to the younger children about having a "game night" and invited some neighbors over to join them. Gabriela put on music and made snacks to help create a party atmosphere.

To get the most benefit out of her experiment, Gabriela filled out the Experiments to Test an Underlying Assumption worksheet. As you can see in Figure 11.4, her predictions were "If I don't worry, something bad will happen to Angelina. Whether something bad happens or not, I will feel like a terrible mother for not worrying." Gabriela recognized she might have difficulty stopping herself from worrying. She wrote this on her worksheet, along with her plans to cope with any worried thoughts by bringing her attention back to the games and focusing on the younger children and the fun they were having.

Gabriela was successful in reducing her worry and enjoying the game night. Despite her predictions, nothing bad happened to her daughter just because Gabriela worried less. Instead of feeling like a bad mother, Gabriela actually felt proud of herself for being able to have fun instead of being upset the whole evening. She concluded that worrying every minute your children are gone is not a required part of being a good parent. In fact, Gabriela began to think that she was a good mother, because she was available if any of her children needed her, and she had spent some enjoyable time with her younger children that night. She also realized that she had taught her children over the years how to be responsible when they were on their own. She began to form a new underlying assumption: "I don't need to worry constantly to be a good mother. If I've taught my children to make good choices and be safe, then that is part of being a good mother."

ASSUMPTION TESTED	If I don't worry, something bad will happen to Angelina. If I don't worry, then I'm not being a good mother.				
Experiment	**Prediction**	**Possible problems**	**Strategies to overcome these problems**	**Outcome of experiment**	**What have I learned from this experiment about this assumption?**
Instead of worrying while Angelina is out with her friends, I'm going to enjoy myself at a game night party with my other children and neighbors.	If I don't worry, something bad will happen to Angelina. Whether something bad happens or not, I will feel like a terrible mother for not worrying.	Even though I am at the party, I'll still start to worry about Angelina.	When I start to worry, I can bring my attention back to the games. If I focus on the younger children and how much fun we are having, it may help me stay focused on the party.	I worried a lot less than usual. When horrible images came to mind, I was able to focus my attention back on the games. When Angelina came home, she said she had a good time. Nothing bad seemed to have happened. I did not feel like a terrible mother. In fact, I felt proud of myself.	When I don't worry, it doesn't make the children more vulnerable. I don't need to worry all the time to be a good mother. If something bad happens, my worry doesn't protect her. I was home if Angelina needed me, and I've taught Angelina how to make good choices and be safe. So it is OK for me to relax when she is gone.
ALTERNATIVE ASSUMPTION THAT FITS WITH THE OUTCOME(S) OF MY EXPERIMENT(S)	I don't need to worry constantly to be a good mother. If I've taught my children to make good choices and be safe, then that is part of being a good mother.				

FIGURE 11.4. Gabriela's Experiments to Test an Underlying Assumption worksheet.

EXERCISE: Experiments to Test Your Underlying Assumptions

Earlier in this chapter, you identified a series of underlying assumptions that guide your behavior (see pp. 140–141). Choose one of those assumptions that you think it would be helpful to test. Think of what kind of experiment you would be willing to try to test your assumption:

1. Does "then . . . " always follow "If . . . "?
2. Observe others and see if your "If . . . then . . . " rule applies to them.
3. Do the opposite and see what happens.

Or maybe you will think of a different type of experiment to test your assumption. For example, instead of observing other people, you might decide to interview some close friends and find out if they follow the same "If . . . then . . . " rule as you do.

The important thing about experiments is that you either make observations or do something to test whether or not your underlying assumption's predictions come true in a variety of situations. In order to make a fair test, it's usually best to do at least three behavioral experiments before drawing a conclusion. So it is helpful to think of small experiments that are easy to do on a daily basis.

On Worksheet 11.2, write the underlying assumption that you are testing at the top of three copies of the worksheet. There are two additional copies of Worksheet 11.2 in the Appendix. In the first column of each page, describe one of the experiments you plan to do. You might do the same experiment three times or describe three different experiments on the three worksheets. In the next column of each worksheet, write your predictions of what will happen, based on your underlying assumption. Then identify any possible problems that might interfere with your doing the experiment, as well as your plan for what you can do to overcome these problems.

Once you have completed these first four columns, do the experiments and write down in as much detail as possible what actually happens, so you can compare these outcomes to your predictions. Answer the following questions in the "Outcomes . . . " column:

- What happened (compared to your predictions)?
- Do the outcomes match what you predicted?
- Did anything unexpected happen?
- If things didn't turn out as you wanted, how well did you handle it?

After doing each experiment, write what you learned in the final column.

WORKSHEET 11.2. Experiments to Test an Underlying Assumption

ASSUMPTION TESTED					
Experiment	**Predictions**	**Possible problems**	**Strategies to overcome these problems**	**Outcome of experiment**	**What have I learned from this experiment about this assumption?**
				What happened (compared to your predictions)? Do the outcomes match what you predicted? Did anything unexpected happen? If things didn't turn out as you wanted, how well did you handle it?	
ALTERNATIVE ASSUMPTION THAT FITS WITH THE OUTCOME(S) OF MY EXPERIMENT(S)					

From *Mind Over Mood, Second Edition*. Copyright 2016 by Dennis Greenberger and Christine A. Padesky. Purchasers of this book can photocopy and/or download additional copies of this worksheet (see the box at the end of the table of contents).

In Chapter 9, you learned to develop an alternative thought to your original hot thought after gathering and reviewing the evidence. In a similar way, after you do experiments, you can see if an alternative assumption fits your experiences better than your original assumption. For example, after Mike did his experiments talking to store clerks (see Figure 11.2, p. 143), he wrote an alternative assumption: "If I talk to people, some of the time they seem genuinely interested, and they don't look like they are criticizing me." When Claudia observed the other waitresses for her experiment (see Figure 11.3, p. 145), she concluded: "It is possible for something to be less than perfect and still have worth. If I make a mistake, then it doesn't mean I'm a failure." Gabriela came up with the following alternative assumption based on her experiment (see Figure 11.4, p. 147): "I don't need to worry constantly to be a good mother. If I've taught my children to make good choices and be safe, then that is part of being a good mother."

Once you have done your experiments, consider whether they support your underlying assumption or not. Look over your copies of Worksheet 11.2. If your predictions did not all come true, try writing an alternative assumption that more closely matches the outcomes of your experiments. You can write this alternative assumption at the bottom of Worksheet 11.2.

We often learn our original underlying assumptions from our families or from the communities and cultures we grow up in. We are usually not fully aware of our assumptions, and it is often surprising to learn that not everyone operates under the same set of rules.

Sometimes assumptions that once served a good purpose no longer work very well, or they even act as barriers to positive changes we want to make. The good news is that because assumptions are learned, we can learn new assumptions. Identifying our underlying assumptions and doing experiments to test them are steps than can help us discover new assumptions – ones that can lead to meaningful change and greater happiness. Some people spend a month or more testing out various assumptions they hold. Alternatively, you can return to this chapter whenever you want to test out additional underlying assumptions in your life.

MOOD CHECK-UP

Before going on to the next chapter, measure your moods again and write your scores on the relevant score sheets.

- Depression/unhappiness: *Mind Over Mood* Depression Inventory
    Worksheet 13.1, page 191, and Worksheet 13.2, page 192
- Anxiety/nervousness: *Mind Over Mood* Anxiety Inventory
    Worksheet 14.1, page 221, and Worksheet 14.2, page 222
- Other moods/happiness: Measuring and Tracking My Moods
    Worksheet 15.1, page 253, and Worksheet 15.2, page 254

Chapter 11 Summary

▶ Underlying assumptions are "If . . . then . . . " beliefs that guide our behavior and emotional reactions at a deeper level than automatic thoughts do.

▶ Underlying assumptions can be identified and tested, just as automatic thoughts can.

▶ To identify underlying assumptions, put a behavior or situation that triggers a strong emotion into a sentence that begins with "If . . ."; follow that by "then . . . " and let your mind complete that sentence.

▶ Underlying assumptions can be tested by using behavioral experiments.

▶ There are many types of behavioral experiments, including doing the "If . . ." part of your assumptions and seeing if the "then . . . " occurs, observing other people to see if the rule applies to them, and trying the opposite behavior and noticing what happens.

▶ It is usually necessary to do a number of behavioral experiments in order to fairly test existing assumptions and to develop alternative assumptions that fit your life experiences.

▶ Developing new underlying assumptions can lead to meaningful change and greater happiness.

12

Core Beliefs

In many ways, automatic thoughts are similar to flowers and weeds in a garden. Thought Records (Chapters 6–9), as well as Action Plans and acceptance (Chapter 10), are tools that enable you to cut the weeds (negative automatic thoughts) at ground level from your garden, making room for the flowers. With practice, these tools will work for you for the rest of your life. Whenever the weeds flourish in your garden, you will know how to cut them back. For many people, the skills learned in Chapters 1–10 are sufficient for coping with problems effectively.

Other people find that even after they use these tools, there are still more weeds than flowers, or that every time they get rid of one weed, two others take its place. In Chapter 11, you learned to identify underlying assumptions and test them with experiments. When you discover that your assumptions are not accurate and discard them, this is like pulling up the weeds by their roots. New assumptions can be planted and nurtured to support more flowers in your garden. It often takes many weeks or months before you can really believe new assumptions, so it is important that you spend whatever time is necessary on Chapter 11 to strengthen your belief in your new assumptions. Usually people will need to spend several months doing the experiments described in Chapter 11 before they have a high degree of confidence in new assumptions.

Many people notice a big mood improvement once they integrate and apply the skills taught in the mood chapters (Chapters 13–15) and the earlier chapters of this book (Chapters 1–11). It takes time and repeated practice for these skills to affect your life in a meaningful way. Once you spend this time, the reward is that alternative thoughts and assumptions will become your new automatic responses, and many areas of your life may improve as a result. You may notice improvements in your moods, your relationships, and your overall sense of well-being. If this has been the case for you, this current chapter is optional. Even if you decide you do not need to complete this entire chapter, you may still find it interesting to read and complete the sections later in the chapter on gratitude and acts of kindness (pp. 175–186), because these sections teach ways to boost your positive moods.

However, if you have spent the time needed to develop proficiency with Thought Records (Chapters 6–9), Action Plans and acceptance (Chapter 10), and experiments (Chapter 11), and you are still struggling with your moods, then the solution may lie in learning to identify and work with your "core beliefs."

The following diagram illustrates the connections among three different levels of thought: automatic thoughts, underlying assumptions, and core beliefs. Automatic thoughts, which you have worked with in Chapters 6–9, are the easiest level to identify. Automatic thoughts are the parts of the weeds or flowers that are above ground. Automatic thoughts are rooted beneath the surface in underlying assumptions and core beliefs. Notice that the arrows in the diagram go in each direction. This is because each of the three levels is connected to the other two. Therefore, when you work on any level of thought, you are also affecting the other two levels. This is why it makes sense to work on the simpler levels (automatic thoughts and underlying assumptions) first. For a lot of people, once they change the top two levels, the core beliefs take care of themselves, and that is all they need to do to bring about enduring positive changes in mood.

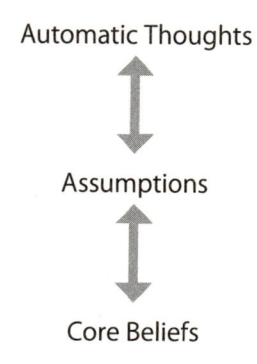

Automatic Thoughts
⇅
Assumptions
⇅
Core Beliefs

Automatic thoughts can be described as words or images that come into our minds automatically. As you learned in Chapter 11, underlying assumptions are not as obvious, but you can identify them when you put a behavior or situation that triggers a strong emotion into a sentence that begins with "If . . . ," follow that by "then . . . ," and let your mind complete that sentence.

Core beliefs are all-or-nothing statements about yourself, others, or the world. Marissa's core beliefs about herself included "I'm worthless," "I'm unlovable," and "I'm inadequate." Her core beliefs about others included "Others are dangerous," "People will hurt you," and "People are mean." She also believed that "The world is full of insurmountable problems." All of these beliefs are "all-or-nothing" beliefs – there are no qualifications. Marissa did not think, "I'm sometimes worthless"; she believed, "I am worthless" (absolutely).

Everybody has both negative and positive core beliefs. This is normal. Our core beliefs get activated when we experience strong moods or have life experiences that are either very positive or negative. When we are feeling good, our positive core beliefs are active ("I'm clever"). When we have negative moods, our negative core beliefs are activated ("I'm stupid"). Once activated, our core beliefs affect how we see things, giving rise to related (either positive or negative) automatic thoughts and assumptions. For example, when we have positive moods and we make a mistake, we might think, "If I make a mistake, I can fix it because I'm clever." When we make the same mistake on a day we are in a negative mood, we might think, "If I make a mistake, it shows how stupid I am."

Generally we work with automatic thoughts and underlying assumptions first, because changes in these levels of thought occur more quickly and will usually lift our moods. That is why Thought Records, Action Plans, acceptance, and experiments are the best first steps to improve mood. When changes at the levels of automatic thoughts and underlying assumptions don't create the mood changes you hope for, this may be a sign that your positive core beliefs are much weaker than your negative core beliefs and need to be strengthened.

Just as you learned to identify and evaluate your automatic thoughts (Chapters 6–9) and underlying assumptions (Chapter 11), you can learn to identify and evaluate your core beliefs. If you have negative core beliefs that are active most of the time, then you will usually want to identify and strengthen your positive core beliefs. Once your positive core beliefs are more active, you are likely to feel better and enjoy a more rewarding life. For example, as long as Marissa saw herself as unlovable (a negative core belief), she did not allow people to get to know her. She behaved in withdrawn and protective ways. As Marissa developed a new positive core belief, "I am likable," she was more willing to get close to people. With this new belief, Marissa became more relaxed over time and had more positive interactions with others.

Where do core beliefs come from? Very often we have had them since childhood. We first learn about ourselves and the world from our family members and other people around us. They teach us things like "The sky is blue. This is a dog. You are worthless." So many of the messages we are given are correct ("The sky is blue," "This is a dog") that we believe all the things we are told, even things that may be wrong ("You are worthless").

Children also reach their own conclusions based on what they experience in life. Some children may not be told, "You are worthless," but they may notice that an older child in the family is given special favors, that boys are valued more than girls, or that athletic children are more popular than bookworms. They may make sense of these experiences by deciding, "I'm not as good as [an older child, a boy, or an athletic child]." Over time, this idea may be stored in their minds as "I'm no good," "I'm defective," or "I'm a loser."

Not all core beliefs are about ourselves. Based on experience, children acquire many core beliefs such as "Dogs bite," or "Dogs are friendly," which guide their behavior (they learn to stay away from or approach an unfamiliar dog). Children also learn rules from other people around them ("Big boys don't cry," "Stoves are hot").

The rules and beliefs a child develops are not necessarily true (e.g., boys and men of all ages do cry), but a young child does not yet have the mental ability to think in more flexible ways. Rules take on an absolute quality for a child. A three-year-old girl may believe, "It's bad to hit someone," and be angry with her mother for hitting her brother on the back when he is choking on a piece of food. An older child will be able to see the difference between hitting to hurt and hitting to help.

In most areas of our lives, we develop more flexible rules and beliefs as we grow older. We learn to approach dogs that are wagging their tails and avoid dogs that are growling. We also learn that the same behavior can be "bad" or "good," depending on the context. However, some of our beliefs from childhood stay absolute even into adulthood.

Absolute beliefs may remain fixed if they develop from very traumatic circumstances, or if consistent early life experiences convince us that these beliefs are true even as we grow older. For example, because Marissa was abused as a child, she concluded that she was bad and that other people were dangerous. Young children tend to believe that everything that happens is their responsibility. Therefore, even though no child deserves to be abused, many abused children decide that the abuse is their fault and happens because they are bad. Unfortunately, these beliefs can continue well into adulthood, especially when a person has no significant experiences that teach a different message. Since Marissa was also physically abused in her relationships with both her husbands, her original negative core beliefs became stronger over time.

Vic grew up with an older brother, Doug, who was a star athlete and straight-A student. No matter how well Vic did in school and sports, he was never as successful as Doug. Despite Vic's own successes, he grew up with a core belief that he was inadequate. This belief seemed true to Vic because, in his own mind, no accomplishment was worthwhile unless it was the absolute best (i.e., better than Doug's achievements). In Vic's mind, this belief was supported when he heard parents, teachers, and coaches describe Doug's achievements with pride.

Because core beliefs help us make sense of our world beginning at a young age, it may never occur to us to evaluate whether they are the most accurate or helpful ways of understanding our adult experiences. Instead, as adults, we act, think, and feel as if these beliefs are still 100% true. This is understandable, especially since some of our core beliefs may have been accurate and helpful for us as children. For example, if we grow up in abusive and alcoholic homes like Marissa's home, it may be adaptive to view others as dangerous and to remain constantly alert to signs of aggression. However, these same core beliefs that helped protect Marissa in abusive relationships interfered with her ability to form close, trusting relationships with people who were not hurtful to her. With a fixed core belief that "People are dangerous," Marissa was at risk of misinterpreting everyday behaviors as negative and aggressive.

It would help Marissa to develop new positive core beliefs – for example, that many people are loving and kind. Developing this companion positive core belief would give Marissa the mental flexibility to draw on the core belief that was most accurate and adaptive for the person she was with at any given time ("People are dangerous," "People are kind"). If we hold both types of core beliefs (positive and negative), then we are able to experience our lives on a full continuum – from very negative to neutral to very positive. When we hold only negative core beliefs, then every life experience becomes negative in some way, because it is viewed through these negative, inflexible lenses.

IDENTIFYING CORE BELIEFS: THE DOWNWARD ARROW TECHNIQUE

One way to identify core beliefs is called the "downward arrow technique." In Chapter 7, you learned to ask questions about the meaning of events — such as "What does this mean about me?" — to identify your automatic thoughts (refer to the Helpful Hints on page 54). Once you identify automatic thoughts, you can ask yourself the same or similar questions to help identify core beliefs. For example, you can ask yourself for any given automatic thought, "If this is true, what does this mean about me?"

Sometimes repeatedly asking yourself, "What does this mean about me?" will help reveal core beliefs about yourself that underlie automatic thoughts you have previously identified.

For example, if Marissa had the automatic thought "I don't think Marsha likes me," and this thought contributed to her depressed mood, the downward arrow technique would help her find her core belief in this way:

I don't think Marsha likes me.

(If this is true, what does this mean about me?)

⬇

Whenever I get close, people end up disliking me.

(If this is true, what does this mean about me?)

⬇

I'll never have a close relationship.

(If this is true, what does this mean about me?)

⬇

I'm unlikable.

In this example of the downward arrow technique, the automatic thought ("I don't think Marsha likes me") was about a particular situation. When Marissa identified her core belief related to her depressed mood ("I'm unlikable"), it was an absolute statement that she believed was true for all situations in her life.

The preceding example illustrates how to identify core beliefs about oneself. We also have core beliefs about others and the world. The downward arrow technique can be used to identify core beliefs about others or the world by modifying the questions.

For example, beliefs about other people can be identified with the downward arrow technique by asking this question:

"If this is true, what does this mean or say about other people?"

Assumptions or core beliefs about the world can be identified by asking:

"If this is true, what does this say or mean about the world and how it works?"

Examples of using the downward arrow technique to identify core beliefs about others and the world follow:

Situation: Vic and his colleagues received new sales quotas.
Vic's Automatic Thought: Everyone will be able to meet these quotas but me.
Downward Arrow:
(What does this say or mean about other people?)

⬇

They are able to do the work more easily than I am.
(If this is true, what does this say or mean about other people?)

⬇

Others are more competent than I am.

Situation: Marissa is called in by her supervisor for an evaluation meeting.
Marissa's Automatic Thought: I've made a mistake again. He's going to fire me.
Downward Arrow:
(What does this say or mean about the world and how it works?)

⬇

Bad things are always happening to me.
(If this is true, what does this say or mean about the world and how it works?)

⬇

The world is harsh and punishing.
(If this is true, what does this say or mean about the world and how it works?)

⬇

The world works against me.

Sometimes identifying core beliefs about yourself will be enough to help you understand a recurrent problem in your life. Often, however, core beliefs about yourself tell only part of the story. Identifying core beliefs about others and the world can complete your understanding of why a situation is so distressing. For example, Vic would have been less concerned about failing to meet the sales quota if he had thought others would fail, too. Seeing other people as more competent than he was intensified his distress and added to his perception that he was inadequate.

Marissa's core beliefs that "The world is harsh and punishing," and "The world works against me," certainly added to her depression and hopelessness. She had difficulty putting forth effort day after day because of her belief that eventually the world would crash down on her, despite her best efforts. In fact, it was a testimony to Marissa's courage that she continued to work hard in her life, despite her beliefs about the world.

It is understandable that negative beliefs about the world may develop for people who have witnessed or experienced trauma; have lived through harsh economic conditions without relief; have grown up in chaotic, unpredictable circumstances; have been hurt by persistent discrimination; or have had life experiences of any kind that were often harmful or punishing. Children who have these types of experiences seem particularly vulnerable to developing negative core beliefs about the world. Even so, powerful negative experiences can help create negative core beliefs at any age.

Similarly, negative core beliefs about others usually develop from traumatic or persistently negative interactions with other people. Sometimes, as we have seen with Vic, an indirect experience such as observing a highly successful sibling can help create a view of others that causes distress. Vic's positive view of others ("They are competent"), linked with his negative core belief about himself ("I'm inadequate"), helped explain his high level of anxiety.

It is important to remember that it is healthy to have both negative and positive core beliefs. Negative core beliefs are only problems when they become fixed and we lose our flexibility to see ourselves, others, and the world in positive ways. Similarly, positive core beliefs can be problems if we lose the flexibility to perceive negative aspects of ourselves, others, and the world. For example, if somebody is trying to take advantage of you, it is helpful to be able to recognize this person's negative intention. It is helpful to be aware that some dogs do bite.

Several exercises follow (Worksheets 12.1, 12.2, 12.3, and 12.4) to help you discover some of your core beliefs. See if you can uncover core beliefs about yourself, others, and the world that link to the types of difficulties you are working on as you use *Mind Over Mood*. If you have difficulty identifying a core belief in one of these areas, it may mean that the situations you have chosen do not involve this type of core belief. Worksheet 12.1 is a simple approach to identifying core beliefs. Worksheets 12.2, 12.3, and 12.4 are more detailed approaches that use the downward arrow technique. You can decide which approach (simple or downward arrow) helps you identify your core beliefs most easily.

> **EXERCISE: Identifying Core Beliefs**
>
> Think of a recent situation in which you had a strong mood. Imagine this situation vividly, as if you are reliving it now. As you imagine this situation, with these strong moods activated, how do you see yourself, others, and the world?

WORKSHEET 12.1. Identifying Core Beliefs

1. I am _____

   _____

2. Others are _____

   _____

3. The world is _____

   _____

From *Mind Over Mood, Second Edition*. Copyright 2016 by Dennis Greenberger and Christine A. Padesky. Purchasers of this book can photocopy and/or download additional copies of this worksheet (see the box at the end of the table of contents).

> **EXERCISE: Identifying Core Beliefs about Yourself**
>
> Think of another recent situation in which you had a strong mood. Complete Worksheet 12.2 for that situation. End the exercise when you arrive at an all-or-nothing, absolute statement about yourself. You may have to continue to ask yourself the question "If this is true, what does this say or mean about me?" more times than printed on the worksheet, or you may arrive at a core belief after asking the question only one or two times.

WORKSHEET 12.2. Downward Arrow Technique: Identifying Core Beliefs about Self

Situation (connected to a strong mood)

_____

What does this say or mean about me?

_____

⬇

If this is true, what does this say or mean about me?

_____

⬇

If this is true, what does this say or mean about me?

_____

⬇

If this is true, what does this say or mean about me?

_____

From *Mind Over Mood, Second Edition*. Copyright 2016 by Dennis Greenberger and Christine A. Padesky. Purchasers of this book can photocopy and/or download additional copies of this worksheet (see the box at the end of the table of contents).

EXERCISE: **Identifying Core Beliefs about Other People**

Complete Worksheet 12.3, using either the same situation used in Worksheet 12.2 or another recent situation in which you had a strong mood that was related to one or more other people. End the exercise when you arrive at an all-or-nothing, absolute statement about other people. You may have to continue to ask yourself the question "If this is true, what does this say or mean about other people?" more times than printed on the worksheet, or you may arrive at a core belief after asking the question only one or two times.

WORKSHEET 12.3. Downward Arrow Technique: Identifying Core Beliefs about Other People

Situation (connected to a strong mood)

_____

What does this say or mean about other people?

_____

⬇

If this is true, what does this say or mean about other people?

_____

⬇

If this is true, what does this say or mean about other people?

_____

⬇

If this is true, what does this say or mean about other people?

_____

From *Mind Over Mood, Second Edition.* Copyright 2016 by Dennis Greenberger and Christine A. Padesky. Purchasers of this book can photocopy and/or download additional copies of this worksheet (see the box at the end of the table of contents).

EXERCISE: Identifying Core Beliefs about the World (or My Life)

Complete Worksheet 12.4, using either the same situation used in Worksheets 12.2 or 12.3, or another recent situation in which you had a strong mood. End the exercise when you arrive at an all-or-nothing, absolute statement about the world. You may have to continue to ask yourself the question "If this is true, what does this say or mean about the world?" more times than printed on the worksheet, or you may arrive at a core belief after asking the question only one or two times. If this question about the world doesn't make sense to you, you can ask, "If this is true, what does this say or mean about my life?"

WORKSHEET 12.4. Downward Arrow Technique: Identifying Core Beliefs about the World (or My Life)

Situation (connected to a strong mood)

_____

What does this say or mean about the world (or my life)?

_____

⬇

If this is true, what does this say or mean about the world (or my life)?

_____

⬇

If this is true, what does this say or mean about the world (or my life)?

_____

⬇

If this is true, what does this say or mean about the world (or my life)?

_____

From *Mind Over Mood, Second Edition*. Copyright 2016 by Dennis Greenberger and Christine A. Padesky. Purchasers of this book can photocopy and/or download additional copies of this worksheet (see the box at the end of the table of contents).

Whatever the origins of the core beliefs that contribute to your distress, the next two sections of this chapter teach you methods for changing them. For Marissa, a change in core beliefs meant learning to see that the world was not always hard and punishing, and that sometimes things did go her way. A belief that things could sometimes go her way encouraged Marissa to begin to look for relationships and environments that she could count on to be more consistently supportive. She then learned to use these supports to help her cope with the harsher relationships and situations in her life. For Vic, a change in core beliefs meant learning to feel good about himself even when he was not "the best." Vic also benefited from learning to see a middle ground between being "the best" and being "a complete failure."

TESTING CORE BELIEFS

You might think that, just as we have used Thought Records to test automatic thoughts, we can test core beliefs by gathering evidence that supports and doesn't support the core beliefs. This approach does not work so well for core beliefs, however. Because we see our experiences through the lens of the core belief that is active, we often don't notice or believe experiences that don't support this core belief.

Marissa, for example, believed that she was unlovable. When she tried to test this idea, she did not value evidence like invitations to lunch from people at work, warm greetings from several colleagues when she arrived at work, the love she received from her children, or the high regard from some of her friends — even when they told her how much they loved her. This was important evidence that Marissa was lovable, but Marissa discounted it because she thought, "They were just feeling sorry for me," or "They don't really know me yet." When a core belief is active, we distort our experiences to fit the belief.

Instead of testing our negative core beliefs, it is usually more helpful to (1) identify new core beliefs that we would like to hold, and (2) look for evidence to support or strengthen these new core beliefs. This offers the possibility of viewing our life experiences in fresh ways. If we find there is a lot of evidence to support our new core beliefs, then we will begin to believe them. We do not need to get rid of our negative core beliefs. When new core beliefs are as strong as our negative core beliefs, then we can be more flexible in our thinking. Core beliefs that fit a given situation are more likely to be activated, instead of always understanding our experiences through our negative core beliefs.

IDENTIFYING NEW CORE BELIEFS

The advantage of identifying a new core belief ("I'm lovable"), as an alternative to trying to test and change a negative core belief ("I'm unlovable"), is that having a pair of core beliefs allows us to become more flexible in our thinking and to understand experiences in ways that help us achieve greater satisfaction and happiness. If a single core belief is activated all the time, most of our experience gets viewed through the lens of this core belief. When we have the balance of two core beliefs instead, an interesting thing happens: With two core beliefs, we can evaluate our experiences more flexibly and see which belief fits a situation better. Also, when we have two counterbalancing core beliefs, we can better understand and accept a range of life experiences. For example, when coworkers smiled at her, Marissa could accept and process this as a positive experience, without filtering it through her core beliefs of lovability or unlovability. She could simply enjoy a nice interaction.

In addition to offering us greater flexibility in how we see things, identifying new core beliefs allows us to remember positive experiences more easily. If we don't have a positive core belief, it is a bit like having a storage container with a hole in the bottom. We can pour liquid (positive experiences) into the container and enjoy it for a short time, but the liquid quickly drains away and is lost. Identifying a new core belief creates a new container to store these positive experiences. Once we have a new core belief, we can capture, store, and remember our positive experiences for a long time. This helps us experience and hold onto greater happiness.

For example, if the negative core belief "I'm unlovable" is always activated, whatever happens is understood in those terms and stored in that container. Recall that even when people appeared to like her, Marissa distorted her experience to fit them into her "I'm unlovable" core belief ("They were just feeling sorry for me," or "They don't really know me yet"). Because she was only viewing the world through the lens of her negative core belief, she fitted all her experiences into the "I'm unlovable" container. If Marissa created a new core belief, "I'm lovable," she would have the option of using that belief to understand and store experiences. Over time, as more and more experiences were stored in the "I'm lovable" container, Marissa's new core belief would grow stronger.

Sometimes a new core belief is the opposite of the initial core belief. For example, Marissa shifted her belief from "I'm unlovable" to "I'm lovable." This new belief did not mean that she expected everyone to love her; it simply meant that she was lovable and had many good qualities, whether people liked her or not. At other times, a new core belief may change an absolute belief to a qualified belief. For example, Marissa shifted her belief that "People will hurt me" to "Even though some people are hurtful, most people are kind and giving." At still other times, a new core belief may evaluate experience from a completely different perspective. For example, Vic shifted his belief that his success and worth hinged on being "the best" to a belief that he was acceptable no matter how well he performed.

Sometimes a new core belief will include a perspective of acceptance. For example, you might choose to shift from a core belief of "People are unreliable" to one of "It is OK if people are unreliable, because I am capable and can handle it." In this instance, a positive core belief about yourself helps you accept a negative core belief about others. As shown in these examples, a new core belief does not always involve shifting to an opposite word (for instance, from "unlovable" to "lovable"). It can shift to a new word, as Marissa did in changing her view of others from "hurtful" to "kind and giving," or as Vic did in changing his core belief about himself from "worthless" to "acceptable."

> **EXERCISE: Identifying a New Core Belief**
>
> Use Worksheet 12.5 to identify a new core belief.

WORKSHEET 12.5. Identifying a New Core Belief

Examine the negative core beliefs you identified on Worksheets 12.1 through 12.4. Do you recognize one of these beliefs as one that is frequently active in your life? Write it on the negative core belief line below.

Now identify a new core belief. What word or words best capture how you would like to think about this?

Negative Core Belief   New Core Belief

_____   _____

From *Mind Over Mood, Second Edition.* Copyright 2016 by Dennis Greenberger and Christine A. Padesky. Purchasers of this book can photocopy and/or download additional copies of this worksheet (see the box at the end of the table of contents).

Once you identify new core beliefs, you will want to look for evidence to support them, because it will take some time before you can believe these new core beliefs as strongly as you currently believe your negative core beliefs. In the next section, you will learn how to notice and create experiences, so you can begin to strengthen your new core beliefs.

STRENGTHENING NEW CORE BELIEFS

> **EXERCISE: Recording Evidence That Supports Your New Core Belief**
>
> At the top of Worksheet 12.6, write down your new core belief from Worksheet 12.5.
>
> Over the next few weeks, notice and write down small events and experiences that support your new core belief. Over the next few months, continue to look for and write down experiences that support your new belief.
>
> Keep in mind that the evidence you are looking for may be quite small. For example, evidence Marissa recorded for her lovability included people smiling and appearing happy to see her, people asking her to spend time with them or agreeing to her invitations to spend time together, and compliments given to her.

WORKSHEET 12.6. Core Belief Record: Recording Evidence That Supports a New Core Belief

New Core Belief: _____

Evidence or experiences that support my new belief:

1. _____
2. _____
3. _____
4. _____
5. _____
6. _____
7. _____
8. _____
9. _____
10. _____
11. _____
12. _____
13. _____
14. _____
15. _____
16. _____
17. _____
18. _____
19. _____
20. _____
21. _____
22. _____
23. _____
24. _____
25. _____

From *Mind Over Mood, Second Edition.* Copyright 2016 by Dennis Greenberger and Christine A. Padesky. Purchasers of this book can photocopy and/or download additional copies of this worksheet (see the box at the end of the table of contents).

HELPFUL HINTS To notice these small events, ask yourself questions like these:

- Did you do anything today alone or with others that fits with this new core belief?
- Did other people behave toward you in small or big ways that fit with this new core belief?
- Are there any habits you follow every day that fit with this new core belief?
- Did anything positive happen today that fits with this new core belief?

Write down any experiences, no matter how small, that fit with your new core belief. If you find yourself thinking, "This is so small or unusual that it doesn't count for anything," write it down anyway. The small experiences add up, and you want to make sure that you are not discounting or ignoring any life experiences. Chances are that you are highly aware of small negative events, so it is important for you to become just as aware of small positive events.

To keep track of how your beliefs are changing, it is helpful to rate the your confidence in your new belief on a scale similar to the one you used in Chapter 3 to rate your moods. For example, when Marissa started looking at the belief that she was lovable, she did not think it was true for her at all, so her lovability scale looked like this:

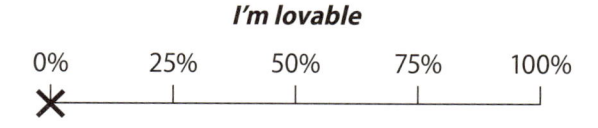

I'm lovable

0%   25%   50%   75%   100%
 ✗

After she completed the Core Belief Record (Worksheet 12.6) for her new core belief for 10 weeks, Marissa's scale looked like this:

I'm lovable

0%   25%   50%   75%   100%
       ✗

While this may look like a small change to you, it was very important to Marissa. This was the first time in her life that she had felt at all lovable. Even this small amount of confidence in her lovability allowed her to begin to experience love from her children and friends. She kept track of small and large signs of her lovability for a year, and her rating eventually reached 70%. As her new core belief became stronger, she began to notice more and more positive experiences that had always been part of her life, but that she had never really noticed or had discounted or distorted in the past. As she began to notice and appreciate these positive experiences, Marissa felt greater joy and happiness in herself and her relationships.

EXERCISE: **Rating Confidence in New Core Beliefs over Time**

On the first line of Worksheet 12.7, write the new core belief you identified and have been strengthening on Worksheet 12.6. Then enter the date and rate the new core belief by placing an ✕ on the scale below the number that best matches how much you think this new belief fits with your current experiences. If you don't believe the new core belief at all, mark your ✕ below 0 on the scale. If you have total confidence in your new core belief, put your ✕ below 100 on the scale. To measure your progress in strengthening your new core belief, rerate the new core belief every few weeks.

WORKSHEET 12.7. Rating Confidence in My New Core Belief

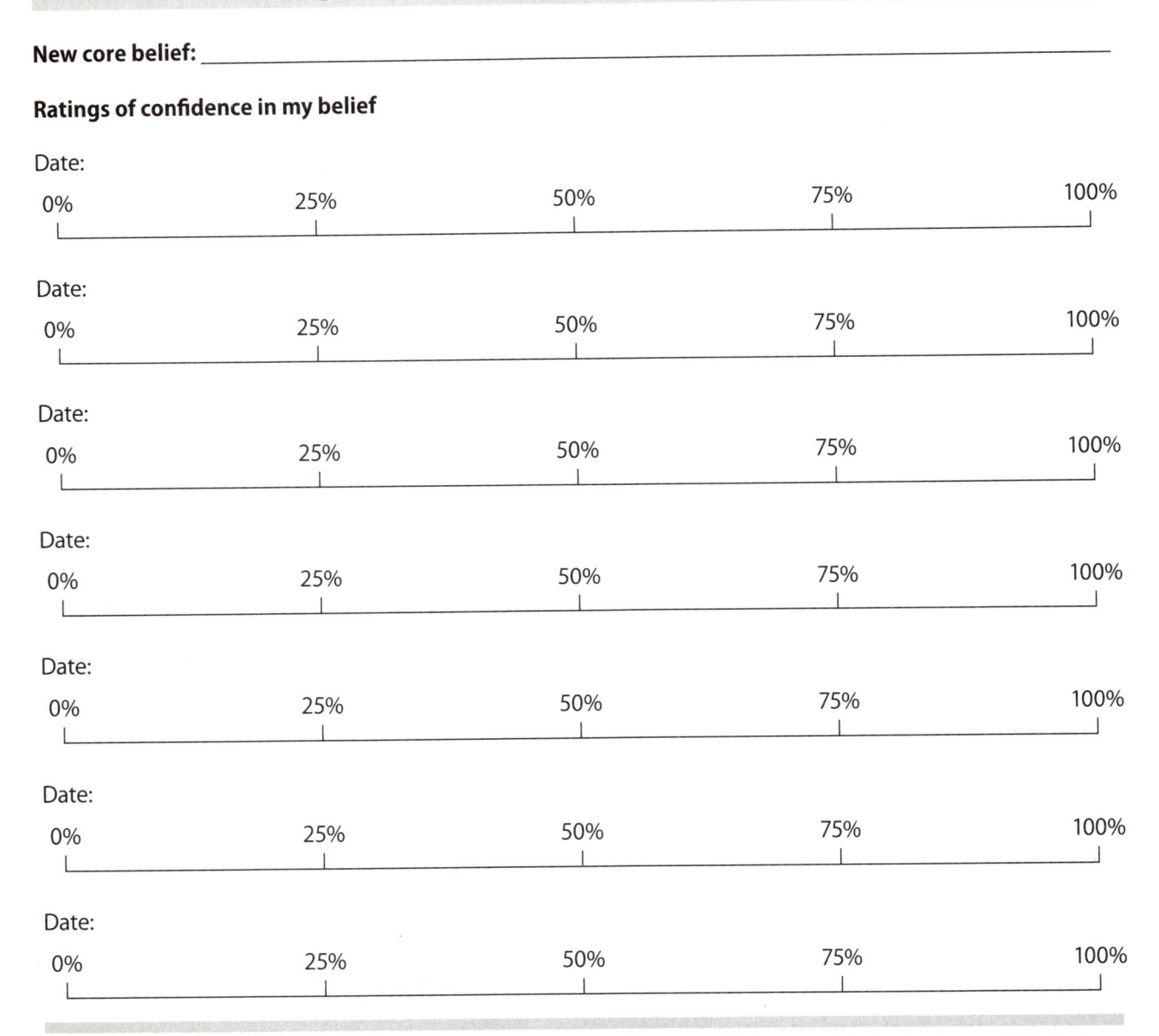

New core belief: _____

Ratings of confidence in my belief

Date:

0%   25%   50%   75%   100%

Date:

0%   25%   50%   75%   100%

Date:

0%   25%   50%   75%   100%

Date:

0%   25%   50%   75%   100%

Date:

0%   25%   50%   75%   100%

Date:

0%   25%   50%   75%   100%

Date:

0%   25%   50%   75%   100%

From *Mind Over Mood, Second Edition.* Copyright 2016 by Dennis Greenberger and Christine A. Padesky. Purchasers of this book can photocopy and/or download additional copies of this worksheet (see the box at the end of the table of contents).

As you record more experiences on Worksheets 12.6 and 12.7, and do the remaining exercises in this chapter, your new core belief will probably become more believable to you. Confidence in a new core belief usually takes months to develop, so don't be discouraged if your confidence rating increases at a very slow pace – or even remains in one spot for a long time. The more experiences you notice and write down to support the new belief, the more likely it is that you will begin to have confidence in it. With this new confidence, you may begin to feel better across many areas of your life. Over time, it often gets easier to see more and more positive experiences, which can increase your life satisfaction and happiness.

It is not necessary to be 100% confident in your new core belief. In fact, most people begin to feel better when their confidence in the new belief reaches a midpoint on the scale. As you rate yourself on the scales in Worksheet 12.7, be sure to give yourself credit for partial success and for progress.

HELPFUL HINTS This chapter introduces you to a variety of exercises that can help you build new core beliefs so you can achieve greater happiness and life satisfaction. Unlike the worksheets presented in earlier chapters, most of the core belief worksheets (Worksheets 12.5–12.9) require you to keep records for weeks or months to gather enough evidence to strengthen your new core beliefs. Don't expect to do all of these worksheets simultaneously. Work on one worksheet for a while, write down what you learn, and then move to another one. The exception to this rule is that it is helpful to do Worksheets 12.6 and 12.7 at the same time.

Since you may be spending a number of weeks doing the worksheets in this chapter, remember to complete your mood measures every week or two so you can track your progress. See page 150 for Mood Check-Up instructions.

VIC: *Using scales to rate positive changes in behavior.*

Sometimes we can strengthen our new core beliefs more quickly if we practice new behaviors or make changes consistent with our new core beliefs. For example, Vic wanted to believe that he was acceptable, regardless of how well he did something. He noticed that he felt badly when he "failed" at something or didn't do a task perfectly. It made sense to Vic that he should be able to feel acceptable about doing a task at work or home less than perfectly. However, he was not so sure he shouldn't feel guilty and unacceptable whenever he exploded in anger at his wife, Judy. He did not want to behave in this way, and he knew that his anger was a problem, because his angry explosions were destructive to his marriage and his self-esteem. Vic knew that if he could positively change his angry behavior, he would begin to see himself as more acceptable. More importantly, he was certain that changing it would improve his relationship with Judy.

Vic set a goal to change his behavior when he was angry. He wanted to stay in control of his behavior and not use threatening behaviors or words. Instead, he wanted to stay connected with Judy and talk through disagreements in a respectful way. This meant that he wanted to listen more to Judy even when they disagreed, and also express his views assertively without putting her down. Because he tended to be perfectionistic, Vic learned to use rating scales to reduce his perfectionism. For example, his therapist taught Vic to rate his anger at work and at home on an "anger control" scale. The following scale shows how Vic rated his anger control in a conversation with Judy.

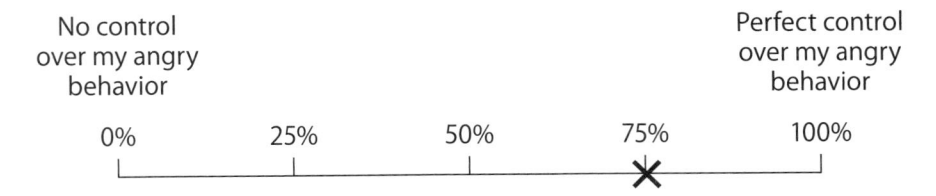

```
   No control                                    Perfect control
  over my angry                                   over my angry
    behavior                                        behavior

      0%        25%        50%        75%        100%
      |—————————|——————————|——————————|——————————|
                                      ✗
```

In the conversation, Vic became irritated and raised his voice several times. He even pounded the table with his fist once. But he did not criticize Judy, leave the house, or behave in any way she considered threatening. He stayed on topic and took one three-minute timeout to cool down when his anger started to feel out of control.

Before learning to rate his experiences, Vic would have judged the conversation as an anger control "failure," because he was not perfectly in control all the time. Evaluating this experience as a "failure" would have discouraged Vic and perhaps added to his hopelessness about learning to control his angry behavior. Using the scale shifted Vic's perspective. He was able to see that he was not a failure: He was 75% successful instead of 0% successful. Even though he was very angry, he did not explode, withdraw, or hurt Judy. He listened to what she had to say, and also talked to her about what was important to him. Even when his anger built up, he was able to return to the conversation after a three-minute timeout. For these reasons, he and Judy considered his efforts worthwhile, even though he showed less than perfect control. Recognizing his partial success showed Vic that he was making progress and helped him feel good about what he was doing well.

Rating your experiences on a scale may be equally helpful in your life. If you have changes you are trying to make, or experiences that you tend to discount or see as "failures" if they are not perfect, try rating them on a scale. See what difference it makes if you focus on the partial positive aspects of the experience, instead of looking solely at the negative aspects.

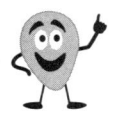

REMINDERS Use a scale to rate experiences you tend to see in "all-or-nothing" or "success-or-failure" terms. Also use a scale to track your progress in changing a behavior or mood. Notice how it feels to look at the positive portion of the scale. Try to give yourself credit for any progress represented on the scale.

EXERCISE: Rating Behaviors on a Scale instead of in All-or-Nothing Terms

On Worksheet 12.8, identify some of your own behaviors related to your new core belief. For example, if you are trying to develop a new core belief that you are lovable, you might rate your social behavior or things you do that you think would make you lovable. If you are trying to develop a new core belief that "I am a worthwhile person," you could focus on behaviors that you think demonstrate your worth. Choose behaviors that you tend to evaluate in all-or-nothing terms. For each scale, describe the situation and write what behavior you are rating. Notice how it feels to rate your behavior on a scale instead of evaluating yourself in all-or-nothing terms. After you have rated several behaviors on these scales, summarize what you have learned at the bottom of Worksheet 12.8. For example, Vic wrote, "I am acceptable even when I have partial successes, because these are steps in the right direction. My efforts to improve myself are a sign of acceptability, even though I am less than perfect."

WORKSHEET 12.8. Rating Behaviors on a Scale

Situation: Behavior I am rating:

0%   25%   50%   75%   100%

Situation: Behavior I am rating:

0%   25%   50%   75%   100%

Situation: Behavior I am rating:

0%   25%   50%   75%   100%

Situation: Behavior I am rating:

0%   25%   50%   75%   100%

Situation: Behavior I am rating:

0%   25%   50%   75%   100%

Situation: Behavior I am rating:

0%   25%   50%   75%   100%

Summary: _____

_____

_____

_____

From *Mind Over Mood, Second Edition*. Copyright 2016 by Dennis Greenberger and Christine A. Padesky. Purchasers of this book can photocopy and/or download additional copies of this worksheet (see the box at the end of the table of contents).

STRENGTHENING CORE BELIEFS WITH BEHAVIORAL EXPERIMENTS

In Chapter 11, you learned to use behavioral experiments to test your underlying assumptions. Behavioral experiments can also help strengthen new core beliefs. It is hard to develop confidence in a new core belief just by thinking about it. Usually our confidence in a new core belief increases only after we begin to experiment with new behaviors that are linked to the new core belief. For example, Vic developed confidence that he could control his anger only after he began experimenting with behaviors that helped him stay in control.

One woman, Carla, saw herself as unacceptable and unimportant. Carla believed that others were more important than she was, and therefore she always did what other people wanted and put their needs above her own. She also avoided conflict in her relationships, because she felt bad when others were upset with her. This was especially true because whenever there was conflict, she assumed that it was her fault, and she felt horrible. As she worked her way through the worksheets in this chapter, she decided she wanted to build three new core beliefs: "My needs are also important," "Conflict is normal in relationships, because different people often want different things," and "If I stand up for myself and tolerate my discomfort, I'll feel better in the long run." She decided to do one or more of several behavioral experiments each day:

1. "I will pay attention to what I want and speak up for myself."

2. "When I disagree with someone, I will express my point of view. I will tolerate my discomfort and not compromise with someone else just to avoid conflict."

3. "I will spend some time every day doing something for myself that is important to me."

Carla made predictions based on her old and new core beliefs about what would happen in these experiments. Her old core beliefs predicted that people would get upset or criticize her when she did these things, and she would feel worse. Her new core beliefs predicted that although there might be discomfort in the short term, she would feel better about herself in the long term.

Since Carla was especially concerned about what her closest friends and family would think about her if she made these changes, she practiced her experiments the first few weeks with strangers. Several things surprised Carla when she behaved in these ways with shopkeepers, clerks, and new people she met. First, contrary to her predictions, most of the time people did not even seem to react when she spoke up for herself and made it clear what she wanted. Some people even responded favorably and said things like "Oh, I can see what you mean."

With these encouraging results, Carla decided to begin doing similar behavioral experiments with family and friends. In these relationships, she sometimes received positive or neutral responses, but she noticed that certain family members got quite upset with her when she asserted herself. When she continued to speak up for herself, Carla was surprised that even though she felt discomfort at first, she sometimes felt a bit better even when the disagreement continued. She was beginning to realize that it was OK to express her needs, whether all family members agreed with her or not. Also, she recognized that she could be acceptable and expressing her needs was important, even when others in her family did not agree with her.

As she thought about her experiments, Carla realized that some family members had come to expect that she would always give in to their opinions and preferences. When she did not, they reacted negatively. Therefore, she decided to talk to them and explain that she wanted to be more direct in expressing her own wants and needs. It took some time, but she gradually changed her role in her family. As Carla more regularly voiced her opinions, she discovered that others often were willing to compromise and resolve differences in ways that met her needs as well as their own.

These experiments required Carla to tolerate discomfort, especially in the beginning. She was pleasantly surprised to learn that her discomfort didn't last, and that it decreased as she did more and more experiments. Once she did her experiments, it increased her confidence when people paid attention to her and went along with what she wanted. When people did not respond to her requests, she was able to see that differences of opinion did not mean she was unimportant. She was able to understand that conflict is a normal part of relationships, because even people who care about each other often want different things.

EXERCISE: Behavioral Experiments to Strengthen New Core Beliefs

At this point, you may be ready to do some behavioral experiments to strengthen some of your new core beliefs. Use Worksheet 12.9 to do the following:

1. Write out two or three new behaviors that are linked to your new core belief. You are likely to feel a bit nervous or hesitant about doing these behaviors. That's a sign that you are probably on the right track.

2. Make predictions about what will happen, based on your old and new core beliefs.

3. If possible, try these behaviors out with strangers first (e.g., shop clerks, people in town you don't know). This can be helpful, because strangers don't expect you to act in any particular way.

4. Once you have done the experiments a number of times with strangers, try out these new behaviors with people you know. If appropriate, you can tell your family and friends what new behaviors you are trying and why this is important for you.

5. Write down the outcome of your experiments and what you learn from them, especially as they relate to your new core beliefs and your predictions (see item 2 above). Do your new behaviors and the outcomes support your new core beliefs even partially?

WORKSHEET 12.9. Behavioral Experiments to Strengthen New Core Beliefs

Write down the core belief(s) you want to strengthen: _____

List two or three new behaviors that fit with your new core belief. These might be behaviors you would do if you had confidence in your new core belief. They might be behaviors that you feel reluctant to do and yet they would strengthen your new core belief if you did them: _____
_____

Make predictions about what will happen, based on your old and new core beliefs.

    My old core belief prediction:
_____
_____

    My new core belief prediction:
_____
_____

Results of my experiments with strangers (write down what you did, who you did it with, and what happened):

Results of my experiments with people I know (write down what you did, who you did it with, and what happened):

What I learned (do the results support my new core beliefs even partially?):

Future experiments I want to do:

From *Mind Over Mood, Second Edition*. Copyright 2016 by Dennis Greenberger and Christine A. Padesky. Purchasers of this book can photocopy and/or download additional copies of this worksheet (see the box at the end of the table of contents).

GRATITUDE

So far in this chapter, you have been working on identifying and strengthening new core beliefs. You may recall that core beliefs come in pairs. Once you have both a positive and a negative core belief, either one may be active in any given moment. You may be wondering if there is some way you can influence your mind so that your positive core beliefs and positive moods are active more often than your negative core beliefs and moods. Adding more gratitude to your life is one approach that can be a path to strengthening positive core beliefs and moods.

A lot of recent research shows that an attitude of gratitude can lead to greater happiness, improvement in a variety of moods, and even improved physical well-being. It is interesting to note that gratitude plays a role in every major religion. It seems that gratitude can be considered a universal human value that cuts across cultures and has been important throughout time. "Gratitude" means thinking about and being thankful for experiences or qualities in ourselves, other people, and the world. When we can identify things to be grateful for or things we appreciate, we are more likely to have our positive core beliefs activated and strengthened. Therefore, one thing each of us can do to improve our mood is to develop a regular practice of gratitude. Gratitude provides a pathway to recognizing and capturing positive experiences. When we follow this path and cultivate this mindset, we tap into the better parts of our nature and experience more positive moods.

Focusing on things we appreciate often results in a shift in perspective from negative to positive. Consider Louisa, who is having lunch with a friend. Louisa's food is not as hot as she would like, and the flavors are a bit disappointing to her. If she focuses on these aspects of her experience, she is likely to experience a negative shift in her mood. However, if Louisa is grateful that someone else has cooked lunch for her, that the food is generally OK, and that she enjoys being with her friend and having a lively conversation, then Louisa is likely to experience a better mood.

Gratitude does not have to mean ignoring negative things. Louisa could ask the restaurant to reheat her food or bring her something else. However Louisa chooses to handle these and other negative aspects of her life, practicing gratitude means accepting the negative aspects and actively looking beyond them to notice positive dimensions of her experiences that she values.

The worksheets in this part of the chapter are designed to help you develop a practice of gratitude in your life. Some people experience the impact of this exercise immediately, and others may not notice any effects until they have used the worksheets for several weeks. If this exercise is helpful for you, you may decide to develop the habit of gratitude as a regular practice for the rest of your life.

EXERCISE: Beginning a Gratitude Journal

For the next six weeks, take five minutes once a week to focus your attention on things you are grateful for. These may be small things like noticing the strength in your arms or the warmth of the sun, or bigger things like experiencing the love of a child or even the election of a good leader. Write these down on Worksheets 12.10, 12.11, and 12.12. Since you are only doing this exercise once a week, it may be helpful to make a note on your calendar or in an electronic diary to remind you to do it. If you run out of space on the worksheets provided in this book, continue in a paper journal or in an electronic file.

As examples, here are some of the items Louisa wrote in her gratitude journal:

I live in a safe neighborhood. I appreciate that my neighbors know me and wave when they see me. I enjoy watching the children play and hearing their laughter. [World]

I enjoyed walking with my dog. She is always excited when I get out her leash to walk her. It helps me after a hard day to know that she will be happy to see me. She cuddles with me on the couch, and I enjoy petting her. [Others]

I took time to help my elderly neighbor. He was trimming some plants and couldn't reach the highest ones. I value helping others, and it made me feel good to do something kind without expecting anything in return. I actually enjoyed doing it. I also felt happy that his mood seemed to lift because I was there, and that we had a nice chat while we worked together. [Myself]

Use the categories in Worksheets 12.10–12.12 to help you. These ask you to think about gratitude in three areas linked to the core beliefs you have been working on in this chapter: the world and your life, other people, and yourself. Notice things you are grateful for, review what you've already written, and add new items to these gratitude worksheets each week.

As in Louisa's example above, it is more helpful to write about a few things in depth than to try to make a long list of things you are grateful for. So try writing about a few things in detail each week, even if it is just one item per worksheet. Some weeks you might write about several items on one or two worksheets instead of on all three worksheets. This is also OK.

Remember to use these three worksheets for at least six weeks (Worksheets 12.10, 12.11, and 12.12). Then, after filling them out for six weeks, answer the questions in Worksheet 12.13.

WORKSHEET 12.10. Gratitude about the World and My Life

Things in the world and my life that I am grateful for and appreciate:

1. _____
2. _____
3. _____
4. _____
5. _____
6. _____
7. _____
8. _____
9. _____
10. _____
11. _____
12. _____
13. _____
14. _____
15. _____
16. _____
17. _____
18. _____
19. _____
20. _____

From *Mind Over Mood, Second Edition*. Copyright 2016 by Dennis Greenberger and Christine A. Padesky. Purchasers of this book can photocopy and/or download additional copies of this worksheet (see the box at the end of the table of contents).

WORKSHEET 12.11. Gratitude about Others

Things about others (family, friends, coworkers, pets, etc.) that I am grateful for and appreciate:

1. _____
2. _____
3. _____
4. _____
5. _____
6. _____
7. _____
8. _____
9. _____
10. _____
11. _____
12. _____
13. _____
14. _____
15. _____
16. _____
17. _____
18. _____
19. _____
20. _____

From *Mind Over Mood, Second Edition.* Copyright 2016 by Dennis Greenberger and Christine A. Padesky. Purchasers of this book can photocopy and/or download additional copies of this worksheet (see the box at the end of the table of contents).

WORKSHEET 12.12. Gratitude about Myself

Things about myself (qualities, strengths, values, good deeds, etc.) that I am grateful for and appreciate:

1. _____
2. _____
3. _____
4. _____
5. _____
6. _____
7. _____
8. _____
9. _____
10. _____
11. _____
12. _____
13. _____
14. _____
15. _____
16. _____
17. _____
18. _____
19. _____
20. _____

From *Mind Over Mood, Second Edition.* Copyright 2016 by Dennis Greenberger and Christine A. Padesky. Purchasers of this book can photocopy and/or download additional copies of this worksheet (see the box at the end of the table of contents).

WORKSHEET 12.13. Learning from My Gratitude Journal

1. Did keeping this journal change my outlook about my life, other people, or myself in any way? If so, how?

2. How has it affected my mood, if at all?

3. Were there benefits to reviewing what I had already written, even if I didn't add much that week?

4. Did it become easier over time to notice things to be grateful for?

5. How did keeping this journal affect my awareness of gratitude throughout the week?

6. Did the effects seem to last longer as I continued this practice?

7. Did keeping this gratitude journal inform my work on strengthening my new core beliefs? If so, how?

8. Would it be helpful for me to continue practicing gratitude? If so, how and why?

From *Mind Over Mood, Second Edition.* Copyright 2016 by Dennis Greenberger and Christine A. Padesky. Purchasers of this book can photocopy and/or download additional copies of this worksheet (see the box at the end of the table of contents).

If your gratitude journal has helped boost your positive moods, you may choose to continue writing in this journal after six weeks. The advantage of a written journal is that you can read and review what makes you grateful on days when your mood is a bit low, and this can help you feel better. Some people prefer simply to think about what makes them grateful, and if this is helpful for you, that is also OK.

EXPRESSING GRATITUDE TO OTHERS

Most people find genuine benefits in keeping a gratitude journal. Being aware of things in our lives for which we can be grateful is an important step. Sometimes it can have added value if we express our gratitude to others. There are several potential advantages to expressing our gratitude to other people. First, it gives us more time to focus on gratitude, because it extends the moment of gratitude. Second, when we talk about the things we feel grateful about to others, they may tell us about things that make them grateful. This can lead to more positive conversations, which can help lift our mood. Third, telling people directly that we are grateful to them for something they have done, or just for being in our lives, may deepen our gratitude experience and improve our relationships. Having more positive relationships with other people is another pathway to happiness. In general, expressions of gratitude keep us in a more positive frame of mind.

EXERCISE: Expressing Gratitude to Others

Therefore, as you continue to keep your weekly gratitude journal, look over what you have written and consider which of these things you could express to other people. There are two different kinds of gratitude you might express to others. First, you can comment (even to strangers) about things you appreciate in the world and your life (Worksheet 12.10). For example, "I feel so lucky we are having nice weather today when other people are experiencing those bad storms." Second, you can look over your Gratitude about Others worksheet (Worksheet 12.11) and choose someone in your life you have written about there. Then either talk directly to this person or write the person a letter/email to express gratitude. Take some time to think through the ways this person has positively affected your life. You can write about what you appreciate in letter form, even though you may or may not choose to send the person what you have written.

If you do decide to tell someone about how you appreciate her or him, there are many ways to do this: face to face, over the telephone, or in an appreciation letter. You could even visit the person to read a letter or to talk about how you feel.

Write down which people you expressed gratitude to and what happened as a result. Here are some of Louisa's examples:

I thanked the shop clerk for being so helpful in finding me the shampoo I was looking for.

What happened?
She seemed really pleased that I appreciated her help. I felt good for cheering her up with such a small thing.

I mentioned during lunch break that I appreciated our nice weather.

What happened?
This got everyone talking about fun things they planned to do outdoors this weekend. It was a more positive conversation than we usually have at lunchtime.

I wrote a letter to the woman who was my piano teacher years ago. I told her how much I still enjoy playing the piano, and I thanked her for her patience and kindness to me.

What happened?
I felt a lot of positive emotion as I was writing the letter. I haven't heard back from her, but I imagine it brightened her day to get this unexpected letter.

Worksheet 12.14 provides a place for you to write down any expressions of gratitude you make and what happens. Be sure to notice any effects these have on your mood, other people, and/or your relationships. Sometimes the effects may be quick and in the moment; at other times, the effects may be more lasting.

WORKSHEET 12.14. Expressing Gratitude

1. Who I expressed my gratitude to: _____

   What I said or wrote: _____

   _____

   What happened? _____

   _____

2. Who I expressed my gratitude to: _____

   What I said or wrote: _____

   _____

   What happened? _____

   _____

3. Who I expressed my gratitude to: _____

   What I said or wrote: _____

   _____

   What happened? _____

   _____

4. Who I expressed my gratitude to: _____

   What I said or wrote: _____

   _____

   What happened? _____

   _____

5. Who I expressed my gratitude to: _____

   What I said or wrote: _____

   _____

   What happened? _____

   _____

From *Mind Over Mood, Second Edition*. Copyright 2016 by Dennis Greenberger and Christine A. Padesky. Purchasers of this book can photocopy and/or download additional copies of this worksheet (see the box at the end of the table of contents).

ACTS OF KINDNESS

In addition to being grateful for the positives in our lives, another way to activate and support our new positive core beliefs is to do kind things for other people. When we are kind to others, we often experience a mood boost and greater happiness. In one study, people who performed kind acts toward others every day for four weeks felt happier and more satisfied with their relationships. The types of kind acts that led to these changes included small things like opening the door for someone, buying lunch for a friend, smiling at a stranger, letting someone go ahead in a line, visiting an ill friend, giving a compliment, and helping a neighbor with shopping or home repairs. When we do these kind acts toward others, we tend to feel better about ourselves, more positively connected to other people, and happier over time.

Christine did an experiment with acts of kindness. When she began going to a new post office, she noticed that everyone there seemed unhappy and irritable about waiting for service. She decided to take each visit as an opportunity to smile at people, greet the clerks warmly, and engage others in line with pleasant conversation. After a few weeks, she noticed that the postal clerks greeted her with a warm smile when she arrived. This warmth extended to other customers. Over time, the post office became a place of good humor, friendliness, and smiles rather than unhappiness. Christine's experiences demonstrate an important idea: Acts of kindness help others feel better as well as ourselves. They also can help transform the places we go into opportunities for improved mood and positive connection with others.

EXERCISE: Doing Acts of Kindness

For the next several weeks, plan to do regular acts of kindness. These can be small things that you do for family, friends, coworkers, neighbors, strangers, or animals. Write down what you do on Worksheet 12.15. After several weeks, you can write at the bottom of the worksheet what you notice about the effects of these acts on your mood and relationships. Also, notice if your positive core beliefs about yourself, other people, or the world are activated when you do these kind acts.

WORKSHEET 12.15. Acts of Kindness

My acts of kindness:

1. _____
2. _____
3. _____
4. _____
5. _____
6. _____
7. _____
8. _____
9. _____
10. _____
11. _____
12. _____
13. _____
14. _____
15. _____
16. _____
17. _____
18. _____
19. _____
20. _____
21. _____
22. _____

How did these kind acts affect my moods (both negative and positive)?

How did these kind acts affect my relationships?

Which of my positive core beliefs were active (self, other people, world)?

From *Mind Over Mood, Second Edition*. Copyright 2016 by Dennis Greenberger and Christine A. Padesky. Purchasers of this book can photocopy and/or download additional copies of this worksheet (see the box at the end of the table of contents).

The learning experiences in this chapter plant the seeds for new positive core beliefs. Positive core beliefs help you feel happier, and as they become stronger, you will have fewer negative automatic thoughts. However, there may still be times in your life when you feel greater levels of depression, anxiety, anger, or other distressing moods. During times of distress, negative thoughts and negative core beliefs may return. At those times, it is helpful to review the worksheets you have completed throughout this book, especially your new positive core belief records and ratings (Worksheets 12.6 and 12.7), your gratitude journal (Worksheets 12.10–12.12), and records of your expressions of gratitude to others and acts of kindness (Worksheets 12.14 and 12.15). During difficult times, it can be helpful to resume exercises that have been helpful in the past. Even better, see how many of these helpful practices you can make a daily part of your life. Over time, these may become familiar habits to you, and you may notice that you automatically notice positive experiences, feel and express gratitude, and act on opportunities to be kind to others.

MOOD CHECK-UP

Use the same measures and worksheets to mark your mood scores as you used before:

- Depression/unhappiness: *Mind Over Mood* Depression Inventory
    Worksheet 13.1, page 191, and Worksheet 13.2, page 192

- Anxiety/nervousness: *Mind Over Mood* Anxiety Inventory
    Worksheet 14.1, page 221, and Worksheet 14.2, page 222

- Other moods/happiness: Measuring and Tracking My Moods
    Worksheet 15.1, page 253, and Worksheet 15.2, page 254

It is especially important to rate your happiness, as many of the exercises in this chapter are likely to affect your level of happiness.

WHAT TO DO NEXT?

Since there are many different orders to read the chapters in *Mind Over Mood,* by the time you finish this chapter, you may have read almost the entire book. If you have reached your goals and feel better now, this is a good time to proceed to Chapter 16, Maintaining Your Gains and Experiencing More Happiness.

If you have been working on one mood and still struggle with it or other moods, this is a good time to review the relevant mood chapters (Chapter 13 for depression; Chapter 14 for anxiety; and Chapter 15 for anger, guilt, and shame). These mood chapters guide you to the *Mind Over Mood* skills most helpful for each mood.

Even if your moods have improved, if you have not yet read all the chapters in this book and want to learn additional skills, this is a good time to read those remaining chapters.

Chapter 12 Summary

- If you are still struggling with your moods after practice with Thought Records (Chapters 6–9), Action Plans (Chapter 10), and behavioral experiments (Chapter 11), then you may need to identify and work with core beliefs.

- Core beliefs are all-or-nothing statements about ourselves, other people, or the world.

- Core beliefs are the roots of our underlying assumptions and automatic thoughts.

- Core beliefs come in pairs. When we have negative core beliefs that are active most of the time, it is helpful to identify and strengthen new positive core beliefs.

- Core beliefs can be identified either by using the downward arrow technique or by completing the sentences "I am . . . ," "Other people are . . . ," and "The world is . . .".

- New positive core beliefs can be strengthened by recording experiences that are consistent with the new core belief, rating your confidence in your new belief, rating behaviors linked to the new core beliefs, and conducting behavioral experiments to try out the new belief.

- Core beliefs shift gradually, but over time they become stronger and more stable, and they exert a powerful influence over the way we think, behave, and feel.

- Keeping a gratitude journal and expressing gratitude can strengthen our positive core beliefs and lead to greater happiness.

- Performing acts of kindness can increase our happiness and improve our relationships.

13

Understanding Your Depression

If you are reading this chapter early in your use of *Mind Over Mood*, it is probably because you are feeling depressed. Throughout this book, you learn about ways to help depression by following the stories of Ben, Vic, and Marissa. Each of them became depressed in a different way.

Ben lived for most of his life without ever being seriously depressed. Ben's depression began during a hard year in which one of his best friends died and his wife, Sylvie, was diagnosed with cancer. Even though Sylvie's treatment went well and she recovered fully, Ben began to feel discouraged and hopeless about his future, and to have more and more negative thoughts about himself and his activities. Over time, he lost his appetite, stopped doing things he enjoyed, and some days found it hard even to get out of bed. Ben's depression started out slowly and gradually grew and grew until it put a dark veil over each day.

Vic, on the other hand, had experienced a sense of worthlessness and low self-esteem since childhood. Most of his life he had struggled with alcoholism, but he had been able to stay sober for most of the last few years with the support of his wife and AA. Vic was never totally knocked down with depression. Instead, most of the time he had a low level of depression, which mostly consisted of self-doubt and a sense that he was inadequate.

Marissa had experienced serious depression many times throughout her life. She had been sexually abused by her father as a young child, and was later abused by two different husbands. When Marissa's depression was especially severe, she struggled with impulses to hurt herself, and she even made two suicide attempts. She learned to think about herself negatively at an early age. Her depression was quite disruptive to her life and made it difficult for her to concentrate at work. Sometimes her depression was so bad that she showed up late to work and had trouble concentrating when she was there; as a result, she was in danger of losing her job.

As these three people illustrate, depression can have different faces: It can start fast or slow, can be mild or severe, may happen once or many times throughout life, or may even be always present in the background. Think about your own depression:

Did it start fast, or slowly build over time? _____

Does it have a mild, moderate, or severe impact on your life? _____

Is this the first time you have felt this way, have you felt this way before, or has depression been with you most of your life? _____

Whatever your answers are to these questions, this chapter will help you understand your depression and begin to take the first steps toward feeling better.

IDENTIFYING AND ASSESSING SYMPTOMS OF DEPRESSION

Although emotions generally enrich our lives, too much emotion can be disruptive. When we are sad about something, it can help us understand what is important to us and gives our lives meaning. For example, if we are dating someone we like and the relationship ends, we usually feel sad. Our sadness helps us realize how important this person was to us and how much we wanted the relationship to continue. These emotions lead us to think about what went wrong and what we could do differently next time to help our relationships succeed. However, if after a relationship breakup our sadness develops into depression, we may begin to feel unlovable and hopeless that anyone will ever care for us again. We may begin to stay in bed and avoid contact with other people. At the extremes, our emotions can disrupt our lives and actually make things worse.

Everyone experiences depression a bit differently. Therefore, a first step toward understanding your depression is to rate how often you experience particular symptoms that often occur with depression. Many people find it interesting to learn that these varied experiences all can be part of depression. Of course, if we are not severely depressed, we may only experience a few of these symptoms occasionally. But when depression gets worse, it is common to have many of these signs of depression active nearly every day.

EXERCISE: Measuring Symptoms of Depression

To track the symptoms of depression you are experiencing, rate each item listed on the *Mind Over Mood* Depression Inventory (Worksheet 13.1). Fill out this inventory periodically as you use this book, to assess how your depression is changing and which *Mind Over Mood* skills are most worthwhile.

Score the inventory by adding up the numbers you circled or marked for all the items. For example, if you circled or marked 3 for each item, your score would be 57 (3 × 19 items). If you couldn't decide between two numbers for an item and circled or marked both, add only the higher number. Compare your scores once or twice each week, to see if any of your symptoms are decreasing (and, if so, which symptoms are decreasing and which are not).

Record your progress on *Mind Over Mood* Depression Inventory scores on Worksheet 13.2. Mark each column at the bottom with the date you completed the Depression Inventory. Then put an × in the column across from your score. It is best to fill out the inventory at fairly regular intervals, such as weekly or twice a month, rather than just filling it out when you feel particularly down. That way, the graph of your scores will be a more representative snapshot of your mood over time.

You may find that your scores fluctuate from week to week, or that they do not improve each and every time you fill out the inventory. Some weeks your score may be higher (more depressed) than the week before. This is not unusual, nor is it a bad sign; in fact, it reflects a pattern of recovery experienced by some people. A general pattern of decreasing scores over time is a sign that the changes you are making are contributing to your improvement.

Two different decreasing patterns are shown in the Epilogue of this book (Figures E.1 and E.2, pp. 293 and 294) for Ben and Marissa. If your scores keep going up or don't change at all over a six-week period, even though you are doing the exercises in this book, this can be a signal that you might need to try a different approach or get help from a health care professional.

WORKSHEET 13.1. *Mind Over Mood* Depression Inventory

Circle or mark one number for each item that best describes how much you have experienced each symptom over the last week.

	Not at all	Sometimes	Frequently	Most of the time
1. Sad or depressed mood	0	1	2	3
2. Feelings of guilt	0	1	2	3
3. Irritable mood	0	1	2	3
4. Less interest or pleasure in usual activities	0	1	2	3
5. Withdrawing from or avoiding people	0	1	2	3
6. Finding it harder than usual to do things	0	1	2	3
7. Seeing myself as worthless	0	1	2	3
8. Trouble concentrating	0	1	2	3
9. Difficulty making decisions	0	1	2	3
10. Suicidal thoughts	0	1	2	3
11. Recurrent thoughts of death	0	1	2	3
12. Spending time thinking about a suicide plan	0	1	2	3
13. Low self-esteem	0	1	2	3
14. Seeing the future as hopeless	0	1	2	3
15. Self-critical thoughts	0	1	2	3
16. Tiredness or loss of energy	0	1	2	3
17. Significant weight loss or decrease in appetite (do not include weight loss from a diet plan)	0	1	2	3
18. Change in sleep pattern – difficulty sleeping or sleeping more or less than usual	0	1	2	3
19. Decreased sexual desire	0	1	2	3
			Score (sum of item scores)	

From *Mind Over Mood, Second Edition*. Copyright 2016 by Dennis Greenberger and Christine A. Padesky. Purchasers of this book can photocopy and/or download additional copies of this worksheet (see the box at the end of the table of contents).

WORKSHEET 13.2. *Mind Over Mood* **Depression Inventory Scores**

Score														
57														
54														
51														
48														
45														
42														
39														
36														
33														
30														
27														
24														
21														
18														
15														
12														
9														
6														
3														
0														
Date														

From *Mind Over Mood, Second Edition.* Copyright 2016 by Dennis Greenberger and Christine A. Padesky. Purchasers of this book can photocopy and/or download additional copies of this worksheet (see the box at the end of the table of contents).

Again, the *Mind Over Mood* Depression Inventory and its score sheet (Worksheets 13.1 and 13.2) are tools you can fill out periodically (e.g., weekly or twice a month) to track changes in your mood. The first time you complete the inventory, you get your baseline or starting score. You may notice changes in your scores (improvement or worsening) over time and as you try different strategies to improve your mood. For example, you might start exercising, take steps to solve a problem that has been bothering you, begin taking medication, or enroll in cognitive-behavioral therapy (CBT). With each of these interventions, you would hope and expect that your depression symptoms would go down, resulting in lower *Mind Over Mood* Depression Inventory scores. This is one way to measure the helpfulness of different approaches you try.

Mind Over Mood Depression Inventory scores are not used to diagnose depression. If you believe you are depressed, you can bring your completed *Mind Over Mood* Depression Inventory to a health care provider or mental health professional. Your answers on the inventory can help you tell this person about your experiences, so he or she can determine a diagnosis and discuss available treatments with you.

The symptoms you rate on the *Mind Over Mood* Depression Inventory are cognitive (thought), behavioral, emotional, and physical changes, just as in the model described in Chapter 2. Notice that cognitive symptoms of depression include self-criticism, hopelessness, suicidal thoughts, difficulty concentrating, and negative thoughts. Common behavior changes associated with depression include withdrawal from other people, not doing as many activities that are enjoyable or pleasurable, and having difficulty "getting started" with activities. Physical symptoms include insomnia, sleeping more or less than usual, being tired, eating less or more, and weight change. The emotional symptoms of depression can include feelings of sadness, irritability, anger, guilt, and nervousness. Figure 13.1 illustrates the profile of depression symptoms.

Thoughts
- Negative thoughts about oneself (self-criticism)
- Negative thoughts about life experience (pessimism)
- Negative thoughts about the future (hopelessness)

Moods
- Depressed
- Sad
- Irritable
- Guilty

Behaviors
- Withdrawing from other people
- Doing fewer activities
- Difficulty getting started doing things
- Low motivation

Physical
- Difficulty sleeping
- Eating less or more
- Being tired

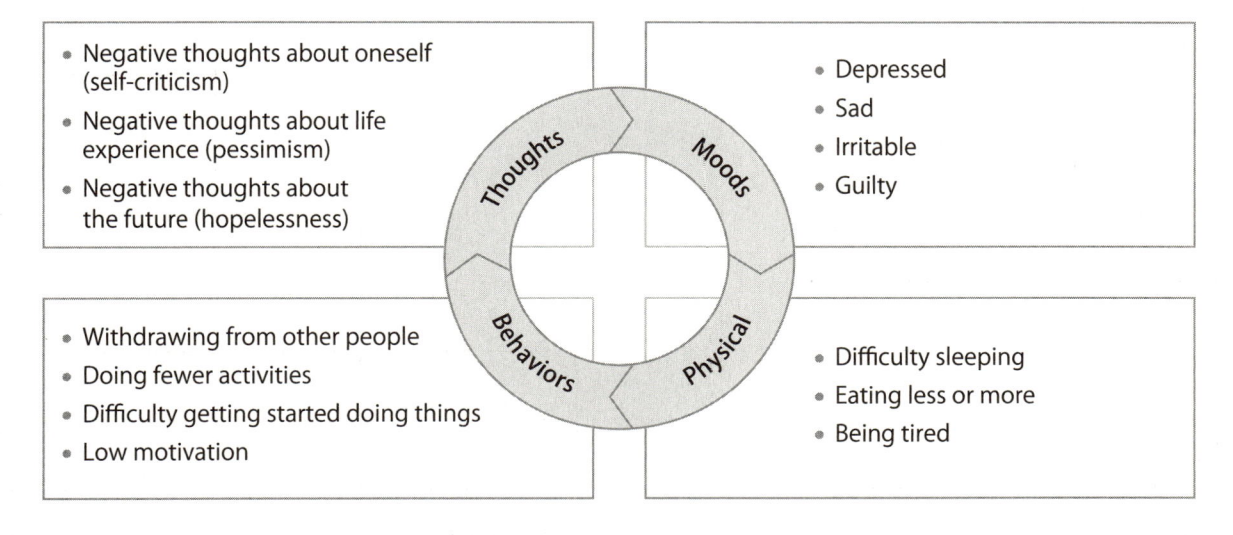

FIGURE 13.1. Profile of depression symptoms.

Does it surprise you to learn that some of these symptoms are characteristic of depression? Some people don't realize that problems with sleep, appetite, motivation, concentration, or anger can be part of depression. But for many people, successful treatment of depression leads to improvement in all these symptoms.

THOUGHTS AND DEPRESSION

Aaron T. Beck has pioneered our modern understanding of depression. In the 1960s, Beck demonstrated that depression was characterized by thought patterns that actually maintained depressed mood. For example, Beck noted that when we are depressed, we have negative thoughts about ourselves (self-criticism), our experiences (general negativity), and our future (hopelessness). The following sections describe these three aspects of depressed thinking in detail.

Negative Thoughts about Myself

Before Marissa began CBT, she was extremely self-critical. For example, she thought, "These awful things happened to me because I'm bad," "I'm an awful mother and a terrible person," and "It's my own fault that I was beaten by my husbands." The themes underlying these thoughts were "I'm worthless," "I'm unlovable," and "I'm no good."

Almost everyone who is depressed has self-critical thoughts. These thoughts are damaging because they contribute to low self-esteem, low self-confidence, and relationship problems, and because they can interfere with our willingness to do things to help us feel better.

To demonstrate how self-criticism plays a role in your life, remember a time when you felt particularly low. It may have been a time when you felt worthless or unlovable. Picture in your mind the moment you were feeling most depressed, and remember or guess what you may have been thinking. Did you have any negative thoughts about yourself? If so, write them here:

_____

_____

_____

_____

These thoughts illustrate the self-critical thoughts associated with depression.

Negative Thoughts about My Life Experiences

Thinking about your current experiences in a negative way is another characteristic of depressive thinking. We often do not take events at face value: We interpret or misinterpret events that occur around us. For example, when a friend, relative, or coworker is talking, we might think that this person is negative, mean, or critical, even though we might not see it that way when we are not depressed.

Negative thinking about our experiences is also a style of thinking in which we notice and remember negative aspects of our lives more vividly than positive or neutral ones. For example, when we are depressed, we tend to look at and remember the negative things that happened during the day and not the positive ones. Focusing on the two out of ten chores that did not get done on a Saturday, rather than the eight that did get done, would be another example of negative thinking about our experiences.

Think about a recent time when you felt particularly depressed. Write down any examples of thoughts you had in which you either (1) focused on the negative and ignored the positive, or (2) interpreted events in a negative way.

_____

_____

_____

_____

_____

_____

_____

Negative Thoughts about My Future

During his first therapy session, Ben's hopelessness was revealed in this statement: "What's the use? The rest of my life will be filled with illness and death." After his wife's successful battle with cancer and the death of his good friend Louie, Ben had come to believe that his own life and the lives of people he was close to would be one tragedy after another, culminating eventually in his own death. He was unable to envision anything other than a bleak future.

When we are depressed, we imagine that the future will be very negative. This prediction or anticipation that events will turn out negatively is called "hopelessness." Examples of this type of thinking include "I'll blow it," "Nobody there will like me," and "I won't be good at it." A negative attitude toward the future may also manifest itself in thoughts like "I'll never get out of this depression," or "What's the use in trying? I'll never get any better." We may anticipate that a conversation will go poorly, that a new relationship won't work out, that a problem can't be solved, or that there is no way out of your depression. In its most extreme form, hopelessness can contribute to thoughts of suicide.

To demonstrate how negative thinking about the future functions in your life, write down some of the negative predictions you make about your future. For example, you may identify an activity you sometimes enjoy but do not do when you are depressed, because you predict it will not turn out well.

_____

_____

_____

_____

_____

_____

_____

EXERCISE: Identifying Cognitive Aspects of Depression

Worksheet 13.3 lists some negative thoughts that people frequently have when they are depressed. To see if you've had these types of negative thoughts, and to help you distinguish among them, mark each thought you have had and indicate whether each thought is negative toward yourself, your future, or your experiences.

WORKSHEET 13.3. Identifying Cognitive Aspects of Depression

Mark each thought you have had:

Is the thought negative toward myself, my future, or my experiences?

- ☐ 1. I'm no good. _____
- ☐ 2. I'm a failure. _____
- ☐ 3. Nobody likes me. _____
- ☐ 4. Things will never get better. _____
- ☐ 5. I'm a loser. _____
- ☐ 6. I'm worthless. _____
- ☐ 7. No one can help me. _____
- ☐ 8. I've let people down. _____
- ☐ 9. Others are better than I am. _____
- ☐ 10. (S)he hates me. _____
- ☐ 11. I'm always making mistakes. _____
- ☐ 12. My life is a disaster. _____
- ☐ 13. (S)he dislikes me. _____
- ☐ 14. This is hopeless. _____
- ☐ 15. Others are disappointed in me. _____
- ☐ 16. I can't change. _____

From *Mind Over Mood, Second Edition*. Copyright 2016 by Dennis Greenberger and Christine A. Padesky. Purchasers of this book can photocopy and/or download additional copies of this worksheet (see the box at the end of the table of contents).

Following are the answers to Worksheet 13.3. Review the relevant sections of this chapter to clarify any differences between your answers and the ones given. When two answers are given, either one is correct.

Answers to Worksheet 13.3

1. I'm no good .... Self
2. I'm a failure .... Self
3. Nobody likes me .... Self/experiences
4. Things will never get better .... Future
5. I'm a loser .... Self
6. I'm worthless .... Self
7. No one can help me .... Experiences/future
8. I've let people down .... Self/experiences
9. Others are better than I am .... Experiences/self
10. (S)he hates me .... Experiences
11. I'm always making mistakes .... Self
12. My life is a disaster .... Self
13. (S)he dislikes me .... Experiences
14. This is hopeless .... Future/experiences
15. Others are disappointed in me .... Experiences
16. I can't change .... Self/future

TREATMENT FOR DEPRESSION

The good news is that depression can almost always be helped. Most of the strategies taught in this book were originally developed to help people overcome depression. This section summarizes the treatment approaches that have been shown to be most effective: cognitive therapy, medication, improving relationships, and behavioral activation. Research suggests that behavioral activation and cognitive therapy are two of the most effective methods for helping people get better and stay better. Together, these two approaches are often referred to as CBT. Although we describe cognitive and behavioral approaches separately, you will learn to use them simultaneously. As with other skills, it is helpful to learn to use them one at a time and combine them once you feel confident in using each. Because they are so effective, we emphasize these two approaches in this chapter and the other chapters of this book.

People who take medication alone are at greater risk for future relapse than people who combine medication with cognitive and behavioral interventions. If you have been prescribed medication for your depression, learning *Mind Over Mood* skills can help you minimize the likelihood that you will get depressed again once you get better and stop taking your medication.

The following sections describe each type of intervention for depression. If you are depressed, it is often best to start with behavioral activation. We want you to read an overview of all these methods first. We describe behavioral activation last, so that when you get to that section, you can do the exercises described there for a few weeks before proceeding to other chapters of this book.

Cognitive Therapy

When we are depressed, we tend to notice and remember the negative aspects of our experiences more readily than we do the positive or neutral aspects. We also are more likely to interpret events in our lives with a negative bias when we are depressed. When we are not depressed, we tend to interpret events with a positive bias. For example, suppose you invite three people to join you for lunch, and two agree to come. If you are depressed, you will tend to focus on the one person who didn't come and maybe even conclude, "No one likes me." If you are not depressed, you are more likely to think, "Most people like me. The one who couldn't come to lunch might have had other plans but they missed out on a good time."

Cognitive therapy teaches people how to identify, test, and perhaps change their negative thoughts by reviewing all the information in their lives – positive and neutral as well as negative. Chapters 6–9 and 11–12 teach you how to think in more adaptive ways to reduce your depression. As you might imagine, this book is called *Mind Over Mood* because many of the chapters show you how to make changes in your thinking that will help you feel better.

Medication

Although medication can sometimes help depression, not everyone who is depressed will benefit from it. Your therapist or another health care provider may recommend a consultation with a psychiatrist or another physician who can evaluate whether or not medication might be helpful for you. Some people worry about the effects of antidepressant medication. Some of the most common concerns are addressed here.

"How Do I Know If Medication Will Help?"

There can be a trial-and-error process to prescribing antidepressants. Currently there are dozens of antidepressants available, so you and your physician can't know with certainty if an antidepressant will work for you until you've taken one for a few weeks. Different antidepressant medications may be prescribed, depending on the particular symptoms you have and the specific effect you and your physician want to achieve. If the first antidepressant prescribed for you does not produce a beneficial effect, then your physician will try others to see if the desired effect can be obtained. Unlike many other medications, antidepressants often take two to four weeks to reach their beneficial effect. And because you may not respond positively to the initial medication prescribed for you, it may take eight weeks or longer to achieve therapeutic levels of the right antidepressant.

One drawback to antidepressants is that many have annoying side effects, especially when a person first begins to take them. The side effects may include dry mouth, drowsiness, and weight changes, although these often diminish or disappear after the medication is taken for a period of time.

"Does Taking Medication Mean I'm Crazy?"

Almost everyone gets depressed sometimes. Being depressed does not mean you are crazy. If you have been stuck in depression for a long time, or if your depression is quite severe, it makes sense to try to find things that will help you feel better. If medication is something that helps you, then it can be a worthwhile addition to your plan to feel better. Taking medication doesn't mean you are crazy. It means you are willing to try different things to help yourself feel better. You can discuss with your physician any concerns you have about medications, and can also ask how long you might need to take them.

"How Long Will I Need to Take Antidepressant Medication?"

Once you and your physician find an effective antidepressant, you will probably take it for one to two years, although some people benefit from taking antidepressant medication longer. You and your physician can evaluate together how long you should take medication. In any case, when your physician recommends that you decrease antidepressant medication, she or he will want you to decrease them gradually and systematically. It is important for you to follow your physician's directions in taking and stopping antidepressant medications. Doses sometimes need to be increased and decreased slowly to achieve the desired effects and to minimize side effects.

Improving Your Relationships

Some treatments for depression emphasize the importance of improving close relationships. Family and friends can provide positive support and help you recover from depression. You can use the strategies taught in this book to make your relationships better. One of the people you follow in this book, Vic, used the skills he learned to improve his relationship with his wife, Judy. Another self-help book that uses a cognitive therapy approach for couples' problems is Beck's *Love Is Never Enough* (New York: HarperCollins, 1988). Gottman's *The Seven Principles for Making Marriage Work*, now in its second edition (New York: Harmony Books, 2014), is another worthwhile self-help guide for improving your marriage or committed relationship.

If you are in an abusive relationship or a relationship with someone who criticizes you constantly, it can be harder to recover from depression. Couple therapy or family therapy can help you improve relationship conditions that may be feeding your depression. If you are being physically or sexually abused, almost all communities have special programs nearby to help you. You can contact your local community mental health center or a health professional for recommendations of programs near you.

Behavioral Activation

If you track your activities and feelings of depression, you may discover that when you are depressed, you are less active. For this reason, an important part of recovering from depression is to increase the number of activities that you do each day. Even more important than just the number of activities are the types and quality of the activities that we do. In general, we get the biggest mood boost from activities that bring us pleasure and a sense of accomplishment, that lead to approaching rather than avoiding life's challenges, and that are connected to what we value most. Each of us needs to discover the right personal mix of these different types of activities to improve our mood. This section of the book helps you discover the right mix for you.

You can use an Activity Record to track your activities and discover how they affect your mood. When you keep this record for one week, it will help you identify what you are doing when you feel most and least depressed. In addition to identifying your activities and moods, the Activity Record can be used as a guide to see what changes in your behavior might help you feel better.

Look at Ben's filled-in Activity Record in Figure 13.2. Notice that Ben wrote only a word or two to describe his activity – just enough to remind him what he was doing when he looked back at the record. When he did more than one activity in a time period, he wrote down the one or two most important ones (e.g., "walk," "breakfast"), or a word that described the overall experience ("shopping").

Although Ben thought the Activity Record would be hard to keep, he found that he needed just a few seconds each hour to put down an activity and a depression rating. Notice that on Thursday from 10:00 to 11:00 A.M., when his depression changed a lot during the hour, he wrote both a low and a high rating to show the change.

Write in each box: (1) Activity. (2) Mood ratings (0–100). (Mood I am rating: __Depression__)

Time	Monday	Tuesday	Wednesday	Thursday	Friday	Saturday	Sunday
6–7 A.M.	Wake up 60	Wake up 70	Wake up 60	Wake up 50	Wake up 60	Wake up 40	Wake up 60
7–8 A.M.	Shower, dress 60	Lie in bed 80	Shower, dress 50	Shower, dress 50	Dress 60	Shower, dress 30	Dress 60
8–9 A.M.	Walk, breakfast 40	Get dressed 80	Breakfast 50	Breakfast 40	Breakfast 40	Breakfast 20	Serve breakfast at church 20
9–10 A.M.	Golf 40	Breakfast 80	Hardware store 40	Walk 30	Clean garage 40	Drive to Bob's 20	Walk 30
10–11 A.M.	Golf 40	Sit in chair 80	Fix door 30	Phone call (Bob) 30–60	Clean garage 30	Visit with Bob and kids 10	Shopping 40
11 A.M.–12 noon	Golf 60	Read 80	Fix door 30	Talk with Sylvie 60	Clean garage 30	Look at photos on the computer with Greg 10	Shopping 30
12 noon–1 P.M.	Lunch with Sylvie 40	Lunch with Sylvie 70	Lunch with Sylvie 20	Lunch 60	Lunch 20	Lunch 0	Lunch out 20
1–2 P.M.	Shopping with Sylvie 40	Wash dishes 80	Wash dishes 30	Therapy 50	Sweep garage 20	Go to park 0	Drive around with Sylvie 20
2–3 P.M.	Shopping 40	Sit in chair 80	Walk 20	Call Bert 40	Walk with Sylvie 20	Play soccer with grandkids 0	Home with Sylvie – relax 20

3–4 P.M.	Shopping 50	Pay bills 80	Read mail 20	Clean up workbench 40	Read news online, write email 20	Walk Bob's dog 0	Relax with Sylvie 10
4–5 P.M.	Unpack shopping bags 50	Drive Sylvie to doctor's office 70	Help cook 20	Help cook 40	Help cook 20	Drive home 10	Make dinner 10
5–6 P.M.	Sit in chair 60	Dinner out 60	Dinner with Sylvie 20	Dinner 30	Dinner 20	Dinner 10	Dinner 10
6–7 P.M.	Dinner 60	Walk at shopping mall 60	Wash dishes 20	Wash dishes 30	Wash dishes 20	Wash dishes 10	Wash dishes 10
7–8 P.M.	TV 60	Movie 50	Play cards 20	TV 30	Phone call with Bob 10	Sit in chair 30	TV 20
8–9 P.M.	TV 60	Movie 50	Play cards 20	TV 40	TV 10	Look at photo album 30	TV 20
9–10 P.M.	TV 60	Drive home 50	Talk to Sylvie 20	TV 40	TV 10	Talk to Sylvie 20	TV 20
10–11 P.M.	TV 60	TV 50	TV 20	TV 40	TV 10	TV 30	TV 30
11 P.M.–12 midnight	Bed 70	Bed 60	Bed 20	Bed 60	Bed 10	Bed 30	Bed 20
12 midnight–1 A.M.	Sleep	Sleep	Sleep	Sleep	Sleep	Sleep	Sleep

FIGURE 13.2. Ben's Activity Record.

The connection between activities and moods is important enough to suggest that you pause in reading this chapter until you have had a chance to fill out an Activity Record for a full week. Then continue reading this chapter. The remainder of the chapter will be more valuable to you once you have a better understanding of the connection between your activities and moods. Worksheet 13.4 on pages 206–207 is the first in a series of worksheets that help you learn how activities can improve your mood.

REMINDERS **How to Use the Activity Record**

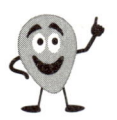

- Name the mood you will rate.

- Write down your activities for each hour of the day.

- For each hour, rate your mood from 0–100 with 0 showing you did not experience that mood and 100 indicating the most you have ever experienced that mood. Write your rating on the chart.

- After filling out an Activity Record for one week, look for connections between what you do and your mood.

Pause here until you have had a chance to fill out an Activity Record for a full week.

EXERCISE: Using the Activity Record

First, choose a mood (depression or low mood, if that is why you are reading this chapter) that you want to improve, and write this mood here:

Mood:

During this week, you will be rating this mood on a 0–100 scale:

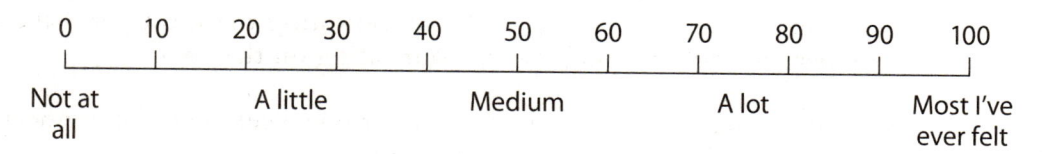

```
    0    10    20    30    40    50    60    70    80    90   100
    |     |     |     |     |     |     |     |     |     |     |
  Not at       A little         Medium              A lot        Most I've
   all                                                          ever felt
```

Fill in your Activity Record (Worksheet 13.4 on pp. 206–207) for one week. For each hour, write in the activity you were doing, and rate your mood on the 0–100 scale. You may forget to do it for some hours, but the more hours you fill in for the week, the more you will have a chance to learn about the mood you are rating. Therefore, if you forget to do it one day, don't give up – just continue the ratings when you remember.

To help you remember to fill out the Activity Record, carry a copy with you or make a digital reminder to take notes on your activities and moods as you go through the day. It is not necessary to fill it out every hour. Most people can remember their activities and moods for several hours, so you may be able to fill it out several times a day rather than hourly. For example, at lunchtime, you can write in all your morning activities and mood ratings. At dinnertime, you can do the afternoon hours. At bedtime, you can fill in the evening hours.

WORKSHEET 13.4. Activity Record

Write in each box: (1) Activity. (2) Mood ratings (0–100). (Mood I am rating: _____)

Time	Monday	Tuesday	Wednesday	Thursday	Friday	Saturday	Sunday
6–7 A.M.							
7–8 A.M.							
8–9 A.M.							
9–10 A.M.							
10–11 A.M.							
11 A.M.–12 noon							
12 noon–1 P.M.							
1–2 P.M.							
2–3 P.M.							

3–4 P.M.									
4–5 P.M.									
5–6 P.M.									
6–7 P.M.									
7–8 P.M.									
8–9 P.M.									
9–10 P.M.									
10–11 P.M.									
11 P.M.–12 midnight									
12 midnight–1 A.M.									

From *Mind Over Mood, Second Edition*. Copyright 2016 by Dennis Greenberger and Christine A. Padesky. Purchasers of this book can photocopy and/or download additional copies of this worksheet (see the box at the end of the table of contents).

Your answers to Worksheet 13.5 can help you identify activities you might need to change in order to feel better. Refer to Ben's Activity Record (Figure 13.2, pp. 202–203), and see how he answered the questions on Worksheet 13.5 (Figure 13.3 on the next page).

> **EXERCISE: Learning from My Activity Record**
>
> Now that you have charted your moods and activities for one week, analyze your Activity Record to look for patterns. Worksheet 13.5 lists some questions that will help you learn from your Activity Record.

WORKSHEET 13.5. Learning from My Activity Record

1. Did my mood change during the week? If so, how? What patterns do I notice?

2. Did my activities affect my mood? If so, how?

3. What was I doing when I felt better? Are these activities in my best long-term interest? What other activities could I do that might also make me feel better?

4. What was I doing when I felt worse? Are these activities in my best interest? If so, is there a way I could do them that would help me feel better while I was doing them?

5. Were there certain times of the day (e.g., mornings) or week (e.g., weekends) when I felt worse?

6. Can I think of anything I could do to feel better during these times?

7. Were there certain times of the day or week when I felt better? Can I learn anything helpful from this?

8. Looking at my answers to these questions, what activities can I plan in the coming week to increase the chances that I will feel better this week? Over the next few weeks?

From *Mind Over Mood, Second Edition.* Copyright 2016 by Dennis Greenberger and Christine A. Padesky. Purchasers of this book can photocopy and/or download additional copies of this worksheet (see the box at the end of the table of contents).

1. Did my mood change during the week? If so, how? What patterns do I notice?

    Yes, my mood changed. Once I get down, it seems to last for hours. Some days were not so bad.

2. Did my activities affect my mood? If so, how?

    Yes. On busy days I usually felt a little better. When I'm with people I care about, like my wife, children, and grandchildren, I usually feel better. When I'm alone and just sitting around, I tend to dwell on things and feel worse.

3. What was I doing when I felt better? Are these activities in my best long-term interest? What other activities could I do that might also make me feel better?

    Doing things with Sylvie — she is a happy person and she means so much to me. Fixing the door — I felt useful. Serving breakfast at church is enjoyable because I talk to people and get a chance to help out. Yes. Spend time with grandchildren. Play more golf. Volunteer more time with church activities. Take Sylvie out to dinner.

4. What was I doing when I felt worse? Are these activities in my best interest? If so, is there a way I could do them that would help me feel better while I was doing them?

    Sitting in my chair thinking — worried about our money running out.

    Phone call from Bob on Thursday — my granddaughter Nicole broke her arm.

    Yes, in my best interest — it is necessary to deal with difficult situations or figure out what to do. Maybe rather than just worrying, I could talk it over with Sylvie and decide how to handle it.

5. Were there certain times of the day (e.g., mornings) or week (e.g., weekends) when I felt worse?

    Felt worse in the mornings until I got going.

    Felt worse early in the week.

6. Can I think of anything I could do to feel better during these times?

    I guess it helps when I shower, get dressed. Walking seems to help, although I don't feel like it when I'm down. Getting out of the house helps on bad days. Being around or helping other people tends to lift my mood.

7. Were there certain times of the day or week I felt better? Can I learn anything helpful from this?

    Generally, later in the day I felt better. This week I felt better on Friday, Saturday, and Sunday. This shows me that my worst moods don't last forever. I tend to be around people more on the weekends, which helps. Maybe I can figure out some ways to see more people during the week.

8. Looking at my answers to these questions, what activities can I plan in the coming week to increase the chances that I will feel better this week? Over the next few weeks?

    Fix up things around the house. Plan more activities — especially things that involve people I care about.

    Visit my grandchildren. Walk Bob's dog. Spend less time sitting alone. Volunteer more at church.

FIGURE 13.3. What Ben learned from his Activity Record.

As you can see, Ben learned a lot from his Activity Record. Depending on the mood you tracked, you might have learned a variety of things from observing your own shifting moods. Depressed people often observe that as they become more active, it helps them feel better. Write one or more ideas here about why you think activities might improve your mood.

_____

_____

_____

_____

_____

_____

_____

We don't know for sure why depressed people often feel better when they are more active. Here is a list of possible reasons:

- Some types of activities, like walking, increase brain chemicals connected to feeling better.

- When we are doing nothing, we are often thinking about negative things over and over again. Activity helps distance us from negative thoughts.

- Activities can give us the opportunity to succeed (e.g., organize a room or desk), to do something enjoyable (e.g., talk with someone we like), or to approach a problem (e.g., begin working on something that has to get done). Each of these experiences – success, enjoyment, approaching things we want to avoid – can help us feel a little better. Doing things that are important to us, or connected to things or people we value, helps create meaning in our lives. Generally, people feel better when their lives have meaning or purpose.

As a first step toward treating depression, it is often helpful to increase activities – especially pleasurable activities, those that lead to a sense of accomplishment, activities that help us approach rather than avoid things, and activities that reflect our values. When we do these types of activities, we usually feel better.

To see if this works for you, fill out the *Mind Over Mood* Depression Inventory (Worksheet 13.1) again, and write down your current score on Worksheet 13.2. It may be higher, lower, or the same as when you filled out this inventory the first time. Then use Worksheet 13.6, on pages 214–215, to schedule some of the types of activities you have identified on Worksheet 13.5 as ones that are likely to improve your mood. Notice that Worksheet 13.6 is just like an Activity Record, but it is called an Activity Schedule, because you are going to write down planned activities ahead of time in the hope of doing more things that help you feel better.

Plan to schedule a number of activities every day. Try different mixes of types of activities. If you are a person who stays very busy mostly doing things that accomplish something, then you may benefit the most from adding pleasurable activities. On the other hand, if you are someone who already does a lot of pleasurable activities, you may get the biggest mood boost from adding activities that accomplish something or overcome avoidance. Figure 13.4 shows the activities Ben wrote down during his Activity Scheduling.

Pleasurable activities: Take a walk with Sylvie, visit the grandchildren, play golf, throw a ball with Bob's dog, invite a friend to lunch, organize a card game, go to a movie, take Sylvie to dinner, go to my granddaughter's recital, play music while I'm driving, pay attention to birds singing and flowers when I am outside, watch the children playing in the neighborhood, look at the stars at night, enjoy the smell of food cooking.

Activities that accomplish something: Fix the dripping faucet, build a bird house, pay bills, organize my digital photos, clean the garage, do laundry, call to get the announcement of volunteer jobs that are not yet filled at church.

What I can do to begin to approach things I have been avoiding: Call to make a doctor's appointment, get out of bed right away and take a shower (especially when I'm feeling down), talk to Sylvie about some of my worries, ask Sylvie to help me figure out activities to put on my schedule when I feel too depressed to do it myself.

Activities that fit with my values: Take on more volunteer work at church, help the grandchildren with their homework, offer to fix my neighbor's gate, say something positive to someone every day, visit my friend who is in the hospital.

FIGURE 13.4. Ben's list of activities for his Activity Schedule.

Schedule Activities That Are Enjoyable or Accomplish Something

By scheduling and doing activities that are enjoyable or accomplish something, you will be making behavioral changes that can reduce your depression.

- Doing ten enjoyable activities in a week are likely to help you more than doing only five.

- Doing activities that are highly enjoyable are likely to help you more than doing activities that are mildly enjoyable.

- Different people enjoy different activities. Choose activities that fit your interests and values.

- Pleasurable activities need not be expensive or time-consuming.

- Examples of enjoyable activities include talking to a friend, listening to music, playing a computer game, taking a walk, going out for lunch, watching a favorite TV show or sporting event, or playing with your child. They are everyday, enjoyable events.

EXERCISE: Activity Scheduling

Before filling out Worksheet 13.6 on the next page, write down at least several activities you want to plan for each day. You might find it helpful to review Worksheet 13.5, on page 208, especially your answers to questions 3, 6, and 8. It is helpful to think of several activities in each of the following categories and spread them out throughout the week.

Pleasurable activities: _____

_____

_____

_____

_____

Activities that accomplish something: _____

_____

_____

_____

_____

What I can do to begin to approach things I have been avoiding: _____

_____

_____

_____

_____

Activities that fit with my values: _____

_____

_____

_____

_____

Some activities could fit in a variety of categories. For example, walking or exercising may be pleasurable for one person, may be an accomplishment for someone else, and may fit with a value of doing healthy activities for yet another person. If you have been avoiding exercise for some time, it may even be overcoming avoidance. Put activities in whatever category makes sense to you. The important thing is to do activities in each of the four areas throughout the week.

WORKSHEET 13.6. Activity Schedule

Referring to the "Activity Scheduling" exercise (p. 213), use this worksheet to schedule some activities. Write down the times and days of the week you plan to do these activities. If something more enjoyable or more important comes along, you can do that activity instead during that time period. If you do something different during any time period, put a line through what you had planned and write down what you actually did. For each time period in which you planned an activity, write down: (1) Activity. (2) Mood ratings (0–100).

(Mood I am rating: _____)

Time	Monday	Tuesday	Wednesday	Thursday	Friday	Saturday	Sunday
6–7 A.M.							
7–8 A.M.							
8–9 A.M.							
9–10 A.M.							
10–11 A.M.							
11 A.M.–12 noon							
12 noon–1 P.M.							
1–2 P.M.							

2–3 P.M.	3–4 P.M.	4–5 P.M.	5–6 P.M.	6–7 P.M.	7–8 P.M.	8–9 P.M.	9–10 P.M.	10–11 P.M.	11 P.M.–12 midnight	12 midnight–1 A.M.

From *Mind Over Mood, Second Edition*. Copyright 2016 by Dennis Greenberger and Christine A. Padesky. Purchasers of this book can photocopy and/or download additional copies of this worksheet (see the box at the end of the table of contents).

Once you have done the activities on your Activity Scheduling Worksheet over the course of one week, fill out the *Mind Over Mood* Depression Inventory (Worksheet 13.1) again, and write down your score on Worksheet 13.2. By comparing your scores before and after this week of activities, you will be able to see if activity scheduling makes a difference in how you feel. Even small changes in your scores demonstrate that small behavioral changes can lead to improvements in your mood. Depending upon your level of depression, it may be necessary to do activity scheduling for a number of weeks before you get a noticeable mood boost in your depression scores.

Questions about Activity Scheduling

The following questions and answers can help you if your mood doesn't improve when you add activities to your week.

"What if I don't feel like doing the activities I scheduled?"

If you don't feel like doing an activity, see if you can do it partially, even for a few minutes. Often we don't feel motivated to do things until we actually get started. You may be surprised to learn that motivation often follows doing something rather than coming first, especially when we are depressed.

If you have skipped one or more activities on your schedule, try not to get discouraged or to criticize yourself. Just pick up where you are and do the next activity on your schedule. If you like, you can reschedule the activities you missed for another time during the week. The goal of the Activity Schedule is to increase the number and types of activities you do, not to perfectly complete every activity you plan. If you do activity scheduling for several weeks, you may find it easier to do more activities as the weeks go by.

"What if I don't enjoy the activities as much as I used to?"

If you decide to try activity scheduling as a first step in reducing your depression, do not expect to find activities as enjoyable or as satisfying as you did before you became depressed. Ben, for example, enjoyed golfing a lot before he became depressed, and yet he found that golfing was not as satisfying when he was depressed. If Ben compared his golfing pleasure when he was depressed to his earlier enjoyment of this activity, he might conclude, "This is no good. I'm not having fun like I used to." As a result of these thoughts, Ben might actually have felt more depressed after golfing. However, if Ben compared his golfing enjoyment to sitting at home doing nothing, he might think, "It's good that I went golfing. At least I enjoyed myself a little bit. It was better than sitting at home feeling glum."

"What if I don't enjoy the activities at all?"

Notice what is going through your mind while you do activities. If you are doing something that you thought would be enjoyable (like walking through a park), and yet you are thinking about negative things at every step, you are not likely to enjoy yourself. When you find yourself dwelling on negative things while you do activities, gently encourage yourself to focus on the activity itself and look for something to feel good about (pleasure, accomplishment, overcoming avoidance, acting on your values). Don't get discouraged if you keep returning to negative thoughts, because this is common in depression. You may need to pull yourself back to look for good parts of the activity hundreds of times each day. Being aware that you are drifting into negative thinking is a really good thing, because it gives you a choice to try to do something different.

Some people, especially those who have been depressed for a long time, have difficulty experiencing positive moods. If this is the case for you, try capturing very tiny positive experiences. A helpful strategy for many people who want to experience more enjoyment is to practice "capturing enjoyment." This involves not only doing activities, but actively looking for pleasure while you do them.

It often helps to start with noticing your sensory experiences (sight, smell, touch, hearing, and taste). Pay attention to all five of your senses as you go through your day. Notice textures, sounds, smells, and sights that you find even a little bit enjoyable. When you eat something, savor the flavors that you taste. When you go outside, stop and smell the air, looking for any smell that might be pleasant. Feel the air on your skin. Is the temperature warm or cool? Listen for sounds that are interesting or pleasant, such as birds or even the sounds of an engine running. Look at the colors that surround you; notice people who seem pleasant or even humorous. It is helpful if you can experience even a tiny moment of positive reaction to something. Such tiny moments can be captured throughout the day.

Over time, it will become easier to experience positive moods more regularly and for longer periods of time. Get into a mindset of savoring small parts of your experiences. Once you can do this, you can add layers to your enjoyment of activities by searching for positive aspects of your experiences. For example, you might enjoy overhearing a bit of a funny conversation, or having a friendly interchange with a clerk. When we deliberately make a choice to look for positives in our day, we've cracked a window open to allow positive experiences in. At the same time, when we are actively looking for positives, our minds are less focused on negatives.

It is best to do activity scheduling for several weeks until your scores on the *Mind Over Mood* Depression Inventory (Worksheet 13.1, on p. 191) show some improvement. Once you find it easier to do more activities throughout the day, then you are probably ready to learn and practice the skills taught in Chapters 5–12, which can lead to additional improvements in your mood. When you are feeling better and your depression scores are lower than when you began, go to Chapter 5 and you'll find your next steps. While you master these new *Mind Over Mood* skills, continue to do the types of activities that help you feel better.

Chapter 13 Summary

- Depression does not just describe a mood; it also involves changes in thinking, behavior, and physical functioning.

- The *Mind Over Mood* Depression Inventory (Worksheet 13.1) can be used to rate depression symptoms. Weekly scores on the inventory can be charted on Worksheet 13.2 to track changes in your depression as you master *Mind Over Mood* skills.

- There are many effective treatments for depression, including CBT, improving your relationships, and medication.

- People who learn the skills taught in *Mind Over Mood* have lower rates of relapse for depression than those treated with medication alone.

- When we are depressed, we tend to have negative thoughts about ourselves, our experiences, and the future.

- CBT for depression helps us learn new ways of thinking and behaving in order to improve our moods in a lasting way.

- Tracking and analyzing your activities and moods on an Activity Record can help you discover the connections between behavior and depression (Worksheets 13.4 and 13.5).

- An Activity Schedule (Worksheet 13.6) can be used to plan activities that are pleasurable, accomplish something, help you overcome avoidance, and/or fit with your values. Using an Activity Schedule in this way for several weeks is likely to boost your mood.

14

Understanding Your Anxiety

You may be reading *Mind Over Mood* to get help with anxiety. Even though it is very common, anxiety is one of the most distressing moods that we experience. Some people feel anxious most of the day and other people experience anxiety just in particular situations.

One of the women described and followed in this book, Linda, experienced panic attacks and lots of anxiety when she needed to fly on an airplane. There were many days when Linda did not experience any anxiety; yet, when she did get anxious, it sometimes was so severe that she went to the hospital emergency room. She also considered turning down a job promotion because she didn't want to get on an airplane or have more panic attacks.

Linda was quite aware of the types of situations that made her anxious. For other people, anxiety can seem a bit of a mystery, especially when it seems to come "out of the blue." As you learn more about anxiety and do the exercises in this book, you will probably get better at identifying what triggers your own anxiety.

The word "anxiety" is sometimes used to describe the temporary nervousness or fear we experience before and during challenging life experiences, such as a job interview or medical test. It is also used to describe more persistent types of anxiety, such as phobias (fear of specific things or situations, such as heights, animals, insects, flying in airplanes), social anxiety (fear of appearing foolish and/or being criticized or rejected in social situations), panic disorder (intense feelings of anxiety in which people often feel as if they are about to die or go crazy), posttraumatic stress disorder (repeated memories of terrible traumas with high levels of distress), health worries (persistent worries about having an illness or physical problem, despite being found healthy in medical tests), and generalized anxiety disorder (characterized by frequent worries and physical symptoms of anxiety).

Think about your own anxiety for a minute:

When do you first remember feeling anxious? _____

Do you feel anxious most of the time, or just occasionally? _____

Is your anxiety mild, moderate, or severe? _____

Do you feel anxious throughout the day, or just in particular situations? _____

If you feel anxious in particular situations, write down the types of events or situations:

I feel anxious when _____

I feel anxious when _____

I feel anxious when _____

I feel anxious when _____

Now that you have identified some information about your anxiety, the next exercise helps you better understand the types of symptoms you experience when you are anxious. Everyone has their own particular ways of feeling anxious. Identifying your own patterns can help you target particular experiences that you want to change.

EXERCISE: Identifying and Measuring Symptoms of Anxiety

To specify what symptoms you experience when you are anxious, rate the symptoms listed in the *Mind Over Mood* Anxiety Inventory (Worksheet 14.1). Fill out the inventory once a week while you are learning methods to manage your anxiety, so you can determine which *Mind Over Mood* skills are most effective and to track your progress.

Score the *Mind Over Mood* Anxiety Inventory by adding up the numbers you circled or marked for all the items. For example, if you marked 3 for each item, your score would be 72 (3 × 24 items). If you couldn't decide between two numbers for an item and circled both, add only the higher number.

To track your progress, record your *Mind Over Mood* Anxiety Inventory scores on Worksheet 14.2. Mark each column at the bottom with the date you completed the *Mind Over Mood* Anxiety Inventory. Then put an × in the column across from your score.

WORKSHEET 14.1. *Mind Over Mood* Anxiety Inventory

Circle or mark one number for each item that best describes how much you have experienced each symptom over the past week.

	Not at all	Sometimes	Frequently	Most of the time
1. Feeling nervous	0	1	2	3
2. Worrying	0	1	2	3
3. Trembling, twitching, feeling shaky	0	1	2	3
4. Muscle tension, muscle aches, muscle soreness	0	1	2	3
5. Restlessness	0	1	2	3
6. Tiring easily	0	1	2	3
7. Shortness of breath	0	1	2	3
8. Rapid heartbeat	0	1	2	3
9. Sweating not due to the heat	0	1	2	3
10. Dry mouth	0	1	2	3
11. Dizziness or light-headedness	0	1	2	3
12. Nausea, diarrhea, or stomach problems	0	1	2	3
13. Increase in urge to urinate	0	1	2	3
14. Flushes (hot flashes) or chills	0	1	2	3
15. Trouble swallowing or "lump in throat"	0	1	2	3
16. Feeling keyed up or on edge	0	1	2	3
17. Being quick to startle	0	1	2	3
18. Difficulty concentrating	0	1	2	3
19. Trouble falling or staying asleep	0	1	2	3
20. Irritability	0	1	2	3
21. Avoiding places where I might be anxious	0	1	2	3
22. Thoughts of danger	0	1	2	3
23. Seeing myself as unable to cope	0	1	2	3
24. Thoughts that something terrible will happen	0	1	2	3
		Score (sum of item scores)		

From *Mind Over Mood, Second Edition*. Copyright 2016 by Dennis Greenberger and Christine A. Padesky. Purchasers of this book can photocopy and/or download additional copies of this worksheet (see the box at the end of the table of contents).

WORKSHEET 14.2. *Mind Over Mood* Anxiety Inventory Scores

Score															
72															
69															
66															
63															
60															
57															
54															
51															
48															
45															
42															
39															
36															
33															
30															
27															
24															
21															
18															
15															
12															
9															
6															
3															
0															
Date															

From *Mind Over Mood, Second Edition.* Copyright 2016 by Dennis Greenberger and Christine A. Padesky. Purchasers of this book can photocopy and/or download additional copies of this worksheet (see the box at the end of the table of contents).

The *Mind Over Mood* Anxiety Inventory and its score sheet (Worksheets 14.1 and 14.2) are tools you can fill out periodically (e.g., weekly or twice a month), to track changes in your anxiety. Your first score on the inventory is called your baseline or starting score. You may notice changes in your scores (improvement or worsening) over time and as you try different strategies to reduce your anxiety. For example, you might start learning the strategies in this book, take steps to solve a problem that has been bothering you, or enroll in cognitive-behavioral therapy (CBT). With each of these interventions, you would hope and expect that the frequency and severity of your symptoms would decrease, resulting in lower *Mind Over Mood* Anxiety Inventory scores. This is one way to measure the helpfulness of different approaches you try.

Mind Over Mood Anxiety Inventory scores are not used to diagnose anxiety. If you believe you are anxious, you can bring your completed *Mind Over Mood* Anxiety Inventory to a health care provider or mental health professional. Your answers on the inventory can help inform this person about your experiences, so she or he can determine a diagnosis and discuss available treatments with you.

The symptoms you rate on the *Mind Over Mood* Anxiety Inventory include cognitive (thought), behavioral, emotional, and physical changes, just as in the model described in Chapter 2 (p. 7), which you have used to help understand your problems. Notice that cognitive symptoms of anxiety include **thoughts** about danger or bad things happening, thoughts that you won't be able to cope, and various other worries. These thoughts often occur as images, not just words. When anxious, we tend to avoid situations and places where we might feel uncomfortable or anxious. Avoidance is the most common **behavior** associated with anxiety. There are many **physical symptoms** of anxiety, including shortness of breath, rapid heartbeat, dry mouth, sweating, muscle tension, shakiness, dizziness, nausea or stomach problems, hot flashes or chills, frequent urination, restlessness, and even difficulty swallowing. A number of words are used to describe an anxious **mood**, such as "nervous," "panicky," or "on edge."

Figure 14.1 on the next page summarizes the types of symptoms that are common in anxiety. The good news is that CBT and *Mind Over Mood* skills are highly effective in reducing all these types of anxiety symptoms.

Life experiences can contribute to or trigger anxiety. Trauma (being physically, emotionally, or sexually abused or bullied; being in an automobile accident; being in a war); illnesses or deaths; things we are taught ("Snakes will bite you," "If you get dirty, you'll get sick"); things we observe (an article in the newspaper about a plane crash, "My heart just missed a beat"); and experiences that seem too much to handle (giving a public speech, job promotion or termination, having a new baby) can all lead to feelings of anxiety. Linda's anxiety began after her father's death. At that time, Linda felt overwhelmed and had greater difficulty coping with problems. She began to expect that another catastrophe would occur and that she would not be able to cope with it.

All these physical, behavioral, and thinking changes we experience when we are anxious are part of the anxiety responses called "fight, flight, or freeze." These three responses can be adaptive when we face danger. To see how this is so, imagine that you are in a new town. You decide to go for a walk at night and find yourself lost on a dark

Thoughts
- Overestimating danger
- Underestimating your ability to cope
- Underestimating help available
- Worries and catastrophic thoughts

Moods
- Nervous
- On edge
- Anxious
- Panicky

Behaviors
- Avoiding anxiety situations
- Leaving situations when anxiety begins
- Trying to be perfect or to control everything
- Doing things to feel safe

Physical
- Sweaty palms
- Tight muscles
- Rapid heartbeat
- Dizziness

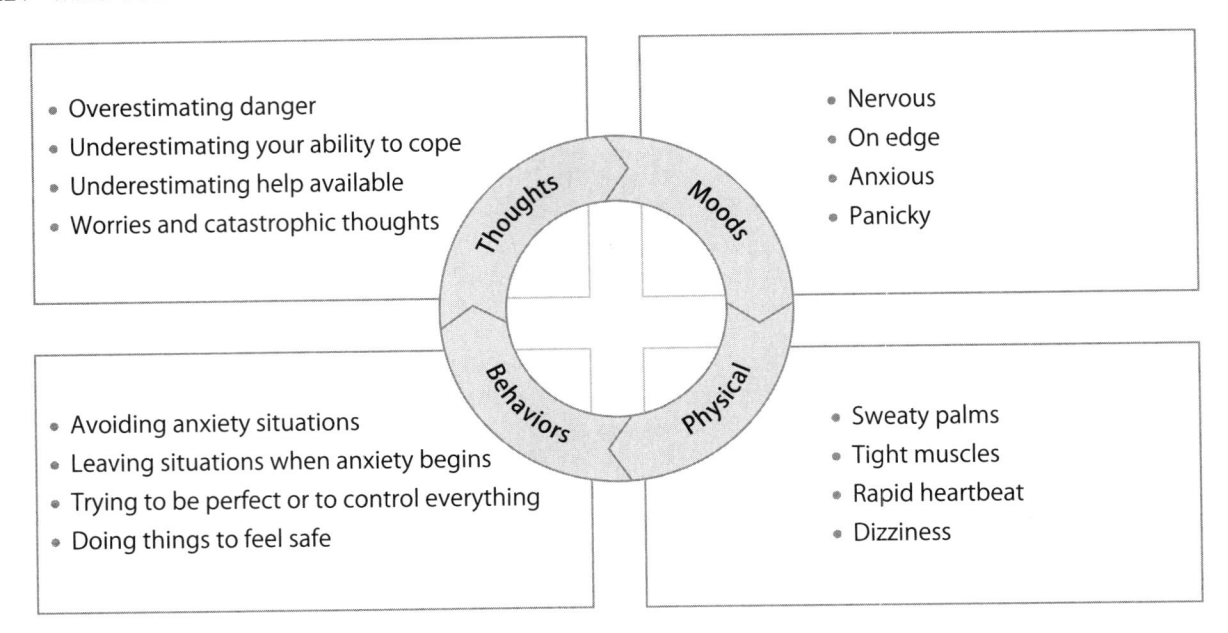

FIGURE 14.1. Profile of anxiety symptoms.

street. You notice a large man approximately 20 yards away walking toward you. You believe that he sees you and think that he is going to attack and rob you. What should you do? One option would be to fight. To do this, your heart would pump faster, your breathing would speed up, and your muscles would tense. Sweating would help cool your body. As you can see, all these body changes would be helpful in this situation. These changes make up the "fight" response.

But maybe you do not think fighting the man is a good idea. Perhaps you think it would be better to run. To run fast, you would also need an accelerated heart rate, plenty of oxygen, muscle tension, and sweating. Therefore, the same physical changes that make up the "fight" response make up the "flight" response. You simply use the extra energy to run rather than to stay and do battle. With a little luck, running may save you from being attacked.

A third response that might work well would be to freeze. Maybe the man has not seen you, and perhaps if you are very still, he will not notice you. In this case, a total freeze would require you to have very tense, rigid muscles. With a tight chest, even your breathing would be invisible to him. These types of physical changes that help you to be very still are part of the "freeze" response.

These three anxiety responses – fight, flight, and freeze – are good reactions to danger. Anxiety is adaptive when dangers are real and serious. So we don't really want to get rid of anxiety completely. Think of anxiety as similar to our pain response: It would be quite risky if we did not experience pain, because then we wouldn't know to pull our hands away from a hot stove. In the same way, we rely on our anxiety responses to alert us to dangers that we might need to face or manage.

Unfortunately, we also experience anxiety when watching a movie about a robbery or when standing in front of a group of people to give a speech. This book teaches methods to reduce your anxiety when danger is not present, when the danger is not as serious as you might think, or when too much anxiety interferes with your good coping. Anxiety treatment's goals are to help you assess the degree of danger more quickly and learn how to reduce your anxiety responses when dangers are smaller than you imagine or can be managed through coping. Often this mean needing to approach what you fear, in order to learn more about the degree of danger and your ability to cope with it.

ANXIETY BEHAVIORS

There are two types of behaviors that characterize anxiety: avoidance and safety behaviors. We avoid and seek safety when we are anxious, because these behaviors help us feel better in the short run. However, these common ways of coping with anxiety also tend to prolong our anxiety, making it worse over time.

Avoidance

Peter needed to take a speech class as a school requirement. He felt really anxious when he imagined speaking in front of his class. As a result, whenever he thought about working on his speech, he procrastinated and did other things so he could avoid feeling anxious. When he went out with his friends instead of working on the speech, he immediately felt better, because thoughts about the speech were replaced with a focus on his friends. As the weeks went by, however, Peter became more and more afraid about the upcoming speech. In addition, Peter did not speak up in class. Each time he had something to say, he felt a surge in his anxiety. When he decided not to speak, his anxiety immediately decreased. Every time Peter avoided speaking, he was rewarded by feeling better, which made it more likely that he would keep avoiding.

Although Peter's avoidance helped him feel less anxious in the moment, it actually made his anxiety worse over time. Avoidance usually leads to an increase in anxiety for four reasons: (1) By not approaching and learning more about what frightens us, we don't have an opportunity to learn ways to tolerate our anxiety; (2) we don't learn ways to cope with the situation that frightens us; (3) we don't have an opportunity to learn that the situation may not be as dangerous as we fear; and (4) we don't have an opportunity to find out if we are already capable of dealing well with the situation.

Mark, another student in Peter's speech class, also felt anxious about giving a speech. Rather than avoiding working on his speech, however, he took steps to reduce his anxiety. First, Mark asked other students about the teacher and speech class, to find out how high the standards would be. He learned that the teacher was a tough grader, but was encouraging as long as students made efforts to participate in class. Mark felt anxious when he sat down to prepare his speech, but stuck with it and learned that his anxiety decreased a bit when he began writing down possible topics and ideas. He began preparing his speech early and practiced dozens of times. He discovered that his anxiety decreased with practice and preparation.

Mark also made comments in class discussions so that he could practice expressing himself in the group. These experiences increased his confidence that he could speak up and cope with everyone looking at him. One day a class member disagreed with one of his ideas and made fun of him. He felt his face flush, but later realized that it was not the end of the world, and he felt good about how he had handled this situation. Another classmate told him that she thought his critic had been rude; this helped Mark realize that even if he made some mistakes or people disagreed with what he was saying, some people might still think positively about him.

One of the things we can learn from the examples of Peter and Mark is that avoidance brings immediate relief but increases anxiety over time. Facing our fears often leads to distress at first, but helps us overcome anxiety in time. If you have been experiencing anxiety, you may have been avoiding a number of situations and experiences. Make a list below of some of the things you have been avoiding because of anxiety.

EXERCISE: What I Avoid Because of Anxiety

1. _____
2. _____
3. _____
4. _____
5. _____
6. _____
7. _____

Safety Behaviors

In addition to avoidance, we often engage in safety behaviors when we feel anxious. What are "safety behaviors"? These are things we do to reduce our sense of risk or keep from being hurt in situations that make us anxious. While these purposes sound like good things, safety behaviors actually often make our anxiety worse, because they increase our perception that this situation is much more dangerous that it may actually be. Here are some examples.

Tyra is afraid of snakes. When she takes her daughter to the zoo, she checks on the map to see where the snake exhibit is housed. Even though she would prefer avoiding this exhibit, her daughter wants to see the snakes, so she goes into the exhibit. While she is there, Tyra keeps one arm on her daughter, just in case she needs to grab her and run out of the exhibit quickly because a snake has gotten loose. Because she keeps her arm on her daughter (safety behavior), Tyra actually thinks even more about danger than usual and feels more anxious, even though the actual danger is close to zero.

Kenji is anxious about a lot of different things. At night, he is nervous that someone will break into his home. He locks his door, and then a few minutes later gets anxious and checks the door (safety behavior) to confirm that it is locked. He repeats this ritual eight or nine times a night, every night. His anxiety goes down briefly each time he sees the door is locked, but his worries quickly return, and he questions his memory that the door is locked. Checking the doors is a safety behavior, and it keeps Kenji focused on the danger of an intruder. His safety behaviors do not have lasting benefit in terms of reducing his anxiety.

Roberta has to attend a weekly office meeting. Each week she becomes very anxious, because she is afraid the manager will ask her a question or assign her a job that she can't do. She attends all the meetings, but sits in the back row (safety behavior). She also refrains from coughing, making eye contact, or volunteering information she does have (more safety behaviors), because she doesn't want to draw attention to herself. These safety behaviors succeed in keeping Roberta out of the manager's awareness, but they do not reduce her anxiety over time. Instead, each week that her manager does not speak to her, Roberta becomes more and more convinced that she could not handle it if he did. Thus, over time, she becomes even more anxious in office meetings.

What Is the Difference between Safety Behaviors and Coping with Anxiety?

When we use safety behaviors, we often think we are doing a good job of coping with our anxiety. But as the examples above show, safety behaviors generally keep us focused on danger and support our belief that situations are highly dangerous, even when they may not be. Like avoidance, safety behaviors help us feel better in the moment, but they actually prolong our struggles with anxiety. This is because safety behaviors prevent us from fully facing our fears and having the opportunity to build our confidence that we can handle things that go wrong or seem dangerous to us.

Good coping, on the other hand, usually involves approaching our fears and managing our reactions and the situations that scare us. When we practice coping with our fears, we build up confidence we can handle them, and our anxiety decreases. There are two ways to tell the difference between safety behaviors and coping behaviors:

1. Safety behaviors are designed to eliminate danger; coping behaviors are designed to help us approach, stay in, and manage situations that frighten us.

2. Safety behaviors maintain or increase anxiety; coping behaviors lead to a decrease in anxiety over time.

Tyra, Kenji, and Roberta are likely to experience a decrease in anxiety after a while if they start to use coping instead of safety behaviors. For example, a good coping behavior for Tyra might be to take her hand off her daughter and watch her daughter's excitement at seeing the snakes. In addition, Tyra can remind herself that all the snakes, even the most dangerous ones, are safely enclosed and not able to escape.

In order to cope, Kenji could focus his attention on the action of locking the door. Then, when he begins to feel anxious, he can stop himself from rechecking the door and instead remind himself that he can tolerate the uncertainty and discomfort. This might be difficult at first, but over time his urge to check will decrease, and he will realize that the checking does not really increase his safety.

Roberta is fearful of being asked questions or assigned jobs that will put her in the spotlight and lead to embarrassment or failure. Good coping might involve speaking out in meetings when she does know information. She could also practice things she might say if her manager asks her a question she does not know the answer to. If she is assigned to a job she does not know how to do, she could ask for help from a coworker to build her skills. The first few times Roberta tries these coping behaviors, she is likely to feel more anxious. However, with experience, she will learn that often nothing bad happens, and that even when it does, she can cope. Over time and with practice, her anxiety will decrease and her confidence will increase.

Just like Tyra, Kenji, and Roberta, you may be using safety behaviors when you get anxious. See if you can identify two or three safety behaviors you sometimes use to try to prevent or reduce anxiety. Remember that sometimes safety behaviors are things you do (e.g., only going to parties if a friend is with you, keeping an antianxiety pill in your pocket in case you start to feel anxious) and sometimes things you don't do (e.g., not making eye contact so people won't talk to you, sitting in an aisle seat instead of the middle of a row so you can make a quick exit if necessary). For this exercise, think of particular situations in which you feel anxious, and recall what safety behaviors you use. There may be more than one safety behavior for each situation.

EXERCISE: Safety Behaviors I Use to Prevent Anxiety

1. Situation: _____

    Safety behavior(s): _____

2. Situation: _____

    Safety behavior(s): _____

3. Situation: _____

    Safety behavior(s): _____

ANXIOUS THOUGHTS

The behaviors associated with anxiety (avoidance and safety behaviors) make even more sense when you understand the thoughts that go along with anxiety. When we are anxious, we have thoughts about *danger, threat*, and our own *vulnerability*. A threat or danger can be physical, mental, or social. A physical threat occurs when you believe you will be physically hurt (e.g., a snake bite, a heart attack, being hit). A social threat occurs when you believe you will be rejected, humiliated, embarrassed, or bullied. A mental threat occurs when something makes you worry that you are going crazy or losing your mind.

In addition to having thoughts about danger, when we are anxious we believe we *can't cope*. In fact, anxiety occurs when our perception is that the danger we face is greater than our ability to cope. Consider how you might feel if someone asked you to dive off a large rock into a lake. There is a certain amount of danger involved, but if you are confident that you know how to dive, the water is deep enough to be safe, and you have watched others make the same dive and they seemed to enjoy it, then you might feel excited instead of anxious. This is because you believe you can cope with the degree of danger involved. Instead of focusing on danger, you can think about the excitement and enjoyment of the moment. However, if you are not convinced that you can dive safely and you are uncertain of your swimming ability, then you are likely to feel anxious rather than excited in the same situation.

We make these judgments about danger and our ability to cope every day of our lives. Our judgments about how fast or slow to drive, our decisions to stay on the curb or walk across the street, our choices to speak up in a group or stay silent — all of these are determined by our assessment of the dangers involved and our ability to cope with them. When we think our ability to cope is equal to or greater than the dangers involved, we do activities with ease. When we think we cannot cope with the risks or dangers in a given situation, then we tend to pull back, avoid, and engage in safety behaviors.

Anxiety is not always a bad thing. If dangers are greater than our ability to cope, it is wise to pull back. However, when we are frequently anxious, we tend to *overestimate danger* and *underestimate our ability to cope* across many situations. This thinking style leads us to experience anxiety in many more situations than necessary. Over time, anxiety can become more severe and begin to affect more and more areas of our lives.

"What If . . . ?" Thinking

Anxious thoughts often predict future or imminent catastrophe. They often begin with "What if . . . ?" and end with a disastrous outcome. Frequently, anxious thoughts include images of danger as well. For example, a man with a fear of public speaking may think before a talk, "*What if* I stumble over my words? *What if* I forget my notes? *What if* people think I'm stupid and don't know what I'm talking about?" He may have an image of himself standing frozen and blushing in front of the crowd. These thoughts are all about the future and predict a negative outcome.

Someone who is afraid of flying in airplanes or driving on the freeway may think, "*What if* the airplane explodes? *What if* I have a panic attack on the airplane? *What if* there's not enough oxygen on the plane to breathe?" or "*What if* I have a traffic accident on the freeway? *What if I* get stuck in rush-hour traffic, have difficulty breathing, and can't get to a freeway exit?" You can see that these thoughts are also future-oriented and predict danger or catastrophe. They would make the person think twice about getting on an airplane or freeway.

Some people feel anxious in close relationships. They may fear intimacy or commitment. They may also be concerned about being judged, rejected, or embarrassed. The thoughts we have when we are fearful about relationships are, like the ones just discussed, oriented toward the future and predict danger or catastrophe. These thoughts include "*What if* I get hurt? *What if* I am rejected? *What* if the other person senses my weakness and takes advantage of me?" Again, these thoughts demonstrate the "something terrible is going to happen" theme that is characteristic of anxiety.

The perception of threat varies from person to person. Some people feel a great sense of safety and security. Other people feel threatened very easily and will often feel anxious. Sometimes this is because of life experiences. For example, if you grew up in chaotic and volatile surroundings, you might conclude that the world and other people are always dangerous. In this case, your ability to anticipate danger and understand your own vulnerability might have helped you survive as a child. If you grew up in a dangerous home, being able to recognize danger or its early warning signs may have been critical to your emotional and perhaps your physical survival. You may have developed a very fine ability to spot and respond to dangerous situations.

At this point in your life, however, it may be important to evaluate whether or not you are overresponding to thoughts about danger and threat. Perhaps the people in your adult life are not as threatening as those in your childhood. You might also consider whether or not your resources and abilities as an adult can open up new and creative ways of coping with threat and anxiety.

Imagery

Our anxious thoughts often occur as images. When we overestimate danger, we don't just think, "What if I have a car accident?"; we actually vividly imagine the scenes that we fear. We might see a car accident in our minds, or hear the sirens of emergency vehicles in our imaginations. When we underestimate our ability to cope, we often see ourselves looking overwhelmed or even shaking uncontrollably. We might imagine other people making fun of us, or hear the sounds of people laughing at us. Sometimes the images in our mind draw on memories of past times when we were anxious or experienced traumatic events. At other times, the images are fictional – creations of our own minds. For example, we might imagine our boss as 10 feet tall and screaming at us with an exaggerated red face. Because these types of images give rise to strong feelings of anxiety, it is important to become more aware of them in order to learn ways to respond to them. Throughout *Mind Over Mood*, whenever an exercise asks you to identify your thoughts, this means thoughts that occur either as words or as images.

LINDA: *Anxious thoughts during a panic attack*

Linda experienced anxiety and panic attacks when she flew on airplanes. "Panic" is extreme anxiety or fear. A "panic attack" consists of a distinct combination of thoughts, emotions, and physical reactions. Often a panic attack is characterized by a change in physical or mental sensations, such as rapid heartbeat, sweating, difficulty breathing, a choking or smothering sensation, shaking, dizziness, pain in the chest, nausea, hot flashes or chills, or disorientation.

Linda had to fly to a city 200 miles away for an impromptu business meeting. She monitored her thoughts and emotional reactions before the flight and summarized them on the partial Thought Record shown in Figure 14.2.

Notice how Linda's anxiety and panic were influenced by thoughts that focused on danger and personal vulnerability. It was not waiting in the airline terminal that caused Linda to panic. Many people wait in airline terminals without feeling anxious or having panic attacks. Linda's thoughts about this situation led her to feel anxious and panicky.

1. Situation Who? What? When? Where?	2. Moods a. What did you feel? b. Rate each mood (0–100%).	3. Automatic Thoughts (Images) What was going through your mind just before you started to feel this way? Any other thoughts? Images?
Waiting in the airport to board my plane.	Anxiety 80% Panic 90%	What if the plane has engine trouble? How safe can this plane be? What if I have a panic attack on the plane?
	List physical reactions you experienced: Sweating Trouble breathing Heart racing	I'll be embarrassed if my boss sees that I'm having trouble breathing and that I'm sweating and panicking. My heart is starting to race already. I think a panic attack is beginning. What if I have a heart attack? Image – I see myself grabbing my chest, sweating, and turning pale. People on the airplane look scared that something is wrong with me.

FIGURE 14.2. Linda's partial Thought Record.

EXERCISE: Identifying Thoughts Associated with Anxiety

To highlight the thoughts that are associated with anxiety or fear in your own life, complete Worksheet 14.3. Think about a recent time when you were anxious, fearful, or nervous. Describe the situation, your mood(s), and any physical symptoms you experienced (e.g., rapid heart rate, dizziness, sweating, tight stomach). Recall the thoughts you had (in words and in images). If you had an image, describe it. If your thoughts began with "What if . . . ?," write down the answer to that question (e.g., the thought or image that made you most anxious).

WORKSHEET 14.3. Identifying Thoughts Associated with Anxiety

1. Situation Who? What? When? Where?	2. Moods a. What did you feel? b. Rate each mood (0–100%).	3. Automatic Thoughts (Images) What was going through your mind just before you started to feel this way? Any other thoughts? Images?
	List physical reactions you experienced:	

From *Mind Over Mood, Second Edition*. Copyright 2016 by Dennis Greenberger and Christine A. Padesky. Purchasers of this book can photocopy and/or download additional copies of this worksheet (see the box at the end of the table of contents).

Were the thoughts you identified in the exercise future-oriented? Do the thoughts reflect a sense of danger, inability to cope, or prediction of a catastrophe? If so, then you have identified anxiety-related thoughts.

Anxiety is often triggered in vague and ambiguous situations. This makes sense because if we tend to be alert to danger, it is hard to decide how dangerous a situation really is if the details are uncertain. People who are anxious sometimes prefer to know a negative thing for sure, rather than remain in a state of "not knowing." This may be one reason why we jump to the conclusion that something is dangerous, even when we don't know for sure. For example, if we have a physical symptom that puzzles us, we sometimes immediately start thinking about serious illnesses rather than less serious explanations.

In addition, anxiety often arises because we don't have control over events. Often when we are anxious, we try to be in control or do things perfectly, in the hope that this will prevent bad things from happening. Since we don't have confidence that we can cope with the dangers that worry us, it makes sense that we try to prevent them. The problem with this approach is that it is really impossible to do things perfectly or have complete control over what will happen in the future. Thus learning to boost our confidence that we can cope when things go wrong is a more helpful approach to managing anxiety than trying to prevent things from going wrong. Did you have any thoughts related to control, perfectionism, or "not knowing" in the situation you described on Worksheet 14.3?

Common Thoughts in Various Types of Anxiety Problems

Figure 14.3 summarizes common thoughts associated with the specific types of anxiety problems mentioned earlier in this chapter. Notice that these thoughts pertain to the danger that is central to each type of anxiety. For example, people with a snake phobia have anxious thoughts and images related to snakes, and people with health worries have thoughts and images about illness. For each category, it is also common to have doubts about our ability to cope with the things we fear.

OVERCOMING ANXIETY

When we have anxiety, we often just want to get rid of it as quickly as possible. We might think it would be wonderful if we never felt anxious again. Actually, eliminating anxiety would not be a good idea. Anxiety is the body's alarm system. It alerts us to danger. If your home had an alarm system that was activated when a dog or cat entered your yard, you would often be on the alert unnecessarily. This wouldn't be a good reason to disconnect your alarm. You would just need either to fine-tune it so it did not go off so easily, or to learn to turn it off quickly as soon as you determined there was no serious danger outside. That is what we try to do in overcoming anxiety. We want to do our best to fine-tune our internal alarm system so it does not go off as often. Furthermore,

Type of Anxiety	Common Thoughts and Images
Phobias	Thoughts and images about specific feared situations (e.g., snakes, heights, insects, elevators).
Social anxiety	"People will judge/criticize me"; "I'll look foolish"; images of blushing, others making fun of me, etc.
Panic disorder	"I'm dying now" (e.g., heart attack, stroke); "I'm losing my mind"; images of paramedics, losing consciousness, etc.
Posttraumatic stress disorder	Flashback memories and images of traumatic events; "I've been damaged forever"; "I'm in danger right now"; thoughts and images triggered by sensory experiences (sounds, smells, sights, and sensations similar to traumatic events).
Health worries	"I have an illness that has not been diagnosed"; "Physical changes or pain are always signs of serious illness"; "When doctors or tests say I'm healthy, they missed something"; "It is important to check or scan often for signs of illness or physical changes."
Generalized anxiety disorder	"What if . . . ?" worries about many different things; "If something bad happens, I can't cope"; images of feeling overwhelmed.

FIGURE 14.3. Common thoughts and images in different types of anxiety.

From *Mind Over Mood, Second Edition.* Copyright 2016 by Dennis Greenberger and Christine A. Padesky. Purchasers may photocopy this box for personal use or use with individual clients.

we can learn to assess the level of threat in a situation and turn off the anxiety response more quickly when we are overestimating danger. And we can increase our confidence in our ability to cope with situations that make us anxious, as well as with anxiety itself.

Fine-Tuning the Anxiety Alarm System

CBT is more successful in treating anxiety than in treating any other type of mood problem. There are specific and effective treatment approaches for every type of anxiety described in Figure 14.3. The following sections briefly describe methods that are commonly used in all these treatments.

Overcoming Avoidance: Exposure

As described earlier in this chapter, avoidance is the most common behavior associated with anxiety. When we avoid a difficult situation, we initially experience a decrease in anxiety. This relief we feel is quite rewarding, and this makes us more likely to want to continue avoiding in the future. Ironically, the more we avoid a situation, the more anxious we become about facing it in the future. In this way, avoidance actually fuels anxiety in the long run, because it helps convince us that the dangers we fear are serious and we aren't capable of coping with them.

To overcome anxiety, we need to learn to approach the situations or people we avoid. Through these experiences, we have an opportunity to increase our confidence in our ability to cope with the situations that frighten us. Learning to approach and cope with situations in which we feel anxious is a lasting and powerful way of decreasing our anxiety. Approaching our fears and coping with them is called "exposure." Generally speaking, the more exposure experiences you have, the less sensitive your anxiety alarm becomes. That is, when you go into anxiety-provoking situations more often, your anxiety alarm system learns not to see these situations as so dangerous. Making your alarm less sensitive by repeated exposure for gradually increasing time periods is called "desensitization." In the next section, you learn to make a Fear Ladder to help you personalize your plans for exposure, so you can overcome your fears as quickly as possible.

Making a Hierarchy or Fear Ladder

When you experience high levels of anxiety, it is helpful to develop a hierarchy of the situations, events, or people you fear. A "hierarchy" is a list, written in order of fear intensity, with the most feared situation or event at the top and the least feared situation at the bottom. You can think of it as a "Fear Ladder" on which the lowest step describes a situation in which you experience a small amount of fear, and each step up the ladder represents situations in which you experience greater degrees of fear. Start to approach situations at the bottom of the ladder first, and work your way up the steps gradually, rising up the ladder as you successfully master events until you can do them with only a medium amount of anxiety. You will stay on each step and continue with exposure practice until you become confident that you can handle that step and you learn to tolerate whatever level of anxiety you experience. By gradually approaching what you fear, you will also gather evidence about the accuracy of your catastrophic expectations and your ability to cope.

As an example, Juanita was nervous when she was asked to give a presentation at the next city council meeting. She usually avoided speaking in front of groups because she felt so anxious. To overcome her anxiety and avoidance, Juanita made a Fear Ladder that looked like the one shown in Figure 14.4 on the next page.

Starting with situation 1 at the bottom of her Fear Ladder, Juanita successfully met the challenges of each situation on her Fear Ladder by combining relaxation methods (described later in this chapter), cognitive restructuring (Chapters 6–9), and Action Plans (Chapter 10) to solve problems that might occur. Juanita did not proceed to the next situation on her Fear Ladder until she could approach the current one with tolerable anxiety and increased confidence. She practiced step 4 – a step that could not be easily repeated numerous times – in her imagination until she felt confident she could do this in person. While Juanita experienced some anxiety when she actually gave her presentation to the City Council, she was not nearly as anxious as she had been in similar situations in the past. She credited her success to her step-by-step practice. Furthermore, as Juanita walked to the podium, she reminded herself how well she had done the speech in practice. By using different methods in combination, Juanita was able to give a public speech, something she had previously avoided.

FEAR LADDER

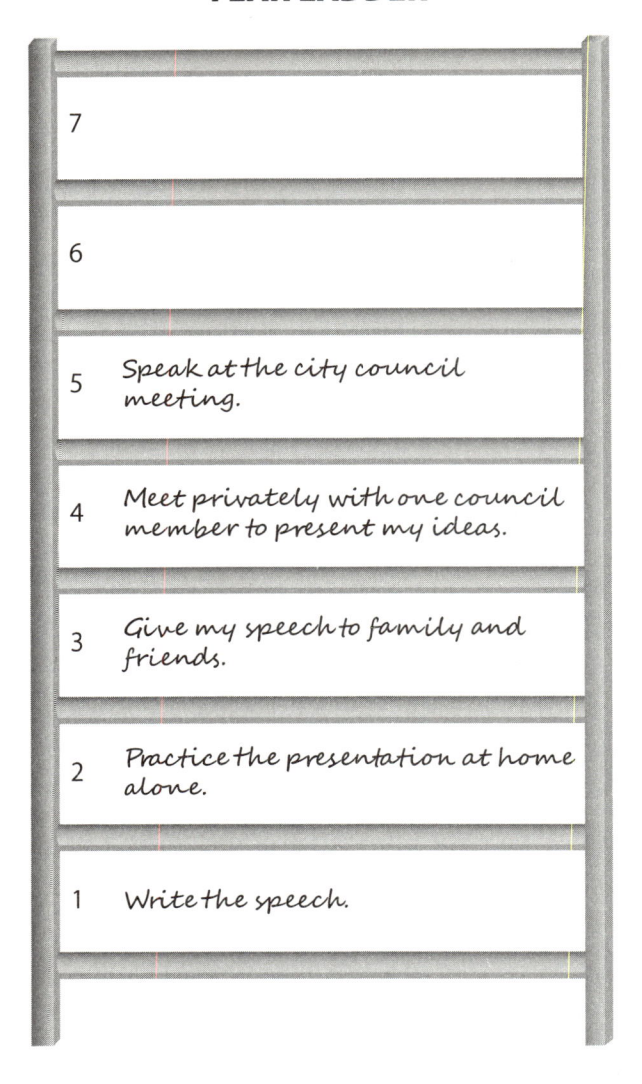

7	
6	
5	Speak at the city council meeting.
4	Meet privately with one council member to present my ideas.
3	Give my speech to family and friends.
2	Practice the presentation at home alone.
1	Write the speech.

FIGURE 14.4. Juanita's Fear Ladder.

Juanita used a Fear Ladder to help her approach public speaking. Sometimes there is not just a single event coming up that makes us anxious, but a whole collection of situations and experiences. For example, Paul avoided a variety of situations in which he feared he might have a panic attack. He avoided driving alone, being too far from home, getting onto elevators, sitting in the middle of a row of seats, and being in crowded places. All these situations made Paul anxious, and he was afraid he would have a panic attack if he approached and stayed in them. Paul thought about which of these situations were the most difficult for him, and then made the Fear Ladder shown in Figure 14.5.

Notice that Paul planned many more steps on his Fear Ladder than Juanita needed to plan. For each of Paul's steps, he planned a variety of exposure experiments that were gradually more challenging for him. For example, when in a movie theatre or at a sports event, he first sat just a few seats from the aisle (step 1) and gradually moved to the center as his confidence grew (step 2). For steps 3 through 7, he began each step at an easier point. Once his exposure was successful (i.e., he was able to stay in the situation as long as necessary to manage his anxiety), he increased the time or intensity of the experience. So, for example, he rode an elevator many times, increasing the number of floors until he could ride to the top of the building. Once he could do this in an uncrowded elevator, he added the challenge of doing this at a busy time when the elevators were quite crowded. It might seem that it would take Paul a very long time to take all these steps on his Fear Ladder, but actually he was able to complete many exposure challenges successfully in a single day – so he reached the top of the ladder in a few months, faster than he expected.

Use Worksheets 14.4 and 14.5 to create your own Fear Ladder.

FEAR LADDER

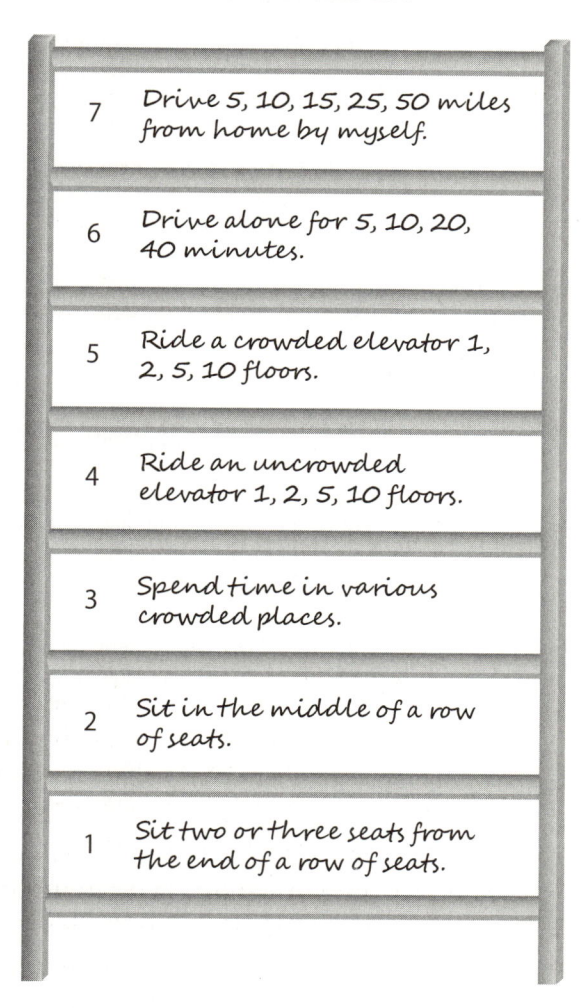

7	Drive 5, 10, 15, 25, 50 miles from home by myself.
6	Drive alone for 5, 10, 20, 40 minutes.
5	Ride a crowded elevator 1, 2, 5, 10 floors.
4	Ride an uncrowded elevator 1, 2, 5, 10 floors.
3	Spend time in various crowded places.
2	Sit in the middle of a row of seats.
1	Sit two or three seats from the end of a row of seats.

FIGURE 14.5. Paul's Fear Ladder.

> **EXERCISE: Making My Fear Ladder**
>
> Make your Fear Ladder by filling out Worksheets 14.4 and 14.5. Worksheet 14.4 helps you brainstorm and rate situations you avoid because of anxiety. Once this is done, put on Worksheet 14.5 the item you rated with the highest anxiety on the top step, and the item you rated with the lowest anxiety on the bottom step. Fill in the other steps from high to low based on your anxiety ratings. If you rated some items equally, put them in the order that makes most sense to you, so that your Fear Ladder steps move from your least feared at the bottom to your most feared situations at the top of the ladder. It's OK if some of your steps are blank.

WORKSHEET 14.4. Making a Fear Ladder

1. First, brainstorm a list of situations, events, or people that you avoid because of your anxiety. Write them in the left-hand column below, in any order.

2. After you complete your list, rate how anxious you feel when you imagine each of the things listed in the first column. Rate these from 0 to 100, where 0 is no anxiety and 100 is the most anxious you have ever felt. Write these ratings next to each item in the right-hand column.

What I avoid	Rate anxiety (0–100)

From *Mind Over Mood, Second Edition*. Copyright 2016 by Dennis Greenberger and Christine A. Padesky. Purchasers of this book can photocopy and/or download additional copies of this worksheet (see the box at the end of the table of contents).

WORKSHEET 14.5. My Fear Ladder

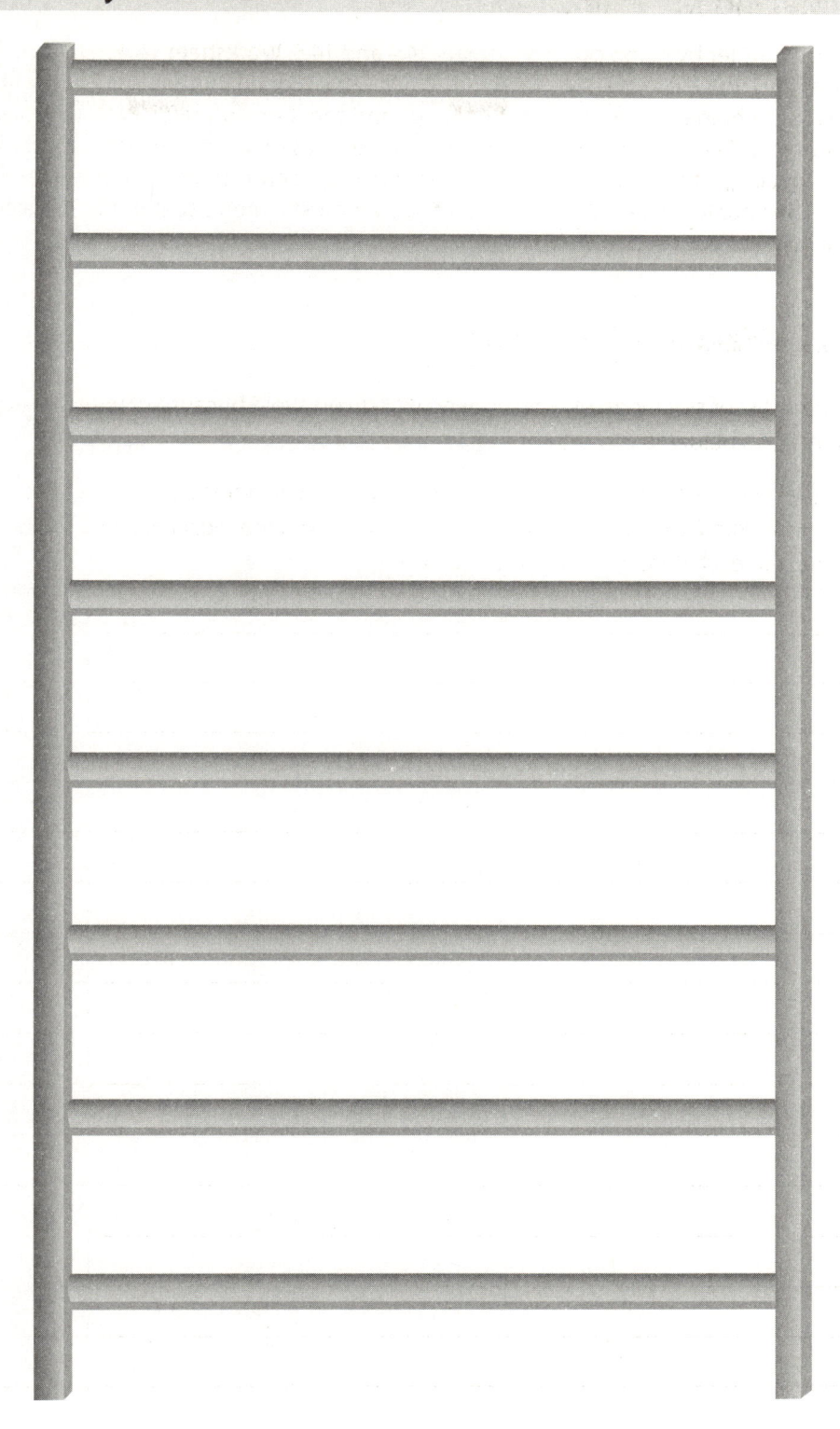

From *Mind Over Mood, Second Edition.* Copyright 2016 by Dennis Greenberger and Christine A. Padesky. Purchasers of this book can photocopy and/or download additional copies of this worksheet (see the box at the end of the table of contents).

Using Your Fear Ladder to Overcome Anxiety and Avoidance

Once you make your Fear Ladder, you are ready to begin to approach your fears (exposure) and learn to manage your anxiety. You have control over how quickly or slowly you proceed up the ladder. Your exposure to each step on the ladder is up to you; you should not feel pushed or pressured to go faster than you believe you can. Having a sense of control over the speed at which you work is likely to help you lower your anxiety and overcome avoidance more quickly.

Moving up a Fear Ladder is never comfortable. But people who are willing to tolerate the temporary discomfort of moving up their Fear Ladders get over their anxiety more quickly. Just as avoidance leads to short-term relief and long-term increase in anxiety, exposure to the steps on your Fear Ladder leads to short-term discomfort and long-term relief from anxiety. Therefore, you should spend as much time as possible working on your Fear Ladder.

If you find that even the least feared situation on your Fear Ladder seems too difficult, you can either break down that step into smaller parts or begin with imagery practice. Imagery practice is simply picturing yourself spending time on the step.

It is often helpful to imagine the situation in great detail. For example, Juanita looked at photos of city council members she planned to visit and thought about the expressions on their faces. She imagined how she would feel shaking their hands and sitting in their offices. She even imagined her voice shaking a bit when she began to speak. She found it helpful to imagine these meetings in two ways: sometimes when everything went smoothly, and other times when she stumbled on her words and felt quite embarrassed. By imagining both easy and difficult circumstances, she was able to plan ways to handle the meetings no matter what happened. This increased her confidence.

Once you are comfortable with the situation in imagination, you can enter the situation in reality. As Juanita's experience demonstrates, it is helpful to use as many of the five senses as possible when doing exposure in your imagination. Imagine what you will see, hear, smell, taste, and touch. It is also helpful to imagine what you might be thinking, feeling, and doing in the situation. Some people find it helpful to write down or digitally record their imagined exposure. In this way, you can either listen to the recording or read what you've written to increase the number of exposures and move up the Fear Ladder more quickly.

How do you know when to move from one step on the Fear Ladder to the next? You don't need your anxiety to go away completely (a rating of 0). In fact, most people will continue to have some anxiety until they have faced the situations they fear many times. The goal is to get your anxiety to a tolerable level. For most people, a good guideline is to stay on each step until the anxiety decreases by more than half or drops below a rating of 40 on the 0–100 scale.

If you have trouble staying in the situation, you can use some of the coping skills described later in this chapter that will help you stay on each ladder step for longer periods of time. Sometimes a supportive spouse/partner or friend can help you become more willing and motivated to face the steps on your Fear Ladder. If you want a helper, choose someone you trust who understands the nature of your fears and avoidance. This person can serve as an empathic source of motivation and support as you do initially difficult activities. Ideally, you will later face your fears on your own as easily as you do with a helper present.

You should expect that your anxiety will increase when you first begin to approach on your Fear Ladder. This is a good sign that you are facing your fears. Alternatively, if there is no anxiety, then either you are not taking big enough steps to face your fears, or you are relying too much on safety behaviors. In addition, for each step of your Fear Ladder, you are learning to tolerate anxiety as you stay in the situation longer. The more you do this, the easier it will become for you to experience anxiety and move up the steps of your Fear Ladder. Ironically, as we become more comfortable with anxiety, our anxiety often decreases. In order to successfully approach and stay in feared situations, use the skills described below to manage your anxiety while you work on your Fear Ladder.

Managing Your Anxiety

It is normal to want to leave or avoid situations when you feel anxious. As you have already learned, it is important to overcome this tendency and stay in situations so you learn to tolerate your anxiety and discover that you are capable of handling the challenges of your fear. In this and other chapters of this book you will learn ways to manage and reduce your anxiety as well as to tolerate increasing amounts of anxiety.

There are a number of things you can do. Once you learn two or three skills to manage and tolerate your anxiety, you will move up your Fear Ladder more quickly. It is important to use these skills to stay in the situations on your Fear Ladder. You don't want to use these skills as safety behaviors to protect you from dangers you fear, or as ways to try to eliminate anxiety. Instead, the goal is to use anxiety management strategies to reduce anxiety to a level you can tolerate and still stay in the situation.

Mindfulness and Acceptance

"Mindfulness" is a practice of learning to stay in the present moment and observe with full attention your experience and immediate surroundings. Part of mindfulness is also accepting your experiences without making judgments about them. For example, you may often walk down a street with your mind focused on what happened earlier in the day or what will happen later, or you may even be scanning texts or emails on a mobile device. Mindful walking means focusing your attention on the motion of your feet, the feel of your muscles as you move, the wind blowing against your skin, the colors and sounds that surround you, and other sensory experiences such as smells or even your own breathing. When there are unpleasant parts of your experience, it can be worthwhile to practice acceptance, which means noticing the unpleasantness without trying to change it into something different or positive.

This is not as easy as it sounds. When you first try to practice mindfulness for even a minute or two, it is quite common for your mind to drift into the future or the past. This is to be expected. Awareness of your mind drifting is a good thing, because this gives you the opportunity to remember to return to your current moment and experience. Part of being mindful is to notice your mental drift without judging it. Instead, gently bring yourself back to the present moment. Mindfulness can be practiced during various activities throughout the day, such as while you eat, walk, or talk with someone. Once you are able to be mindful for even a few minutes in situations that don't make you anxious, you are ready to use this skill in situations that make you anxious.

Linda learned to practice mindfulness effectively in the early phases of her therapy. Linda was on an airplane when the pilot announced that the plane would be delayed on the runway for 20 minutes. Her initial thoughts were "I won't be able to handle this. I'll have a panic attack," and she became anxious. Linda then decided to experiment with mindfulness.

Linda focused her attention on various parts of her current experience. She noticed shades of blue in the sky and the colors and shapes of the clouds. She allowed her eyes to run over the outlines of the clouds and observed closely the texture of each cloud. Linda tuned in to her breathing and noticed that it began to slow a bit as her anxiety decreased. She felt the texture of her clothes and listened to the sounds of passengers nearby. Linda became so absorbed in these scenes that the 20-minute delay went by quickly with tolerable levels of anxiety. It also helped that she accepted the anxiety she felt. She thought, "This is an unexpected delay. I'm still anxious about flying, and I understand and accept that I am feeling anxious. I don't need to change it. I can tolerate it."

Mindfulness and acceptance help with anxiety in several ways. First, most anxiety is about fears that are not currently happening, but about things we fear might happen in the future, even a few minutes from now. If you learn to keep your mind in the present moment, your anxiety will decrease. Second, when you are fully engaged in the moment, your brain is not focused on your fears. Focusing on the present moment occupies your mind and helps you feel grounded in your experience. This generally leads to a feeling of relaxation. Third, one of the long-term benefits of mindfulness and acceptance is that they can help you tolerate and feel less anxiety, because you will learn to see your anxious thoughts as simply mental activity rather than as the truth. With practice, you can begin to understand your personal patterns of thinking and responding to events. You can learn that you don't need to respond to your patterns of thinking and emotional reactions. Instead, you can simply observe them as they occur. People who practice mindfulness on a regular basis generally report greater feelings of calm, well-being, and acceptance of life's difficulties.

If mindfulness sounds like something that would be helpful for you, many communities have classes that teach mindfulness. There are also books, audio programs, and mobile apps that teach and can remind you to engage in mindfulness practice.

Breathing

A related way to manage your anxiety is to practice balanced, deep breathing. Many people breathe shallowly or irregularly when they are anxious or tense. These breathing patterns lead to an imbalance of oxygen and carbon dioxide in the body, which can cause the physical symptoms of anxiety. For example, when we breathe more shallowly, we take in less oxygen. One of the functions of the heart is to pump oxygen throughout the body via the blood stream. If the heart gets less oxygen, it beats faster to try to supply the same amount of oxygen to the body.

In the beginning, it is important to practice balanced, deep breathing for at least four minutes at a time, because this is roughly how long it takes to restore the balance of oxygen and carbon dioxide in your body. The balancing works most effectively if you breathe slowly and deeply in and out for an equal amount of time. If you put one hand on your upper chest and one hand on your stomach, your hand on your stomach should move out as you breathe in.

Try breathing in to a slow count of 4 and out to a slow count of 4 for four minutes right now, and see if you become more relaxed. It doesn't matter whether you breathe through your mouth or your nose; breathe whichever way is comfortable for you. Be sure to breathe gently and not take big gulps of air. Try to keep your attention on your breath and the motion of your hand on your stomach as it moves up and down. When you find your attention drifting elsewhere, just bring it back to your breathing. Again, it helps to practice this skill when you are not highly anxious. If you practice balanced deep breathing four minutes at a time, four times a day for a week, you will get quite skilled at it. Then you are ready to use it to manage your anxiety and help you stay for longer periods of time in situations in which you feel anxious.

Progressive Muscle Relaxation

"Progressive muscle relaxation" is a technique in which the major muscle groups in the body are alternately tensed and relaxed. The process can proceed from the head to the feet or from the feet to the head. Progressive muscle relaxation can lead to deep levels of physical and mental relaxation. The idea is to tense and then relax the muscles in the forehead, eyes, mouth and jaw, neck, shoulders, upper back, chest, biceps, forearms, hands, stomach, buttocks, groin, legs, thighs, calves, and feet. Each muscle group is tensed for 5 seconds and then relaxed for 10–15 seconds, then tensed again for 5 seconds and relaxed again for 10–15 seconds. Generally you want to choose a time to do this exercise when it is relatively quiet, and in a place where you are comfortable and unlikely to be disturbed. It will take about 15 minutes to go through all the muscle groups.

When you use progressive muscle relaxation, it is really important to notice the difference between feelings of relaxation and feelings of tension. For some people, relaxation feels heavier or warmer than feeling tense. Others experience a lighter feeling. Whatever your experience is, notice the difference so you will become better aware of tension and relaxation in your body.

Once you become more aware of your muscle tension, you can use these relaxation exercises throughout your day and particularly when you begin to feel anxious. Different people carry muscle tension in different parts of their bodies, so the particular areas that need emphasis vary from person to person. Most people report increased levels of relaxation and decreased levels of physical tension and anxiety when they do progressive muscle relaxation. Repeated practice of any relaxation method creates even deeper levels of relaxation. Relaxation is a skill that can be developed, much like playing the piano or throwing a ball: The more you practice, the greater your development of the skill will be. When you become more skilled, this is a method that you can use as an alternative to avoidance, to help you manage your anxiety and stay on the steps of your Fear Ladder long enough for your anxiety level to go down.

Imagery

Imagery can be used to help you calm down before you enter a situation that is likely to make you feel anxious. Imagery can also give you the courage to stay in situations long enough to experience the natural reduction in anxiety that occurs over time. It helps to imagine scenes that are tranquil and relaxing to you, or inspirational ideas that increase your commitment to facing anxiety. Relaxing scenes may be actual places you know that feel safe and calming, or they may be tranquil scenes you create in your mind. Inspirational imagery can include people, music, or situations that increase your courage and confidence. The specific scene is less important than how the image makes you feel and whether it helps you face your anxiety.

The more senses you can incorporate into your image, the more helpful your imagery is likely to be. If you can imagine the smells, sounds, sights, and tactile sensations of the scene, you will improve your ability to relax or get inspired. For example, if you imagine yourself walking along a tree-lined mountain path, you may want to focus your attention on the birds singing, the light dancing through the tree branches, the smell of pine, the greenness of the forest, and the cool breeze as it touches your skin. If you have an inspirational scene from a movie, and you want to use this image to help you tolerate a higher level of anxiety, you might imagine how this person looks, the music playing in the background, and the feeling of courage in your chest. Each of your senses can contribute to your experience of relaxation and/or confidence.

Imagery does not need to be about a place or another person. You may find it helpful to vividly recall experiences in which you felt confident and capable. Jolene was nervous about an upcoming meeting with her manager. In the past she had found ways to avoid such meetings, but this was now a step on her Fear Ladder, and she was committed to taking that step. Before the meeting, she decided to use imagery to help calm herself, boost her confidence, and put herself in a better frame of mind. One area of her life where Jolene felt confident was her part-time job as a piano teacher. She decided to imagine vividly how she felt when she worked with her piano students. She remembered and imagined her sense of pride and accomplishment when her students played music well. She heard the music in her mind and felt the cooling air of the window fan in her piano room. She felt her back straighten, and she took on the posture of a successful teacher. After spending five minutes imagining this scene, Jolene felt calmer, more confident, and more capable. When she entered the meeting with her manager, she was able to sit tall in her chair, and she felt more prepared to stay in the situation and tolerate whatever anxiety arose.

EXERCISE: Practicing and Rating Relaxation Methods

So far you have learned how mindfulness and acceptance, breathing, progressive muscle relaxation, and imagery can help you manage your anxiety and stay longer in situations that make you anxious.

- Try each of these relaxation methods once or twice to see which ones work best for you.
- Use Worksheet 14.6 on the next page to rate your level of anxiety or tension on a 0–100 scale before and after each practice session.
- Once you identify the one or two methods that work best for you, start using them regularly.
- If you practice them every day, you are more likely to be able to use them effectively when you need them.

WORKSHEET 14.6. Ratings for My Relaxation Methods

Under "Relaxation Method Used," write "Mindfulness and acceptance," "Breathing," "Progressive muscle relaxation," or "Imagery." For each of your practice sessions, rate your anxiety or tension level on a 0–100 scale, where 0 is none at all and 100 is the most ever, both before and after the exercise. Do a number of practice sessions with each of the methods you want to try. At the bottom of the worksheet, make some comments about what you learn. See if your relaxation skills improve with practice, and also compare the different relaxation methods to learn which ones work best for you.

Relaxation Method Used	Anxiety/Tension Rating at Start (0–100)	Anxiety/Tension Rating at End (0–100)

What I learned (Did my relaxation improve with practice? Which methods work best for me?):

_____

_____

_____

From *Mind Over Mood, Second Edition.* Copyright 2016 by Dennis Greenberger and Christine A. Padesky. Purchasers of this book can photocopy and/or download additional copies of this worksheet (see the box at the end of the table of contents).

Changing Anxious Thoughts

Changing your anxious thoughts is one of the most important things you can do to bring about an enduring reduction in anxiety. Anxiety can be reduced either by decreasing your perception of danger or by increasing your confidence in your ability to cope with the things you fear. Many of the *Mind Over Mood* skills taught throughout this book will help you learn to test and change your anxious thoughts. At the end of this chapter, Figure 14.6 recommends an order in which to read *Mind Over Mood* chapters that will help you learn skills to manage your anxiety.

One main skill that will help with your anxiety is to use behavioral experiments (see Chapter 11) to test your thoughts related to steps on your Fear Ladder. As you have begun to do in this chapter, the fastest way to reduce anxiety is to face it by using a Fear Ladder. You can do experiments on each step of your Fear Ladder to see how you can cope with situations that you have previously avoided. These experiments offer the possibility of learning that you are more capable of coping than you originally believed. Chapter 10 helps you develop Action Plans and use acceptance to help you face situations on your Fear Ladder.

Chapter 11 teaches you about underlying assumptions, which are a common type of belief present in anxiety. For example, a common assumption for anxious people is "If something goes wrong, then I won't be able to cope." In Chapter 11, you learn how to set up behavioral experiments to test these types of anxious assumptions.

If working on your Fear Ladder is proving helpful for you, you can read and use the ideas taught in Chapters 10 and 11 as soon as you finish this chapter. If you decide to read those chapters first, you can read Chapters 5–9 of the book after you finish Chapters 10 and 11.

Chapters 5–9 teach you how to set personal goals, notice improvement, and test your anxious thoughts so that you can more quickly evaluate how dangerous a situation actually is and how well you can cope with it. Your anxiety may decrease if you examine the evidence and discover that the danger you face is not as bad as you thought and your ability to cope is better than you thought.

When Your Anxious Thought Is an Image

As described earlier in this chapter, anxious thoughts often occur in the form of images as well as words. These images can be still pictures, such as your face blushing. Very often, images appear more like a film in which an entire scene plays out. For example, you might imagine a sequence in which you say something embarrassing and then turn a deep shade of red, while people laugh at you and shake their heads as they walk away. Whether in words or images, anxious thoughts are usually either about danger ("Something will go wrong," "I'll die of embarrassment," "My boss will think less of me and I'll be fired") or the inability to cope ("I can't handle this," "I'm weak," "Other people are more confident than me").

Often images are distorted. For example, if you have an image of your boss being upset with you, your image might picture your boss as taller and more frightening than in real life. Or your image might exaggerate how uncomfortable you look to someone else. Such distortions are common in anxious imagery. Thought Records (Chapters 6–9) can be used to test your images and see how closely they fit your actual experience. You can also use experiments to test distorted beliefs. For example, if you imagine your face is deep red, you can take a selfie photo and compare the photo with your imagination.

When your anxious images are accurate descriptions of the dangers you face, it is helpful to figure out what strategies will best help you cope with them (Chapter 10). As you can see, changing anxious thoughts involves both testing your predictions of danger and improving your awareness of and confidence in your coping ability. The approaches you learn in this book will work equally well, whether your thoughts are in words or images.

Medication

Even though medications may offer relief from anxiety, they can interfere with lasting improvement. Research suggests that this is probably because medications often reduce opportunities to learn, practice, and develop new skills, such as those taught in this book. In addition, when people approach their fears while they are on medications, they tend to think that the drugs are the reason for their success. For example, imagine you succeed in staying for a long time on one of the steps of your Fear Ladder. If you do this while you are on a medication, you might think your success is due to the drug and not to your skills and coping practice.

An important part of overcoming anxiety is learning to tolerate feeling anxious. If medications reduce your feelings of anxiety, then you don't have the chance to learn that you are able to tolerate and manage these feelings. To develop skills to manage anxiety, you need to feel anxious and learn how to reduce and/or tolerate it. You cannot fully appreciate the effects of mindfulness and acceptance, breathing, progressive muscle relaxation, imagery, changing anxious thoughts, and overcoming avoidance if you are taking medication. One benefit of an initial high level of anxiety is that this increases our motivation to learn and practice coping skills. When we are very anxious, our desire to learn new methods to manage anxiety is very high.

The effectiveness of any intervention, including medication, is measured by relapse rates as well as by immediate effect. Relapse rates record the number of people helped by an intervention who reexperience the same symptoms when the treatment ends.

People who have been successfully treated for their anxiety disorders with only medication experience high rates of relapse. That is, the majority of people who benefit from medication as their only treatment for anxiety have a return of anxiety within a year after they stop taking the medication. In contrast, studies show that most people treated successfully with CBT for anxiety are still anxiety-free up to one year after the end of treatment. CBT teaches skills for managing anxiety that lead to long-lasting improvement. In other words, once you get better with CBT, you are likely to stay better. The same cannot be said of medication.

One additional caution regarding antianxiety medications is to be aware of their addiction potential. Many of the medications recommended to treat anxiety are tranquilizers. Tranquilizers have addiction potential. People who take tranquilizers for an extended period of time may develop tolerance, which means that it takes greater and greater amounts of the tranquilizer to produce a relaxed effect. In addition, after taking tranquilizers for an extended period of time, many people experience withdrawal symptoms if they suddenly stop taking the medication. Withdrawal symptoms include nausea, sweating, jitteriness, and an intense craving for the medication. Withdrawal and tolerance are two of the primary characteristics of addiction. This is why your physician will monitor you closely if you are on any of these medications. This is also why your physician may recommend this book to help you learn other methods to cope with your anxiety.

This does not mean that medication should never be used in the treatment of anxiety. However, most research suggests that when antianxiety medication is used, it should be used on a short-term basis only – for weeks instead of years. Also, research indicates that medication will rarely be enough to create enduring improvement. Learning anxiety management skills in CBT should be part of a treatment plan to maximize the likelihood of long-lasting results.

MAKING THE BEST USE OF *MIND OVER MOOD* FOR ANXIETY

If you have already read Chapters 1–4 (step A in Figure 14.6 on the next page) and completed all the exercises in this chapter (step B in Figure 14.6), you are now ready to develop other *Mind Over Mood* skills. While all of the skills taught in *Mind Over Mood* can help you with anxiety, it may be best to develop these skills in a particular sequence. For the most rapid relief from anxiety, read the remaining *Mind Over Mood* chapters in the order listed in Figure 14.6.

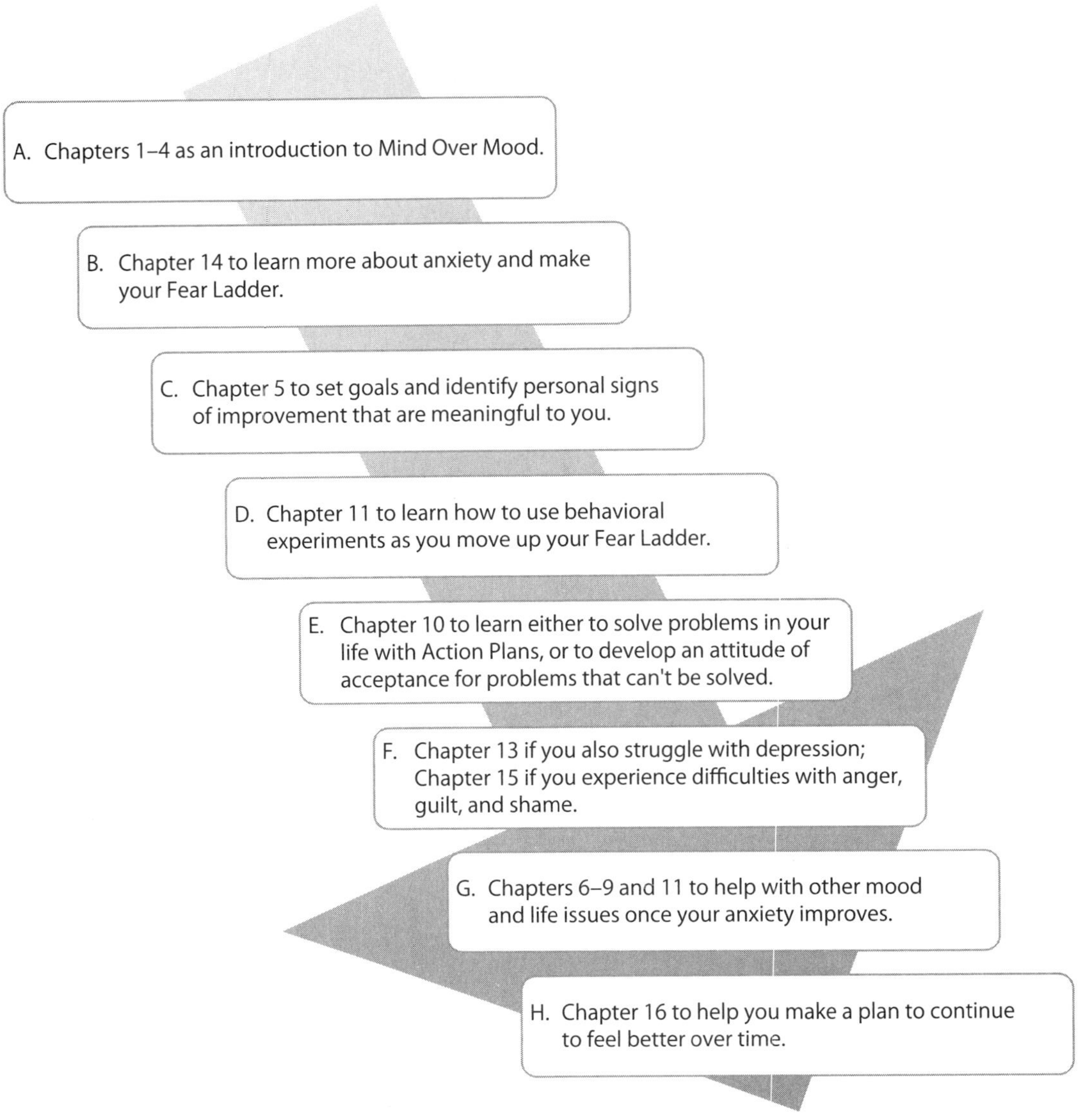

250   *Mind Over Mood*

A. Chapters 1–4 as an introduction to Mind Over Mood.

B. Chapter 14 to learn more about anxiety and make your Fear Ladder.

C. Chapter 5 to set goals and identify personal signs of improvement that are meaningful to you.

D. Chapter 11 to learn how to use behavioral experiments as you move up your Fear Ladder.

E. Chapter 10 to learn either to solve problems in your life with Action Plans, or to develop an attitude of acceptance for problems that can't be solved.

F. Chapter 13 if you also struggle with depression; Chapter 15 if you experience difficulties with anger, guilt, and shame.

G. Chapters 6–9 and 11 to help with other mood and life issues once your anxiety improves.

H. Chapter 16 to help you make a plan to continue to feel better over time.

FIGURE 14.6. *Mind Over Mood* chapter reading order for anxiety.

Chapter 14 Summary

▶ Common types of anxiety include phobias, social anxiety, panic disorder, posttraumatic stress disorder, health worries, and generalized anxiety disorder.

▶ Anxiety symptoms include a wide range of physical reactions; moods that range from nervousness to panic; avoidance of situations or feelings; and worries about danger, as well as thoughts about not being able to cope.

▶ Common behaviors when we are anxious are avoidance and safety behaviors. These types of behaviors reduce our anxiety in the short term, but make our anxiety worse over time.

▶ Anxious thoughts include overestimations of danger, along with underestimations of our ability to cope with the threats we anticipate.

▶ Thoughts that accompany anxiety often begin with "What if . . . ?" and contain the theme that "Something terrible is going to happen, and I won't be able to cope."

▶ Our anxious thoughts often occur as images. It is important to identify these images so we can respond to them in helpful ways.

▶ Different types of anxiety are characterized by different thoughts, depending on the type of dangers anticipated.

▶ One of the best ways to overcome anxiety is to face our fears through exposure to what scares us. A Fear Ladder is often used to help us face our fears one step at a time at a pace we can tolerate.

▶ Many skills can help us manage anxiety as we face our fears, including mindfulness and acceptance, breathing, progressive muscle relaxation, imagery, and changing our anxious thoughts.

▶ Medication may be helpful to some people in the short term, but it does not lead to enduring improvement in anxiety for most people.

▶ Changing our thoughts is an important way to achieve enduring improvement from anxiety.

▶ *Mind Over Mood* chapters can be customized and read in various orders, to help you learn *Mind Over Mood* skills for various purposes. Figure 14.6 describes a helpful chapter reading order for anxiety.

15

Understanding Your Anger, Guilt, and Shame

You may be reading this chapter because you or someone you care about struggles with anger, guilt, or shame. These moods affect almost all of us sometimes. They are a problem when they affect us more days than not, and when they lead us to make decisions or choices in our lives that hurt either us or other people.

Two of the people described in detail throughout this book struggled with these moods. Vic was a salesperson who generally got along well with colleagues and friends. However, he sometimes had explosive anger, especially when he felt disrespected or when people close to him didn't seem to care about him. His difficulties in controlling his anger at home created significant problems in his marriage with Judy. Marissa was a working mother of two teenage children. Despite overcoming many difficulties in her life, Marissa frequently experienced deep shame about having been sexually abused as a young girl. Her shame affected her self-esteem and her relationships.

As Vic's experiences illustrate, anger is a feeling that often leads us to attack and hurt others. When we experience guilt or shame, we may attack and hurt ourselves as Marissa did. This chapter describes anger, guilt, and shame, and details strategies for understanding and dealing with these moods.

If you are using this book to target anger, guilt, or shame, use the scales in Worksheet 15.1 to rate these moods on a regular basis. Positive change will show up as experiencing these moods less often, for shorter durations of time or less strongly. For example, if you are dealing with anger, as you progress through the book you may find that you get angry less often, stay angry for shorter periods of time, and feel it more mildly. Changes in any of these areas can be signs of progress and are important to track and measure over time.

> **EXERCISE: Measuring and Tracking My Moods**
>
> Worksheet 15.1 can be used to track a variety of moods including anger, guilt, shame, and positive moods such as happiness.

WORKSHEET 15.1. Measuring and Tracking My Moods

Use this worksheet to measure and track the frequency, strength, and duration of any mood you want to improve. This worksheet can also be used to measure and track positive emotions, including happiness.

Mood I am rating: _____

FREQUENCY

Circle or mark the number below that most accurately describes how often you experienced this mood this week:

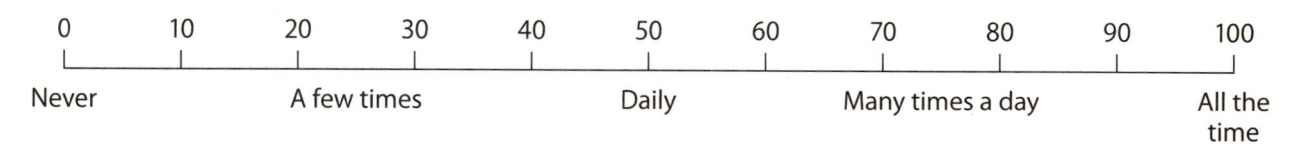

```
0      10     20     30     40     50     60     70     80     90     100
|      |      |      |      |      |      |      |      |      |      |
Never         A few times         Daily         Many times a day    All the
                                                                    time
```

STRENGTH

Circle or mark below how strongly you felt this mood this week. Rate the time when your mood was the strongest, even if most of the time you did not experience it this strongly. A score of 0 would mean that you did not feel the mood this week. A score of 100 would show that it was the strongest you have ever felt this mood in your life. Strongly felt moods will score higher than 70. If you felt the mood at a medium level of strength, give it a rating between 30 and 70. Rate a mild mood between 1 and 30.

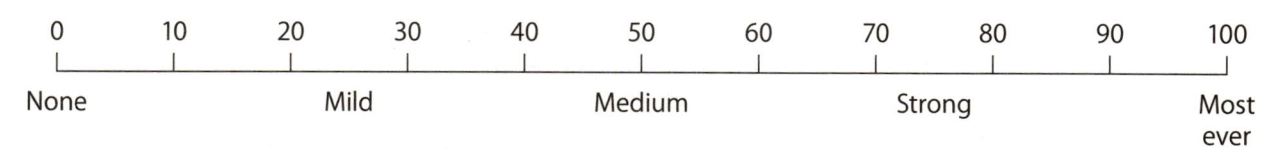

```
0      10     20     30     40     50     60     70     80     90     100
|      |      |      |      |      |      |      |      |      |      |
None          Mild          Medium        Strong                    Most
                                                                    ever
```

DURATION

Circle or mark the number below that matches how long your mood lasted. Again, make this rating for the time during the week when you felt this mood most strongly (think about the rating you gave this mood on the Strength scale above). If you did not experience the mood this week, circle 0.

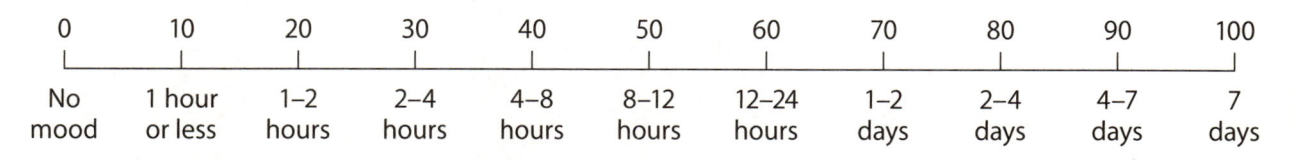

```
0       10      20      30      40      50      60      70      80      90      100
|       |       |       |       |       |       |       |       |       |       |
No      1 hour  1–2     2–4     4–8     8–12    12–24   1–2     2–4     4–7     7
mood    or less hours   hours   hours   hours   hours   days    days    days    days
```

From *Mind Over Mood, Second Edition*. Copyright 2016 by Dennis Greenberger and Christine A. Padesky. Purchasers of this book can photocopy and/or download additional copies of this worksheet (see the box at the end of the table of contents).

EXERCISE: Mood Scores

Use Worksheet 15.2 to record your scores on the frequency, strength, and duration of the mood(s) you are rating on Worksheet 15.1. You can label them F (frequency), S (strength), and D (duration) on Worksheet 15.2, or you can use different colors for each. By tracking all three types of mood ratings on the same chart, you will be able to see your progress as you learn *Mind Over Mood* skills. Use a different copy of Worksheet 15.2 for each mood you are rating. For example, you might be rating both shame and happiness, and you want to track each on a different Worksheet 15.2. There are additional copies of both these worksheets in the Appendix to this book and at *www.guilford.com/MOM2-materials*.

WORKSHEET 15.2. Mood Scores Chart

Mood I am rating:

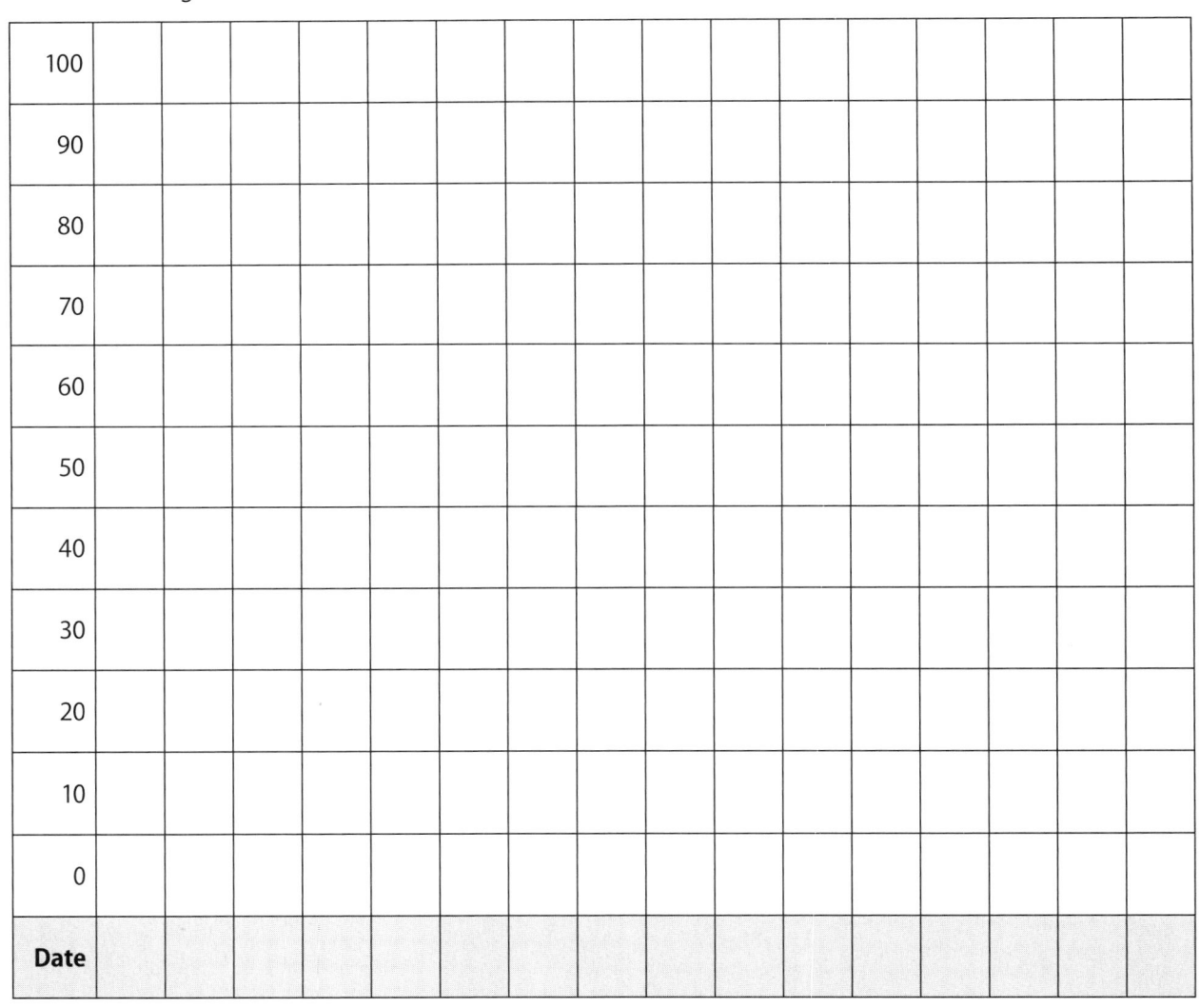

100														
90														
80														
70														
60														
50														
40														
30														
20														
10														
0														
Date														

From *Mind Over Mood, Second Edition.* Copyright 2016 by Dennis Greenberger and Christine A. Padesky. Purchasers of this book can photocopy and/or download additional copies of this worksheet (see the box at the end of the table of contents).

Once you have rated the frequency, strength, and duration of your mood, and marked your scores with today's date on Worksheet 15.2, you are ready to learn more about anger, guilt, and shame and what you can do to feel better for those moods.

ANGER

Rick asked his partner, John, to put his new shirt in the laundry while Rick went grocery shopping. John was happy to do this and put the shirt in the dryer after it was washed. When Rick got home, he asked about the shirt, and John realized he had forgotten to take it out of the dryer. When he removed the shirt from the dryer, it appeared to have shrunk. Rick was furious because he thought John should have been more careful and read the instructions to find out if the shirt could be machine dried. Rick yelled at John, "You don't care about my stuff! You are so careless and thoughtless!" John was hurt. Although he felt bad about Rick's shirt, he thought that Rick's anger was out of proportion. John yelled back, "It's your fault! If your shirt needed special care, you should have told me! I won't do you any more favors!"

You may or may not express anger as Rick and John did, but you probably have experienced similar feelings of anger when you thought that you were being seriously mistreated, or that someone was hurting you or taking advantage of you. As all moods are, anger is accompanied by changes in thinking, behavior, and physical reactions, as shown in Figure 15.1. When we are angry, our bodies mobilize for defense or attack. Our thoughts are often filled with plans for retaliation or "getting even," or we focus on how "unfairly" we have been treated.

Notice that the emotion of anger can range from irritation to rage. How angry we become in a given situation is influenced by our interpretation of the meaning of the event. After their argument about the shirt, John became silent the rest of the day. If

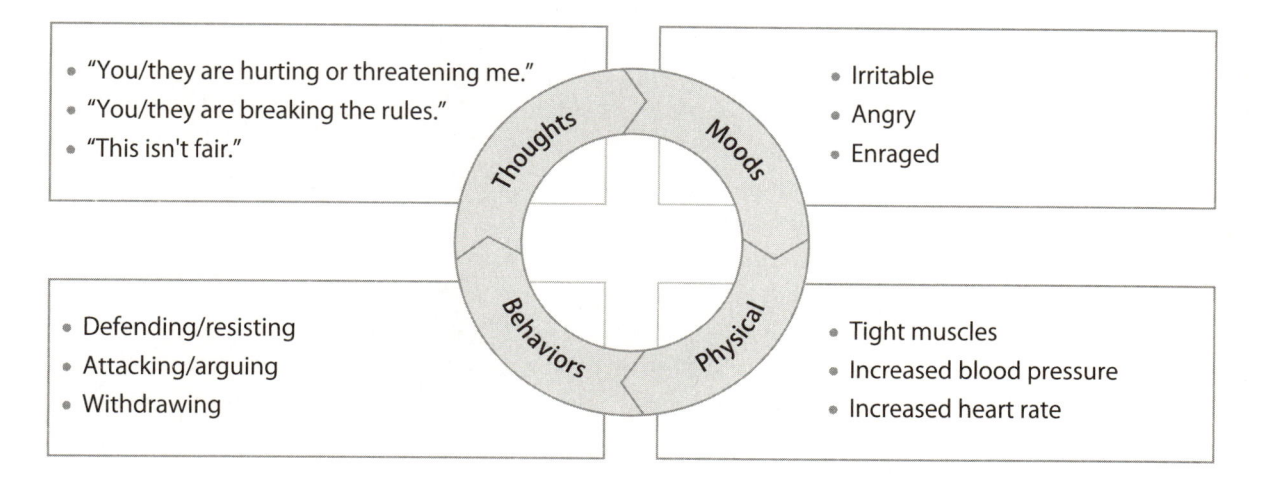

Thoughts
- "You/they are hurting or threatening me."
- "You/they are breaking the rules."
- "This isn't fair."

Moods
- Irritable
- Angry
- Enraged

Behaviors
- Defending/resisting
- Attacking/arguing
- Withdrawing

Physical
- Tight muscles
- Increased blood pressure
- Increased heart rate

FIGURE 15.1. Profile of anger symptoms.

Rick interpreted this reaction as John's having hurt feelings, Rick might be mildly irritated or even concerned for John's feelings. However, if Rick thought that John's silence meant John didn't care about him or was ignoring his concerns, Rick would probably feel much angrier.

There is great individual variation in the types of events that elicit anger. One person may get angry while standing in line, and yet may listen calmly to criticisms of job performance. A different person may be perfectly content to stand in line, and yet may quickly attack anyone who points out work flaws. The types of events that provoke our anger are usually linked to our past, as well as to rules and beliefs that we hold.

For example, if we have been abused frequently or severely in the past, we may have a tendency to be "on guard" against future abuse. Some people who have a long history of abuse or criticism are quick to see current events as abusive and may experience chronic anger, sometimes seemingly out of proportion to the events that provoke their anger.

The pattern of quick and frequent anger goes along with a belief that it is possible to protect ourselves by confronting abuse. What about people who have been frequently abused, but who feel helpless to protect themselves? People who believe they are helpless often react to abuse not with anger, but with resignation or depression. If you feel helpless in the face of abuse, your challenge may be learning to experience anger when someone is hurting you, rather than learning to control it. Therefore, anger can be a problem either because it is too frequent, out of proportion to the event, and expressed in destructive ways, or because it is absent. It is normal to feel angry sometimes, and anger can be a healthy and adaptive response.

EXERCISE: Understanding Anger

To understand what happens when you are angry, remember a recent time when you felt angry or irritated. Describe the situation in column 1 of the partial Thought Record in Worksheet 15.3. Write one word to describe your mood in this situation (e.g., anger or irritation). On a 0–100 scale, with 100 being enraged or the angriest you have ever felt, 50 being a medium level of anger, and 10 being mildly irritated, rate your mood.

At the point when you were most angry, what was going through your mind? Write these thoughts (words, images, memories) in column 3. If you are uncertain what thoughts, images, or memories you had in this situation, Chapter 7 teaches you how to identify these.

If anger is a mood you want to understand better, repeat this exercise for two other recent situations in which you have been angry: Describe the situations; rate the intensity of your mood; and then write down your thoughts, including any images or memories you had. Once you have filled out Worksheet 15.3 for several situations, proceed to the next two sections of this chapter, which will give you a better understanding of anger and outline approaches to help you manage and/or express your anger in constructive rather than destructive ways.

WORKSHEET 15.3. Understanding Anger, Guilt, and Shame

1. Situation	2. Moods	3. Automatic Thoughts (Images)
Who? What? When? Where?	a. What did you feel? b. Rate each mood (0–100%).	a. What was going through your mind just before you started to feel this way? Any other thoughts? Images? Memories? b. Circle or mark the hot thought.

From *Mind Over Mood, Second Edition*. Copyright 2016 by Dennis Greenberger and Christine A. Padesky. Purchasers of this book can photocopy and/or download additional copies of this worksheet (see the box at the end of the table of contents).

Angry Thoughts

Anger is linked to a perception of threat, damage, or hurt, and to a belief that important rules have been violated. We also can become angry if we think we have been treated unfairly or prevented from obtaining something we expected to achieve. In the fight over the damaged shirt, Rick was angry because he expected that John would clean his shirt without any damage. John was angry because Rick's personal attack ("You are so careless and thoughtless!") seemed very unfair. It discounted his love and caring for Rick and his good intentions in laundering the shirt. Notice the emphasis on fairness, reasonableness, and expectation. It is not simply the hurt or damage that makes us angry, but the violation of our rules and expectations.

Imagine a man who loses his job. Does he feel angry? It depends. If the man loses his job and considers this a fair decision (perhaps because the company went bankrupt and all of its employees lost their jobs), he is unlikely to feel angry. However, if he thinks his job loss was unfair (perhaps others were not fired, or only men of a certain race or age lost their jobs), then he may feel very angry.

Similarly, if a child steps on your foot while you are riding on a bus, you feel pain. Whether or not you feel angry depends on your interpretation of the intent and reasonableness of the child's behavior. Your anger is likely to be quick if you think the injury was intentional. But if you think that the child stepped on your foot by accident when a swerve of the bus made the child lose balance, you may wince in pain, but you probably do not feel anger. The probability of anger in response to an injury is related to your judgments of reasonableness or intention. For example, on an overcrowded bus, you may overlook someone's stepping on your foot more easily than you do on a nearly empty bus.

These rules of anger may seem quite straightforward until you consider that people vary greatly in what they consider fair and reasonable. Rick expected John to be attentive and supportive to him, even when Rick was behaving in ways John considered hurtful. John expected Rick to speak calmly to him, even when Rick was feeling enraged. Both Rick and John believed that their own expectations were reasonable and the other's expectations were unrealistic.

As Rick and John discovered, anger is most likely to emerge in close relationships. Anger is rarely so intense as when it is experienced with someone with whom we are in close contact, whether this person is a love partner or a work colleague. The link between anger and intimacy can be best understood by recognizing that each of us has multiple expectations for our friendships, love relationships, work partnerships, and so forth. We are less likely to have specific personal expectations for people we meet casually. We rarely feel intense anger toward a store clerk, because our expectations for this type of relationship are quite low. The closer our relationship with someone, the more likely it is that we have high expectations of this person. To complicate the picture, we may not tell people about our expectations, or even become aware of them ourselves, until they have been broken. Then we feel hurt, disappointed, and often angry.

Anger Management Strategies

Testing Angry Thoughts

How we respond to angry thoughts depends on the role these thoughts play in our lives. If we rarely experience anger, and angry thoughts arise from a clear injustice, our response will be to find out how to use our anger to respond constructively to the situation. When we are frequently angry, especially if our anger creates problems for us and our relationships, then we want to learn to examine our angry thoughts and see if there might be another way of thinking about things. The Thought Record, which you learned to use in Chapters 6–9, is a good tool for learning to think in alternative ways.

When we are angry, we tend to interpret or misinterpret other people's intentions in a personal and negative way. We may think that they are intentionally mistreating us or taking advantage of us, even when this is not the case. For example, suppose you are standing a few feet from the counter in a store, waiting for a clerk to finish with another customer because you need help. As soon as the clerk finishes with that customer, someone else walks up to the counter and begins to talk to the clerk. If you think that this person saw you and deliberately stepped in front of you, you might feel angry. If, on the other hand, you thought that this was an honest mistake and the person did not see you standing there, then you are less likely to feel angry. The difference between these two reactions is whether we personalize the other person's actions. Do we think they did this "to us," or was the other person unaware that we were standing there?

When we get angry, we tend to personalize other people's actions. One of the advantages of Thought Records is that they help you think through these types of situations. You can learn to ask yourself questions that help you consider other people's intentions. Thought Records can help you consider alternative explanations for other people's behavior. Can you remember a time when you stepped in front of someone else who was waiting in line because you didn't see that person standing there? You did not intend to take advantage of the person. Instead, it was a simple mistake that everyone makes from time to time. Learning to interpret other people's actions less personally, to consider the intentions of other people in a kinder way, and to look at situations from different perspectives are helpful ways of responding to anger.

Angry thoughts often put people in boxes, so to speak. In the example earlier in this chapter, Rick became very angry with John when John washed Rick's shirt and it shrank. Rick called John "careless" and "thoughtless." We often label other people like Rick did when we get angry. If these labels are used often enough, they become boxes that block our flexible view of the other person's intentions. If Rick continued to think of John as "thoughtless," then he might start to misinterpret many behaviors as proof of this label. For example, if John walked into the kitchen and poured himself a cup of coffee, Rick might think, "Oh, he's so thoughtless. He didn't offer me a cup." Rick did not consider that John knew that Rick never drank more than one cup of coffee and he'd already had one cup that morning. John was not being thoughtless, but was demonstrating his attentiveness to Rick's habits. In fact, John thought of himself as attentive and caring, and his behavior generally backed this up. Putting a person in a box with a single label on it usually results in lots of misinterpretations and unnecessary upset.

If you find yourself labeling and judging someone in your life in a consistent way, this is often a sign that you have put this person in a box. When you become aware of this, there are several things you can do to reduce your anger and open up the box. First, you can be aware of your "hot button" issues that get pushed. Rick realized he was very sensitive to signs that his feelings and needs are being ignored. When your hot buttons get pushed, instead of reacting in an angry way, you can try to be a nonjudgmental observer and get more information, so you can test your assumptions about other people's intentions.

Rick wanted to improve his relationship with John. So rather than get silently angry about John's getting a cup of coffee for himself, Rick asked John, "Why didn't you get me a cup of coffee?" This gave Rick a chance to test his assumption that John was being thoughtless. John replied, "I saw you already had a cup of coffee this morning, and I know you never drink more than one cup. But if you want another, I'm happy to get you one. I'll make a fresh pot." John's reply gave Rick additional information and helped him realize that John's behavior was not "thoughtless" at all. The advantage of gathering more information when we start to think negatively about others is that it often helps us understand other people's actions in new ways.

Other methods that may help you control your anger include anticipating and preparing for events that place you at high risk for experiencing anger, recognizing the early warning signs of anger, timeouts, assertion training, and couple or family therapy.

Using Imagery to Anticipate and Prepare for Events

It can help to anticipate and prepare for situations in which you are likely to get angry. Calming down before entering these situations prepares you to handle events that might normally trigger anger. The imagery methods described in Chapter 14 (on pp. 244–245) as ways to lower anxiety can also be used to prepare you for situations in which you are at risk for losing your temper. In addition to using imagery to calm yourself, you can use imagery to plan and prepare the types of responses you want to make.

It is best to use imagery before entering a situation in which you are at high risk for losing your temper. You may find it helpful to imagine yourself saying what you want to say, in the manner in which you want to say it, and getting the response you hope to get. Just in case things don't turn out as well as you hope, it may be helpful to imagine how you can handle problems that might occur. Mentally rehearsing responses to challenging situations can help you feel more confident and less threatened if things go poorly. In turn, this confidence can help you respond in effective and adaptive ways, rather than simply erupting in anger when things don't work out. Imagery works, in part, because it helps you think through possible problem areas and design your response in advance. Furthermore, it can be helpful to see yourself as effective and relaxed in a high-risk, stressful situation. Finally, it is helpful to construct an ideal image of how you want to respond; the image can help guide your responses in the actual situation.

If you can identify a situation that is going to be stressful and in which you are at high risk for experiencing anger, you have the opportunity to plan, write out, and rehearse exactly what you want to say and how you want to say it. This script can help you develop a strategy targeted to what you want to achieve and enter the situation with a greater degree of confidence.

Recognizing Early Warning Signs of Anger

In addition to the anticipation of situations in which you are likely to be angry, it can be helpful to recognize the signs that you are becoming angry or that your anger is getting out of control. For many people, early warning signs of anger that might get out of control include shakiness, muscle tension, clenched jaw, chest pressure, yelling, clenched fists, and saying things that are not true. Some anger is OK – but when you recognize that you are beginning to move into a destructive zone of anger, take a moment to remind yourself of your options. You can choose to be angry, or to use timeouts or assertion as described below to calm down.

Timeouts

Timeouts can be an effective way to control your anger. Taking a timeout involves removing yourself from the situation you are in when the early warning signs indicate that your anger might get out of control. Taking a timeout helps you reclaim control over yourself and over the situation. You can remind yourself what is important to you and what you are trying to accomplish.

The effective use of timeouts involves recognizing the earliest signs that your anger is interfering with how you want to handle the situation or is becoming destructive. You can use timeouts as athletes do: to regroup, strategize, relax, or simply rest. Your timeout may be as short as 5 minutes or as long as 24 hours. The timeout is not used to avoid a situation, but rather to enable you to approach the situation from a new angle and with a fresh start. At times, merely getting out of the situation will help you to view it differently. During the timeout, you may also find it helpful to practice the relaxation exercises described in Chapter 14 (on p. 243). You may find that you get the most out of a timeout when you use it to test some of your angry thoughts (as described earlier in this chapter and in Chapters 6–9). Some people try to reenter the situation with a new strategy in mind, to minimize the possibility of an angry blowup. As described earlier, you can use imagery to practice what you plan to say and do before you go back into the situation.

Assertion

Learning to be assertive can reduce difficulties with anger. Assertion is often described as the middle road between being aggressive and passively allowing someone to take advantage of us. When we are aggressive, we attack the other person. When we are overly passive, we allow others to attack us. Assertion describes a middle road in which we stand up for ourselves without attacking the other person. For example, here are three responses to someone who calls us "stupid."

Aggressive: (*shouting*) "If you think I'm stupid, you are an idiot!"

Assertive: (*calm and firm*) "You might think I'm stupid, but let's get back to the real issue, which is *XYZ*."

Passive: (*hanging head, saying nothing*)

Assertion also means expressing wants and needs in a straightforward way. For example, suppose you are coming home from work, and your children all start asking for your attention at once. If you are tired and try to satisfy all their needs (passive), you may start feeling overwhelmed and eventually blow up in anger at them (aggressive). It is often better to be assertive and say something like this: "I'm really tired and need a few minutes to myself before I can play with you." This gives you time to regroup, remember how much you love your children, and prepare yourself for spending time with them and/or setting limits as necessary. In this way, assertion can reduce the frequency of being treated unfairly or being taken advantage of, and therefore can prevent situations that give rise to anger. It also gives you a greater sense of control in your life.

Four Strategies to Help You Plan and Practice Assertive Responses

1. Use "I" statements. Angry statements tend to begin with the word "you" and express blame for problems (e.g., "You always think of yourself first"). Starting a conversation in this way often puts the other person on the defensive, and the person is then less likely to hear what you have to say. Assertive responses often begin with "I" and express your reactions, needs, and wishes (e.g., "I really would like you to listen to what I'm thinking and feeling"). Expressing a need or request is more likely to lead the other person to hear your message, and is thus more likely to lead to a productive conversation.

2. Acknowledge any truth in someone's complaints about you, and at the same time stand up for your own rights. For example, imagine that someone asks you to do something, and you say no. The other person then says, "But I really need you to do this for me, and it seems selfish for you not to help out if you can." You might reply, "I understand you are disappointed, and yet I need to say no, because I am really tired right now. That is not being selfish; it is just taking care of myself."

3. Make clear and simple statements of your wants and needs, rather than expecting other people to read your mind or anticipate what you want. It is assertive to ask directly for help, tell others what you need, and be clear about your expectations. You might tell your partner, "My feet are hurting. Would you please give me a foot massage?" A mother might say to her children, "Please pick up all your toys and put them away. When I come back, I expect the floor to be clear." Or a manager might say, "I need you to have this project done by 3 o'clock today. Please let me know if anything interferes with meeting that deadline."

4. Focus on the process of assertion rather than results. Being assertive doesn't mean that you will always get what you ask for. The goal of assertion is clear communication. Even though there is no guarantee that each assertive statement will lead to a desired outcome, consistent assertive communication is likely to lead over time to more positive relationships.

Thoughts and Assumptions That Interfere with Being Assertive

"If you really like/love me, then you will know what I need."

"People won't like me if I say no."

"Why bother? I'm not going to get what I want anyhow."

"It's not worth the argument it is going to create."

"I can live with this the way it is."

"If someone is not speaking nicely to me, I don't need to respond nicely."

These assumptions can be harmful to relationships. People who care deeply about us often do not know what we want or need. The assumption that people *should* know without our saying anything leads to frequent hurt and anger. Making clear and simple statements about your wants and needs is a good relationship skill and often reduces the hurt and irritation that can lead to anger.

If these types of thoughts interfere with your assertion, you can test them by using the skills taught in Chapters 6–9. You can also test your thoughts and the usefulness of assertion by doing behavioral experiments as taught in Chapter 11.

Forgiving Others

When someone has deeply or repeatedly hurt us, anger can last a long time. Ongoing anger can eat away at our spirit and prevent us from experiencing happiness and joy. In this case, finding a way to let go of anger may be worthwhile. Forgiving others who have hurt us can help us let go of anger and hurt. If the person who hurt us is sorry and apologizes, forgiveness is a bit easier. However, if the person is not sorry for what has been done or said, then forgiveness is often more difficult. It is helpful to keep in mind that forgiveness is about relieving ourselves of the burden of anger. It does not mean overlooking the actions of the other person; it means looking at those actions in a different way. For example, we might accept that the person who hurt us is troubled or has his or her own issues to work out.

Sometimes we may decide not to forgive someone, such as when someone continues abusing us or those we care about. In this case, the only way to let go of anger may be to accept that the other person is abusive, be clear in our own minds that we are not to blame, and figure out ways to protect ourselves from future abuse. Action Plans, described in Chapter 10, can help us design a series of actions and responses to protect ourselves from abuse. Sometimes this includes putting distance between ourselves and the abusive person.

If you decide you want to forgive someone, here are two approaches that can help. Remember that you can engage in this process of forgiveness for your own sake, and not for the benefit of the other person. In fact, you do not even need to communicate your forgiveness to the other person. Option 2 below (writing a forgiveness letter) can foster forgiveness even if you are no longer in contact with the person who hurt you.

1. Directly tell other people how they have hurt you, in order to help them understand why you are angry. If you use "I" statements as described in the section on assertion above, the other person has a chance to consider your perspective and respond. For example, you might say to a spouse or a good friend, "I feel like an outsider when you don't introduce me to your friends. When you continue to do this, even though we have talked about it many times, I get the message that you really don't care about my feelings." If the other person apologizes, you can decide either to forgive the person or to talk about what future changes you need in order to forgive. For example, you might say, "I want to believe you and forgive you. If you introduce me to some of your friends over the next month, this will begin to show me that you really do care, and it will make it easier for me to stop feeling hurt and angry."

2. Write a forgiveness letter describing the hurt or damage that was done to you. This is a letter that you are not going to send. It is important not to censor your thoughts as you write the letter. Also, do not think about how the other person would react if she or he ever read the letter. This letter of forgiveness is for you – not for the person you are forgiving. Therefore, you can write the letter with full freedom, because the person who hurt you is never going to read it.

> **EXERCISE: Writing a Forgiveness Letter**
>
> Use Worksheet 15.4 as a guide to help you write your forgiveness letter. It is not easy to forgive those who have mistreated us, but it can be instrumental in healing deep wounds and letting go of anger. If you are not ready at this point to write a forgiveness letter, that is fine. Just skip over this exercise and section, and perhaps come back to these pages at another time – if you choose to do so.

WORKSHEET 15.4. Writing a Forgiveness Letter

1. This is what you did to me:

2. This is the impact it has had in my life:

3. This is how it continues to affect me:

4. This is how I imagine my life will be better if I'm able to forgive you:

5. (Forgiveness often begins with a compassionate understanding of persons who have hurt you. Write about any life experiences the other person or persons had that might have contributed to the ways they hurt or mistreated you.) This is how I can understand what you have done:

6. (Everyone hurts someone else sometimes. When you hurt someone else, how would you want that person to think about you?) This is how I would want to be viewed if I hurt someone:

7. (Forgiveness does not mean that you approve of, forget, or deny what was done and the pain you have experienced. Instead, forgiveness means finding a way to let go of your anger and understand the events from a different perspective.) This is how I can forgive what you have done:

8. These are the qualities I have that will allow me to move forward:

From *Mind Over Mood, Second Edition.* Copyright 2016 by Dennis Greenberger and Christine A. Padesky. Purchasers of this book can photocopy and/or download additional copies of this worksheet (see the box at the end of the table of contents).

EXERCISE: Rating Anger Management Strategies

So far, you have learned how testing angry thoughts, preparing for events with imagery, recognizing early warning signs of anger, timeouts, assertion, and forgiveness can help you manage your anger. Try some of these anger management methods to see which ones work best for you. To figure this out, use Worksheet 15.5 to rate your level of anger on a 0–100 scale before and after using them. Once you identify the one or two methods that work best for you, start using them regularly. The more you practice, the more likely it is that you will be able to use these strategies effectively when you need them.

WORKSHEET 15.5. Ratings for My Anger Management Strategies

Under "Anger Management Method," write "Testing thoughts," "Imagery preparation," "Recognizing early warning signs," "Timeout," "Assertion," or "Forgiveness." For each of your practice sessions, rate your anger on a 0–100 scale, where 0 is none at all and 100 is the most ever, both before and after the exercise. Do a number of practice sessions with each of the methods you want to try. At the bottom of the worksheet, make some comments about what you learn. See if your anger management skills improve with practice, and also compare the different methods to learn which ones work best for you.

Anger Management Method	Anger Rating at Start (0–100%)	Anger Rating at End (0–100%)

What I learned (Did my anger management improve with practice? Which methods work best for me?):

_____

_____

_____

From *Mind Over Mood, Second Edition*. Copyright 2016 by Dennis Greenberger and Christine A. Padesky. Purchasers of this book can photocopy and/or download additional copies of this worksheet (see the box at the end of the table of contents).

Couple or Family Therapy

For some people, anger mostly occurs with family members. If the anger management strategies described above do not help you handle anger in your closest relationships, couple or family therapy can help. Your perceptions, attitudes, beliefs, and thoughts about your partner, your children, or other family members can fuel your anger. Therapy can teach you how to communicate better, increase positive interactions in your relationships, and to develop negotiation skills. It can also help you learn strategies for identifying and altering expectations and rules. These skills can reduce anger and improve the quality of your relationships.

GUILT AND SHAME

Guilt and shame are closely connected emotions. We tend to feel guilty when we believe we have violated rules that are important to us, or when we have not lived up to standards that we have set for ourselves. We feel guilty when we judge that we have done something wrong. If we think we "should" have behaved differently or that we "ought" to have done better, we are likely to feel guilt.

Shame also involves the sense that we have done something wrong. However, when we feel ashamed, we assume that what we have done wrong means that we are "flawed," "no good," "inadequate," "rotten," "awful," or "bad." Shame is usually connected to a highly negative view of ourselves. Secretiveness often surrounds shame. We may think, "If others knew this secret, they would be disgusted with me or think less of me." For this reason, the source of shame is rarely revealed and remains hidden and destructive. Shame often accompanies a family secret involving other family members – a secret such as alcoholism, sexual abuse, abortion, bankruptcy, or other behavior considered dishonorable in the community.

Marissa was ashamed that she had been sexually abused. Although the abuse had begun when she was 6 years old, Marissa never fully revealed the extent of her abuse until she was 26 years old. She had attempted to tell her mother about the abuse when she was younger, but was scolded and accused of lying. Whenever Marissa had memories of the sexual abuse, she was overwhelmed by feelings of shame. While in therapy, Marissa filled out Worksheet 15.3 on page 257. Her worksheet demonstrated the connection between her thoughts and her shame (Figure 15.2 on p. 268). This example demonstrates the secretive nature of shame ("I could never tell Julie this happened . . ."), as well as how shame was connected to Marissa's view of herself as "awful" and "despicable."

Overcoming Guilt and Shame

Overcoming guilt and shame does not necessarily mean letting yourself off the hook if you believe you have done something wrong. It does mean taking an appropriate amount of responsibility and coming to terms with whatever led you to feel this way.

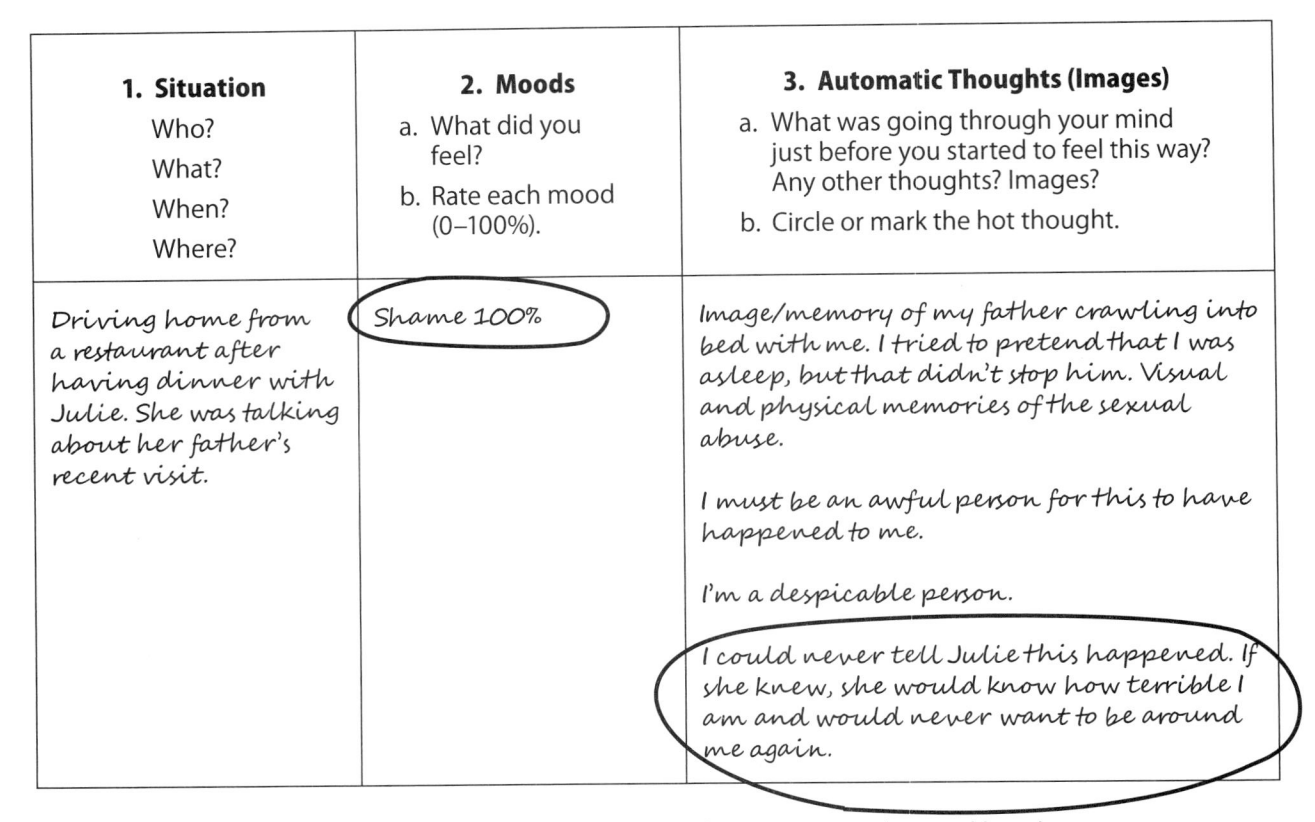

1. Situation Who? What? When? Where?	2. Moods a. What did you feel? b. Rate each mood (0–100%).	3. Automatic Thoughts (Images) a. What was going through your mind just before you started to feel this way? Any other thoughts? Images? b. Circle or mark the hot thought.
Driving home from a restaurant after having dinner with Julie. She was talking about her father's recent visit.	(Shame 100%)	Image/memory of my father crawling into bed with me. I tried to pretend that I was asleep, but that didn't stop him. Visual and physical memories of the sexual abuse. I must be an awful person for this to have happened to me. I'm a despicable person. (I could never tell Julie this happened. If she knew, she would know how terrible I am and would never want to be around me again.)

FIGURE 15.2. Marissa's responses on Worksheet 15.3 to understand her shame.

There are five aspects to overcoming guilt and shame: assessing the seriousness of your actions, weighing personal responsibility, making reparations for any harm you caused, breaking the silence surrounding shame, and self-forgiveness. Often only one or two of these exercises are necessary to help in overcoming guilt. Overcoming shame may require working on all five aspects.

Assessing the Seriousness of Your Actions

We can feel guilty or ashamed about both large and small actions. How would you compare the seriousness of these three actions on Toby's part?

1. Toby was tired at the end of the day. Her phone rang, and she decided not to answer it, because she didn't feel like talking to anyone. She heard her mother's voice on the answering machine saying, "Toby, are you there? I want to tell you about my vacation." Toby didn't answer the phone.

2. After Toby's mother had left her message, the phone rang again. When Toby heard her best friend's voice on the answering machine, she picked up the phone and chatted for 10 minutes.

3. The next day Toby told her mother that she had not been home when her mother called the night before.

Toby's three experiences describe fairly small events. Yet many people would judge the seriousness of these events differently. For which of these three events would you be likely to feel guilty? Why?

Your evaluation of the seriousness of an action or thought depends on your own rules and values. Many people say that they would feel guiltier about lying to their mothers (example 3) than about not answering the phone (example 1). Some people may feel equally guilty in all three examples.

Frequent guilt and shame mean either that you are living your life in a way that violates your principles (e.g., having an affair when you believe in monogamous marriage), or that you are judging too many small actions as serious. To evaluate the seriousness of your actions leading to guilt and shame, you can answer the questions in the Helpful Hints on page 270. These questions encourage you to look at the situation from different perspectives. This will be particularly helpful if you tend to feel guilt or shame in many situations, even when others with similar values do not feel that way. Perspective-shifting questions can help you evaluate the seriousness of your actions. Ask yourself, "How important will this seem in five years?" Having an affair will almost certainly still seem like a big violation of a monogamous relationship in five years. Arriving home late for dinner three nights in a row will not seem important in five years, even if it is a distressing event for you or your partner now. Therefore, lasting guilt about an affair would make more sense than lasting guilt about arriving home late for dinner.

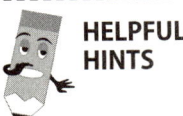

HELPFUL HINTS — **Questions to Evaluate the Seriousness of My Actions**

- Do other people consider this experience to be as serious as I do? Why?
- Do some people consider it less serious? Why?
- How serious would I consider the experience if my best friend did this instead of me?
- How important will this experience seem in one month? One year? Five years?
- How serious would I consider the experience if someone did it to me?
- Did I know ahead of time the meaning or consequences of my actions (or thoughts)? Based on what I knew at the time, do my current judgments apply?
- Did any damage occur? If so, can it be corrected? If so, how long will this take?
- Was there an even worse action I considered and avoided (e.g., I considered lying but instead avoided answering the phone)?

EXERCISE: Rating the Seriousness of My Actions

Using the questions in the Helpful Hints as a guide, rate how serious you think your actions are on the Worksheet 15.6 scales. Since people have different values and beliefs about what is right and wrong, you should first make the endpoints personal to you. At the 100 mark on the scale at the top of the worksheet, write the most serious wrong action you could imagine a person doing. For example, this might be to torture and murder someone. While 0 would not be serious at all, 10 might be something like not returning a small amount of extra change you were overpaid in a store.

Label a few marks on the scale at the top of Worksheet 15.6 so that you see the differences among minor, medium, and serious actions that you might feel guilt or shame about. Then think of the worst thing you have ever done in your life. Assuming that it is less serious than torture and murder, put that action on the scale where you think it belongs.

Once you have created your personal scale, use it to rate the seriousness of actions that prompt you to feel guilt or shame.

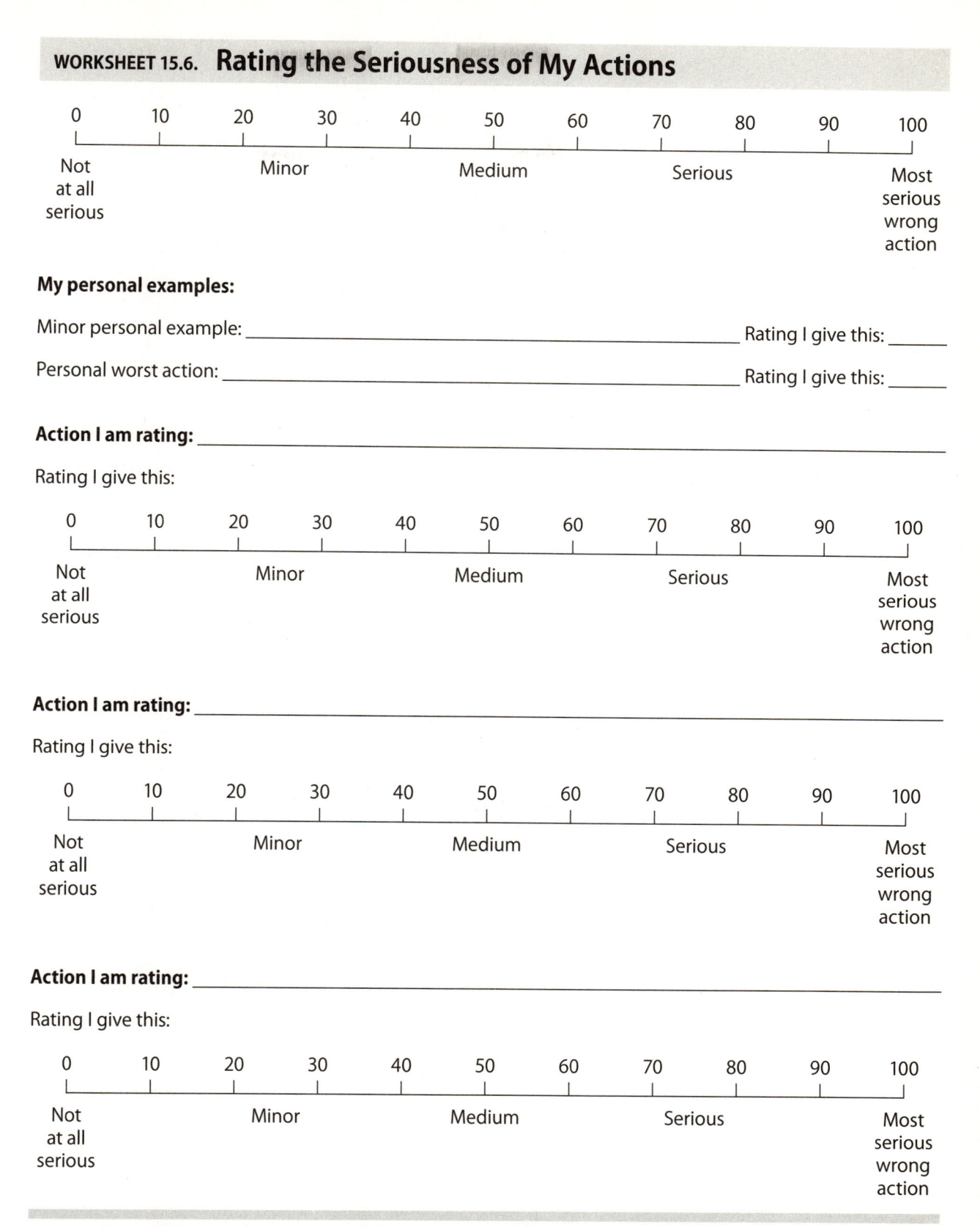

WORKSHEET 15.6. Rating the Seriousness of My Actions

```
0    10    20    30    40    50    60    70    80    90    100
|─────|─────|─────|─────|─────|─────|─────|─────|─────|─────|
Not         Minor         Medium         Serious        Most
at all                                                  serious
serious                                                 wrong
                                                        action
```

My personal examples:

Minor personal example: _____ Rating I give this: _____

Personal worst action: _____ Rating I give this: _____

Action I am rating: _____

Rating I give this:

```
0    10    20    30    40    50    60    70    80    90    100
|─────|─────|─────|─────|─────|─────|─────|─────|─────|─────|
Not         Minor         Medium         Serious        Most
at all                                                  serious
serious                                                 wrong
                                                        action
```

Action I am rating: _____

Rating I give this:

```
0    10    20    30    40    50    60    70    80    90    100
|─────|─────|─────|─────|─────|─────|─────|─────|─────|─────|
Not         Minor         Medium         Serious        Most
at all                                                  serious
serious                                                 wrong
                                                        action
```

Action I am rating: _____

Rating I give this:

```
0    10    20    30    40    50    60    70    80    90    100
|─────|─────|─────|─────|─────|─────|─────|─────|─────|─────|
Not         Minor         Medium         Serious        Most
at all                                                  serious
serious                                                 wrong
                                                        action
```

From *Mind Over Mood, Second Edition.* Copyright 2016 by Dennis Greenberger and Christine A. Padesky. Purchasers of this book can photocopy and/or download additional copies of this worksheet (see the box at the end of the table of contents).

Weighing Personal Responsibility

Once you have assessed the seriousness of your actions, it is helpful to weigh how much of your perceived wrongdoing is your personal responsibility. Marissa felt ashamed that she was molested as a child. The molestation was certainly a serious event in her life, but was she responsible for it? Vic felt guilty that he blew up in anger at his wife, Judy, one night when she started complaining about their overdue credit card bills. Was he responsible for his angry reaction?

A good way to weigh personal responsibility is to construct a "responsibility pie." To do this, list all the people and aspects of a situation that contributed to an event about which you feel guilty or ashamed. Include yourself on the list. Then draw a circle to represent a pie, and assign slices of the responsibility for the event in sizes that reflect relative responsibility. Draw your own slice last, so that you do not prematurely assign too much responsibility to yourself.

Figure 15.3 shows what people and things Marissa identified as partly responsible for her sexual molestation and how she completed her first responsibility pie. Although Marissa had always felt personally responsible for being molested, when she filled out a responsibility pie, she gave herself a very small part of the responsibility. She decided that she felt responsible only for not saying no to her dad. Most of the responsibility for what happened was her father's, and even the slices representing her mother, grandfather, and alcohol were larger than Marissa's.

When Marissa showed her responsibility pie to her therapist, they discussed further her "responsibility" for the molestation. After a number of sessions, Marissa came to understand and believe that she was not at all responsible for being molested. She learned that molestation is entirely an adult responsibility; like most children, she did not have the knowledge or security to say no at age 6 or even at age 13. When she did finally say no at age 14, the molestation stopped. But stopping her father at age 14 did not mean

RESPONSIBILITY PIE

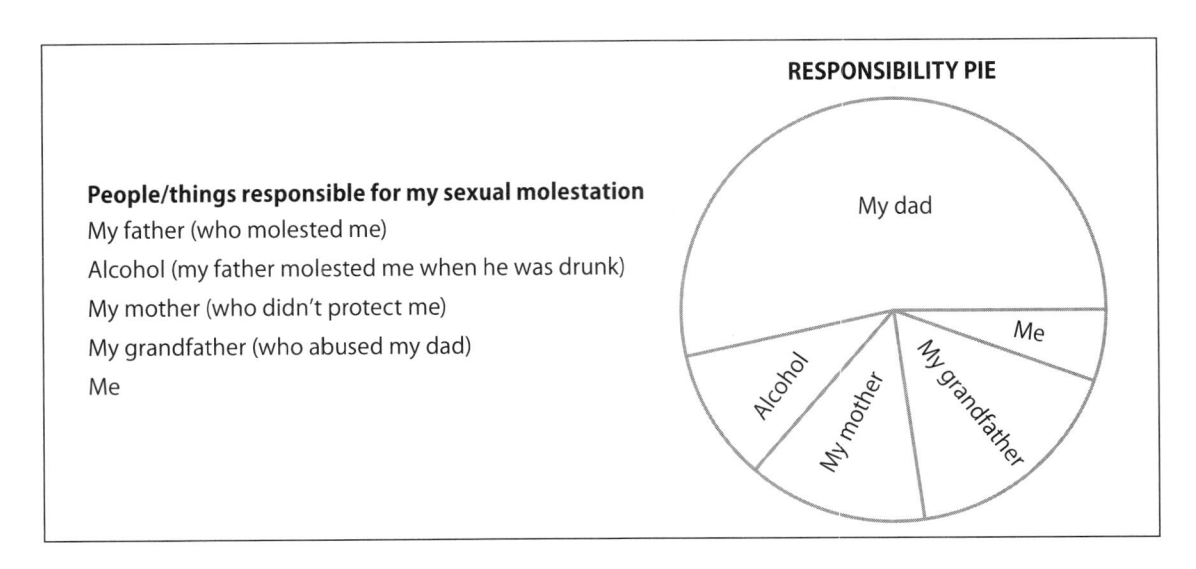

People/things responsible for my sexual molestation
My father (who molested me)
Alcohol (my father molested me when he was drunk)
My mother (who didn't protect me)
My grandfather (who abused my dad)
Me

FIGURE 15.3. Marissa's responsibility pie.

RESPONSIBILITY PIE

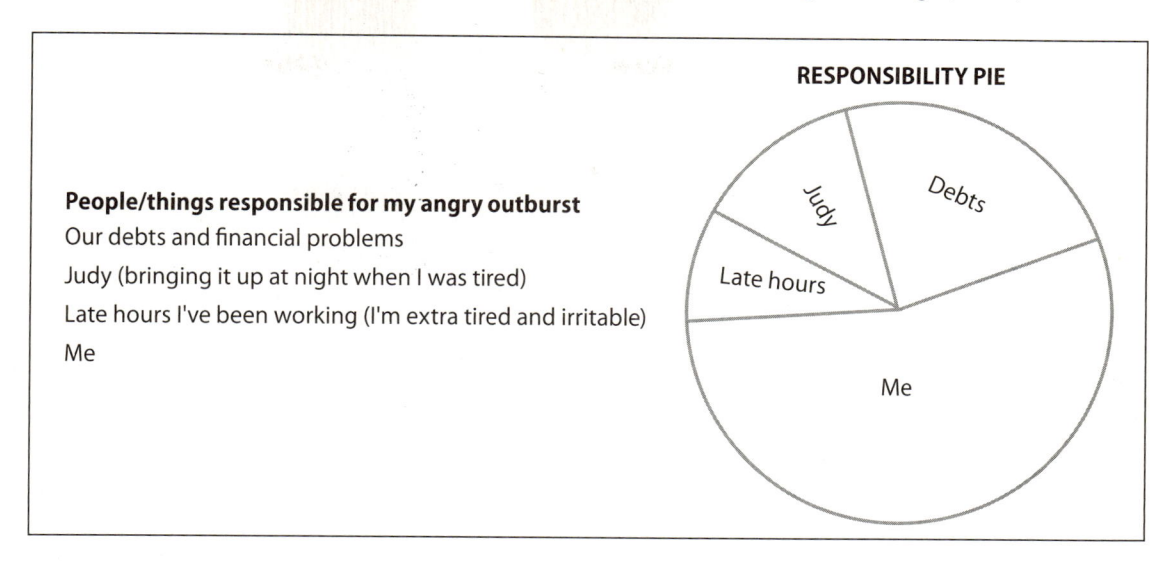

People/things responsible for my angry outburst
Our debts and financial problems
Judy (bringing it up at night when I was tired)
Late hours I've been working (I'm extra tired and irritable)
Me

(Pie chart showing: Debts, Judy, Late hours, Me — with "Me" as the largest slice)

FIGURE 15.4. Vic's responsibility pie.

that she had had the ability to do this all along. Her father might have been unwilling to risk confrontation with her as an older child. But he would have had no trouble overpowering her when she was younger. Even if she had said no when she was younger, it probably would not have stopped him. Even when older children and adolescents say no to sexual molestation, they are often ignored. The responsibility pie helped relieve Marissa of her guilt.

Vic completed a responsibility pie (Figure 15.4) when he felt guilty about yelling at his wife, Judy, after she complained to him about overdue credit card bills. This was a serious violation of his promise to Judy that he would not attack her in anger. Although he did not hit or shove Judy, he physically intimidated her by standing close to her and shouting in her face.

As you see, Vic decided that he was primarily responsible for his angry outburst. Although Judy, their debts, and his late work hours contributed to his anger, he felt that he could have handled the situation in a less intimidating fashion. Therefore, Vic decided that he should make reparations to Judy for what he had done. This incident also confirmed for Vic that he needed to change his anger responses.

As the examples of Marissa and Vic illustrate, responsibility pies can help you evaluate the level of responsibility of each of the contributors to a situation. A responsibility pie is not designed to always reduce guilt. Sometimes it is healthy to feel guilty about what we have done. In these instances, we can take steps to make amends for harm we have done to others. We can also come up with a plan to help ourselves respond in ways that are closer to our values. People who often feel guilty over small things find that responsibility pies help them recognize that they are not 100% responsible for the undesirable things that happen. People who feel guilt or shame when they have caused harm to others can use a responsibility pie to evaluate their role in any damage that was done before making reparations.

> **EXERCISE: Using a Responsibility Pie for Guilt or Shame**
>
> (1) Think of a negative event or situation in your life for which you feel guilt or shame. List this event or situation in item 1 of Worksheet 15.7. (2) In item 2 on Worksheet 15.7, list all the people and circumstances that could have contributed to the outcome. Place yourself at the bottom of the list, so you can rate your portion of the responsibility last. (3) Divide the pie in item 3 of the worksheet into slices, labeling these slices with the names of the people or circumstances on your list. Assign bigger pieces to people or circumstances that you think have greater responsibility. (4) When you are finished, use the questions in item 4 of the worksheet to consider how much responsibility is yours.

WORKSHEET 15.7. Using a Responsibility Pie for Guilt or Shame

1. Negative event or situation leading to guilt or shame: _____

2. People and circumstances that could have contributed to this outcome:

   _____   _____

   _____   _____

   _____   _____

   _____   _____

   _____   _____

3.

4. Are you 100% responsible? How does this responsibility pie affect your feelings of guilt and shame? Is there some action you can take to make amends for the part you are responsible for?

   _____

   _____

   _____

From *Mind Over Mood, Second Edition.* Copyright 2016 by Dennis Greenberger and Christine A. Padesky. Purchasers of this book can photocopy and/or download additional copies of this worksheet (see the box at the end of the table of contents).

Making Reparations

If you have injured another person, it is important to make amends for your actions. Trying to repair the damage you have done can be an important component in healing yourself and the relationship. Making amends involves recognizing what you did, being courageous enough to face the person you have hurt, asking forgiveness, and determining what you can do to repair the hurt you caused.

EXERCISE: Making Reparations for Hurting Someone

Worksheet 15.8 can help you make your personal plan to make amends for hurting someone.

WORKSHEET 15.8. Making Reparations for Hurting Someone

This is who I hurt:

This is what I did that was hurtful:

This is why it was wrong (my values that I violated):

This is what I can do to make amends:

This is what I can say to the person I hurt:

   I realize when I (describe the action or behavior here) _____
   _____,
   this hurt you. This was wrong because _____
   _____.
   I'm sorry I did this. I want to do _____
   _____
   to let you know how truly sorry I am, and I hope that you can forgive me in time.

From *Mind Over Mood, Second Edition*. Copyright 2016 by Dennis Greenberger and Christine A. Padesky. Purchasers of this book can photocopy and/or download additional copies of this worksheet (see the box at the end of the table of contents).

Notice that Worksheet 15.8 focuses on your making amends, not on the other person's forgiving you. You can ask someone to forgive you "in time," but this is no guarantee that the person will do so, especially if you have hurt this person very deeply or many times. However, making amends can help you feel better, especially when you are truly sorry, make some change in your behavior to try to be a better person, and make an effort to make amends to the person you hurt. Your attempts to be a better person brings you closer to acting within your values, and this can help you feel better about yourself.

Breaking the Silence Surrounding Shame

When secretiveness surrounds shame, it may be important to talk to a trusted person about what occurred. The need to keep silent is often based on the expectation that revealing your secret will result in condemnation, criticism, or rejection. It is not unusual for people who have carried a secret for a lifetime to be surprised at the acceptance they receive when they reveal their secret. Acceptance runs counter to the anticipated rejection and forces a reassessment of the meaning of your secret.

Although you may not trust anyone fully, it is important to reveal your secret to the people you trust the most. You may tell people how anxious it makes you feel to reveal your secret and how difficult it is for you to do. Be sure to talk to someone at a time and place when you will have adequate time to say everything you need to say, and to talk about the feedback you get.

Even though Petra was a successful administrative assistant for a large company, she hid the fact that she failed and was kicked out of her university after her first year as a student. This followed a wild period in her youth during which she partied much of the time and was using illegal drugs. Now, as a respected working adult, she told people that she had never had the financial opportunity to study at a university. Petra felt ashamed about her younger behavior and even more ashamed of her school failure. She worried that people would judge her negatively if they knew. This weighed heavily on her, especially when others talked about drug use or their children's university graduations.

One night Petra went out to dinner with her closest friend, Monique. They were talking about mistakes they had made when they were younger. Monique told the story of one man she had dated who was quite scary when he drank. She told Petra that sometimes she had a hard time accepting what poor judgment she had in staying with him for as long as she did. Petra swallowed hard and decided to take a risk. She started out by telling her friend that she had used some drugs when she was a teenager. Petra was surprised that Monique did not seem to judge her for this, but instead said, "So many people our age did that back then." This response encouraged Petra to tell Monique more details about her wild youth. By the end of the hour, she revealed her shame about failing and being kicked out of school. Petra was surprised that Monique was understanding and sympathetic toward her experiences. Instead of being critical, Monique expressed appreciation for how much Petra had accomplished in her life after such a rocky start. After this evening, Petra felt even closer to Monique than she had before. She began to view her youthful failures with less shame.

Self-Forgiveness

Being a good person doesn't mean that you will never do bad things. Part of being human is making mistakes. If, after careful evaluation, you conclude that you have done some things wrong, then self-forgiveness may help alleviate your guilt or shame.

No one is perfect. All of us, at one point or another, have violated our own principles or standards. We feel guilty and ashamed if we believe that what we did means that we are bad. But violations do not necessarily mean that we are bad. Just as in Petra's case, our actions may have been linked to a particular situation or to a specific time in our lives.

Self-forgiveness can lead to a change in interpretation of the meaning of the violation or mistake we made. Our understanding may change from "I made this mistake because I'm an awful person," to "I made this mistake during an awful time in my life, when I didn't care if I behaved this way."

Just as in the forgiveness letter you wrote to someone else in Worksheet 15.4, self-forgiveness does not mean that you approve, forget, or deny whatever pain you have caused others. Instead, self-forgiveness involves recognizing your own imperfections and mistakes and accepting your shortcomings. It can also help if you see that your life has not been one mistake or harmful action after another. Self-forgiveness includes recognizing your good and bad qualities, your strengths as well as weaknesses.

EXERCISE: Forgiving Myself

Some people have great difficulty forgiving themselves; they may have harsh and critical internal voices. If you are able to forgive others for their faults, but you have a hard time forgiving yourself, you can benefit from practicing self-forgiveness. This involves learning to view yourself with the same kindness or compassion with which you view others. Worksheet 15.9 on the next page can guide you through this process.

WORKSHEET 15.9. Forgiving Myself

1. This is what I need to forgive myself for:

2. This is the impact that what I did has had on me and others in my life:

3. This is how it continues to affect me and others:

4. This is how I imagine my life will be better if I'm able to forgive myself:

5. Forgiveness often begins with understanding. What life experiences have I had that might have contributed to what I did?

6. How would I think about someone else who did this?

7. What positive aspects of myself and my life do I tend to ignore when I'm feeling guilt or shame?

8. Forgiveness does not mean that you condone, forget, or deny what was done and the pain you have experienced. Instead, forgiveness means finding a way to let go of your guilt and shame, and understand your actions from a different perspective. Write with a kind, compassionate voice about how I can forgive myself for what I have done:

9. These are the qualities that I have that will allow me to move forward:

From *Mind Over Mood, Second Edition*. Copyright 2016 by Dennis Greenberger and Christine A. Padesky. Purchasers of this book can photocopy and/or download additional copies of this worksheet (see the box at the end of the table of contents).

WHEN YOU COMPLETE THIS CHAPTER

Once you have completed this chapter, return to Chapter 5 to set goals and identify signs of improvement that are meaningful to you. You will learn additional skills to help you manage your anger, guilt, and shame in Chapters 6–12.

Chapter 15 Summary

- As you practice *Mind Over Mood* skills, Worksheets 15.1 and 15.2 help you rate and track your progress in the frequency, strength, and duration of your moods.

- Anger is characterized by muscle tension, increased heart rate, increased blood pressure, and defensiveness or attack.

- When we are angry, our thoughts focus on our perceptions that other people are hurting us, threatening us, breaking the rules, or being unfair.

- Anger can range from mild irritation to rage. How angry we feel is influenced by our interpretation of the meaning of events, our expectations for other people, and whether or not we thought the other persons' behavior was intentional or not.

- Methods that are effective in controlling anger include testing angry thoughts, using imagery to anticipate and prepare for events in which you are at high risk for anger, recognizing the early warning signs of anger, timeouts, assertion, forgiveness, and couple or family therapy.

- We feel guilty when we believe that we have done something wrong or not lived up to the standards we have set for ourselves.

- Guilt is often accompanied by thoughts containing the words "should" or "ought."

- Shame involves the perception that we have done something wrong, that we need to keep it a secret, and that what we have done means something terrible about us.

- Guilt and shame can be lessened or eliminated by assessing the seriousness of your actions, weighing personal responsibility, making reparations for any harm you caused, breaking the silence surrounding shame, and self-forgiveness.

16

Maintaining Your Gains and Experiencing More Happiness

A wise fisherman, while fishing off the end of a pier, was approached by a hungry woman who hadn't eaten anything for several days. Eyeing the basket of fish he had caught, the woman begged him to give her some fish to satisfy her hunger. After thinking for a moment, the fisherman replied, "I'm not going to give you any of my fish, but if you sit down next to me and pick up a pole, I'll teach you how to fish. That way you will not only eat today, but you will learn how to feed yourself for the rest of your life." The woman took the fisherman's advice, learned to fish, and never went hungry again.

Just as learning the skill of fishing helped the woman in this story, the *Mind Over Mood* skills you have practiced and learned can help you today and for the rest of your life. This final chapter asks you to review what you have learned through using *Mind Over Mood*, and to determine how you can use these skills to continue improving your life.

If you have worked this far into the book, it is likely that your moods have improved. You probably can use many *Mind Over Mood* skills with confidence. People learn these skills in three stages. In the first stage, you apply skills in a conscious and deliberate way (writing out Thought Records, filling out weekly Activity Schedules, planning behavioral experiments, etc.). The second stage in the development of *Mind Over Mood* skills begins when you have used the skills often enough that you are now able to carry them out in your head, without the worksheets, but still with deliberate and conscious effort. The final stage begins when you have practiced these skills so much that they begin to occur automatically, without any conscious or deliberate effort. For example, you might have the automatic thought "I'm such a failure," and then quickly think, "Wait a minute. I messed this up, but that doesn't make me a failure." And then later, in this same situation, you might simply think, "Oh, I messed this up," without any thought at all about being a failure. This is when your new ways of thinking and behaving have become ingrained and automatic.

HELPFUL HINTS Often when we start to feel better, we stop using the skills that helped us get to that point. It is actually better to keep deliberately using helpful skills until they become automatic.

Even when you begin to use *Mind Over Mood* skills automatically, you can anticipate that you will still sometimes feel the same moods that led you to use this book. Experiencing a variety and intensity of moods is a normal and valuable part of life. At the same time, you want to be alert to notice if normal mood fluctuations turn into what is called a "relapse." The word "relapse" applies when your moods become more severe, last too long, occur too frequently, or begin to have negative effects on your life or relationships.

Most mood difficulties can be successfully helped. If you are doing the exercises in this book, and you are not improving or you relapse frequently, don't give up hope. Perhaps you will get better when you try alternative forms of help. For example, you may want to consult a mental health care professional for additional guidance. This is also recommended if you feel so poorly that you struggle to use this book because you can't concentrate or remember what you are reading.

If you have improved through using *Mind Over Mood* skills, and then a relapse occurs, you want to be prepared to recognize your setback as soon as possible. It is helpful to view your setback as an opportunity to strengthen your skills. The earlier you apply your *Mind Over Mood* skills to whatever difficulty you are facing, the more quickly you will feel better again. If your moods begin to get worse, it is a good idea to go back to the deliberate and effortful application of the skills that helped you get better in the first place. You may be surprised to find that when you consciously start using skills again, they help more quickly than when you first learned them. This is because you are not learning something new, but refreshing what you already know. This is just like when you ride a bicycle after you have not been on one for a long time: It may seem a little awkward at first, but you quickly remember what you know how to do.

EXERCISE: Reviewing and Rating *Mind Over Mood* Skills

This chapter guides you through steps you can take to continue to benefit from and build on the *Mind Over Mood* skills you have learned so far to prevent and manage relapse. As a springboard for this planning, fill out Worksheet 16.1. This worksheet lists the skills taught in *Mind Over Mood.* Use the 0–3 rating scale at the top of the worksheet to rate each skill on how often you have used it, how often it is helpful when you use it, how often you still use it, and how much you think you might use this skill in the future. Don't worry if you haven't mastered all these skills. You may have forgotten you practiced some of them. There may be some skills you skipped while reading this book. You may be using other skills so automatically now that you forgot you learned them. The Skills Checklist reminds you that there are many different tools available to help you manage your moods.

WORKSHEET 16.1. *Mind Over Mood* Skills Checklist

For each skill listed, there are four rating categories: Used = Did you use this skill?; Helpful = How often was it helpful?; Still use = Do you still use this skill?; Future use = Do you think you will use this skill in the future?

Rate each skill in all four categories using the following scale:

0 = Not at all   1 = Sometimes   2 = Frequently   3 = Most of the time

See chapter	Core Skills	Used?	Helpful?	Still use?	Future use?
2	Notice interactions among thoughts, moods, behaviors, physical reactions, and environment				
4	Identify moods				
4	Rate intensity of moods				
5	Set goals				
5	Consider advantages and disadvantages of change				
6–7	Identify automatic thoughts and images				
6–7	Complete the first three columns of a Thought Record				
7	Identify hot thoughts				
8	Find evidence that supports and does not support a hot thought				
9	Generate alternative or balanced thoughts based on the evidence collected				

(continued on next page)

From *Mind Over Mood, Second Edition.* Copyright 2016 by Dennis Greenberger and Christine A. Padesky. Purchasers of this book can photocopy and/or download additional copies of this worksheet (see the box at the end of the table of contents).

WORKSHEET 16.1 *(continued from previous page)*

See chapter	Core Skills	Used?	Helpful?	Still use?	Future use?
6–9	Fill out a seven-column Thought Record				
10	Gather more evidence to strengthen new thoughts				
10	When evidence on a Thought Record supports a hot thought, complete an Action Plan to solve the problem				
10	Use Action Plans to make a change in your life or reach a goal				
10	Practice acceptance of life situations, thoughts, and moods				
11	Identify "If . . . then . . ." underlying assumptions				
11	Test an underlying assumption with behavioral experiments				
11	Develop alternative assumptions that fit your life experience				
12	Identify core beliefs				
12	Identify new core beliefs				
12	Write down evidence to support and strengthen new core beliefs				
12	Rate confidence in new core beliefs				
12	Use scales to rate positive change				
12	Strengthen new core beliefs with behavioral experiments				
12	Practice gratitude by using a gratitude journal				
12	Express gratitude to others				
12	Act with kindness				

See chapter	Depression Skills	Used?	Helpful?	Still use?	Future use?
13	Rate depression symptoms				
13	Use an Activity Record to notice activities and mood connections				
13	Use an Activity Schedule to schedule activities that are pleasurable, accomplish something, help you approach things you have been avoiding, and fit with your values				

(continued on next page)

WORKSHEET 16.1 *(continued from previous page)*

See chapter	Depression Skills	Used?	Helpful?	Still use?	Future use?
13	Do activities even when you do not feel like it				
13	Notice and enjoy small positive experiences				
6–13	Test depressed thoughts and images				

See chapter	Anxiety Skills	Used?	Helpful?	Still use?	Future use?
14	Rate anxiety symptoms				
14	Recognize when you are avoiding something because of anxiety				
14	Identify your safety behaviors				
14	Make a Fear Ladder				
14	Use a Fear Ladder to face your fears and overcome avoidance				
14	Use mindfulness and acceptance to manage anxiety				
14	Practice breathing to manage anxiety				
14	Practice progressive muscle relaxation to manage anxiety				
14	Use imagery to manage anxiety				
6–9, 11, 14	Test anxious thoughts and images				

See chapter	Anger Skills	Used?	Helpful?	Still use?	Future use?
15	Use imagery to anticipate and prepare for events				
15	Recognize early warning signs of anger				
15	Use timeouts				
15	Use assertive communication				
15	Practice forgiveness				
6–11, 15	Test angry thoughts and images				

(continued on next page)

WORKSHEET 16.1 *(continued from previous page)*

See chapter	Guilt and Shame Skills	Used?	Helpful?	Still use?	Future use?
15	Assess seriousness of your actions				
15	Use a responsibility pie				
15	Make reparations				
15	Break the silence				
15	Practice self-forgiveness				

Mark any of the skills in Worksheet 16.1 that have become automatic for you – the ones that occur without deliberately planning. There may be some skills that are helpful most of the time but are not yet automatic for you. Keep practicing them. It may take several months before a skill becomes automatic.

> **HELPFUL HINTS** One of the purposes of Worksheet 16.1 is to highlight *Mind Over Mood* skills you have learned. The improvement you have made is a result of your effort and the new skills you have developed. You can go forward with confidence that no one can take these skills away from you. In fact, you will learn to use your skills in many more situations over time. As you do, you are less likely to struggle with future mood problems and more likely to experience happiness and find positive purpose and meaning in your life.

REDUCE THE LIKELIHOOD OF RELAPSE

Sometimes we stop using skills because we are feeling better. At other times, old thinking and behaviors return despite our best efforts, and we begin to experience more frequent, severe, longer-lasting, and disruptive negative moods. As bad as this feels, it can be an opportunity to further develop our skills and help them become more automatic. As described earlier in this chapter, if we notice these relapses early and take action, we have a good chance of improving our moods quickly.

The following three steps will reduce the likelihood of relapse:

1. **Identify high-risk situations.** As you have worked through the exercises in this book, you may have noticed that you are more likely to struggle with problematic moods in certain situations. Linda was more likely to feel anxious on airplanes and when

her heart started racing. Ben was prone to feeling depressed when it seemed that his children and grandchildren didn't need him. Vic's anger flared when he thought that people weren't supporting him. Marissa became more depressed when she thought that people didn't care about her or were taking advantage of her. On Worksheet 16.2 (see p. 288), list some situations that may be high-risk for you in terms of the moods you have been targeting.

2. **Identify early warning signs.** Whether you are in high-risk situations or not, it is good to be aware that most of us have early warning signs that we are sinking into deeper and more problematic mood states. For example, Ben became quite active again with friends and family members when his depression lifted. He noticed, however, that whenever his mood dipped for a few days, he ignored phone calls and thought about ways to avoid getting together with friends and family. When Ben stopped answering phone calls and looked for reasons not to see people, he recognized these as early warning signs that his depression might be returning.

Your early warning signs may be behaviors that you do or don't do (e.g., staying in bed longer, procrastinating more, avoiding situations or people), thoughts (negative, worried, self-critical), moods (a rise in *Mind Over Mood* Depression Inventory or Anxiety Inventory scores, increased irritability), and/or physical changes (difficulty sleeping, fatigue, muscle tension, appetite change). Think back over your past experiences. What might be your early warning signs? If you are not aware of any, try asking family members or friends if they have any ideas. Write down your early warning signs on Worksheet 16.2.

For most of us, identifying early warning signs will include regular measurement of our moods, even after we are feeling better. If you were depressed or anxious in the past, you can fill out the *Mind Over Mood* Depression Inventory and/or Anxiety Inventory on a monthly basis as part of your early warning monitoring system. For other moods, you can rate their frequency, strength, and duration periodically on a 0–100 scale, as you learned to do on Worksheet 15.1 in Chapter 15. A good time to put your plan to reduce relapse risk into effect is when your mood scores begin to increase in frequency, strength, and/or duration.

3. **Prepare a plan of action.** One of the advantages of learning mood management skills is that you can use these during challenging times to help you understand, tolerate, and reduce your distress. In the third section of Worksheet 16.2 on page 288, you consider which skills, values, and beliefs you hold that can help you during high-risk situations and when you begin to get early warning signs that certain moods are becoming problematic again. Think about what you have learned in *Mind Over Mood* that helped you get better. The learning that was most important to you is identified on Worksheet 16.1 (pp. 282–285), so review your answers there when you are developing a plan to prevent and/or recover from relapse.

Write down on Worksheet 16.2 the skills and steps you can take in high-risk situations, and when you have early warning signs of worsening moods. For example, when Ben noticed himself withdrawing from his family and friends (his early warning sign), he reviewed Worksheet 16.1 and realized that he had benefited the most from his Activity Schedule (Worksheet 13.6). Therefore, he wrote on his Plan to Reduce Relapse Risk that he would be more active, get out of the house more, and make plans to be around other people. Also, after reviewing Worksheet 16.1, Ben recognized that another important part of his improvement resulted from learning to think differently. This came about from his use of Thought Records and a gratitude journal.

Because Ben had filled out Thought Records for several months, he had developed the ability to respond automatically to negative thoughts with more balanced thoughts, without consciously thinking about it or needing to write anything down. Ben anticipated that he might not be able to automatically respond to his negative thoughts if his depression came back. Therefore, he also made a plan to fill out Thought Records again if his *Mind Over Mood* Depression Inventory scores rose above 15. He planned to continue testing his thoughts on paper until his scores dropped below 10.

When he kept his gratitude journal, Ben recognized the importance of his family and friends. As he realized how fortunate he was to have so many good people in his life, he felt happier, and his activities became more meaningful to him. As part of his relapse management plan, therefore, Ben decided to review and add to his gratitude journal on a weekly basis. He also planned to express his appreciation about something to at least one person every week.

> **EXERCISE: Reducing Relapse Risk**
>
> Worksheet 16.2 helps you reduce your risk of relapse by:
>
> 1. Identifying your high-risk situations.
> 2. Identifying early warning signs that you are sinking deeper into depression, anxiety, anger, guilt, or shame.
> 3. Preparing a plan of action to help you face challenges and periods of distress.

WORKSHEET 16.2. My Plan to Reduce Relapse Risk

1. My high-risk situations:

_____
_____
_____
_____
_____

2. My early warning signs:

_____
_____
_____
_____
_____

Rate my moods on a regular basis (monthly, for example). My warning score is _____

3. My plan of action (review Worksheet 16.1 for ideas):

_____
_____
_____
_____
_____

From *Mind Over Mood, Second Edition*. Copyright 2016 by Dennis Greenberger and Christine A. Padesky. Purchasers of this book can photocopy and/or download additional copies of this worksheet (see the box at the end of the table of contents).

> **EXERCISE: Imagine Yourself Coping**
>
> It can help to practice your plan from Worksheet 16.2 before you need it. One way to do this is to imagine one of your high-risk situations occurring in the future. Imagine this situation in great detail. What is happening? What do you see and hear? Next, imagine you are experiencing several or all of your early warning signs. How do you feel? What are you thinking? What are you doing? Now imagine putting your plan of action into effect. Spend several minutes imagining doing each step of your plan in detail. As you carry out each step in your imagination, pay attention to what you are doing, thinking, and feeling. How does this affect your mood? Thoughts? Behavior? Physical experience?
>
> Based on this imagination exercise, how confident are you (low, medium, or high) that the plan of action you wrote in section 3 of Worksheet 16.2 will be enough to help you feel better again if you start to relapse? If your confidence level is high, then your plan is probably a good one. If you confidence in your plan is low, then you want to think about what else you can add to it that will boost your likelihood of managing future challenges. If you think the plan is a good one, but you lack confidence in your skills to carry it out, the best thing to do is to continue practicing the skills in your plan of action even when you are feeling well. Ideally, you want most of your relapse reduction skills to be fairly automatic when you are doing well, so that you can rely on them to help you if you begin to feel worse.

KEEP *MIND OVER MOOD* WHERE YOU WILL SEE IT

You have probably been using this book and practicing the skills on a regular basis. If you are feeling better now, you may tend to put the book aside, especially if you have completed reading most or all of it. Actually, it is better to continue to refer to this book, even if you are no longer using it as regularly as you were. For example, if you have been using it daily, it is helpful to keep the book somewhere you are likely to see it, so you remember to periodically review what you learned (e.g., once a week for a few months). If you have been using this book once a week, you might refer to it every few weeks or once a month for a number of months. Research shows that people who review and continue to practice what they have learned are less likely to relapse than are those who stop their practice.

USE *MIND OVER MOOD* TO ENHANCE YOUR LIFE AND EXPERIENCE GREATER HAPPINESS

Most people use *Mind Over Mood* skills at first to help with moods that trouble them, such as depression, anxiety, anger, guilt, or shame. These same skills can also help you develop greater happiness. *Mind Over Mood* skills operate like an elevator: They can lift you out of the basement and take you not just to ground level, but up to the top floor.

For example, in Chapter 12 you learned to use a gratitude journal, express gratitude to others, and act with kindness. These practices boost happiness. Chapter 14 describes how to use positive imagery to manage anxiety. Positive imagery can also be used to imagine new ways you would like to be. When you actively imagine new behaviors, you are more likely to carry them out. You can use positive imagery to help create positive change in your life.

When you want to make positive changes, you can use Action Plans (Chapter 10) or behavioral experiments (Chapter 11) to try out new ways of doing things and see what works best for you. Practicing acceptance (Chapter 10) and mindfulness (Chapter 14) are methods that can help you develop a greater sense of well-being. One of our recommended activities to reduce depression is to notice and enjoy small positive experiences (Chapter 13). Savoring positive experiences when you are not depressed can help create greater life satisfaction. You also learned that it is important to engage in a variety of activities when you are depressed (activities that are pleasurable, give you a sense of accomplishment, help in overcoming avoidance, and fit with your values). When you are feeling better, these same types of activities can help you create a life filled with satisfaction and well-being. Even though you may feel good now and may no longer feel depressed, anxious, or angry, consider how you can continue to use *Mind Over Mood* skills to take the elevator to the upper floors.

If you like the *Mind Over Mood* approach and want to find a cognitive-behavioral therapist near you, visit one of the following websites:

www.mindovermood.com

www.anxietyanddepressioncenter.com

www.academyofct.org

www.asiancbt.weebly.com (Asia)

www.aacbt.org (Australia)

www.abct.org (Canada and United States)

www.cacbt.ca (Canada)

www.eabct.eu (Europe)

www.alamoc-web.org (Latin America)

www.cbt.org.nz (New Zealand)

www.babcp.com (United Kingdom)

If you can't find a cognitive-behavioral therapist near you on these websites, ask your medical care provider or someone else you trust to recommend a therapist. If *Mind Over Mood* is helpful for you, many therapists will incorporate your use of this book in your therapy. If you are using this book while you work with a therapist and you are not improving, discuss with your therapist what changes might make therapy more effective. There is likely to be a solution for you. So do not give up until you feel better.

Chapter 16 Summary

- Learning *Mind Over Mood* skills progresses through three stages: conscious and deliberate practice; being able to use skills in your head with conscious effort; and finally having new behaviors and thinking processes occur automatically, without planning or effort.

- People tend to stop using skills once their moods improve, and yet it is better to continue practicing them until their use becomes automatic.

- Everyone can expect normal mood fluctuations. It is important to recognize when these begin to become a "relapse" – that is, when moods become more severe, last too long, occur too frequently, or begin to have negative effects on your life or relationships.

- The *Mind Over Mood* Skills Checklist (Worksheet 16.1) highlights what skills you have used, how often they help you, whether you still use them, and how often you plan to use them in the future.

- The *Mind Over Mood* Skills Checklist also helps you understand that the improvements you have made are the results of your efforts and the skills you have built.

- To reduce your risk of relapse, it is helpful to identify your high-risk situations, learn your warning signs, and make a plan of action based on the skills you now possess.

- It is helpful to practice your relapse risk reduction plan in imagination when you are feeling well, to test how confident you are that it will help you if you need it.

- Even after you finish reading *Mind Over Mood,* keep the book somewhere you will see it, so you can remember what you have learned and continue to practice the skills that help you feel better.

- The same activities and skills than lift you out of depression, anxiety, anger, guilt, and shame can also help lift you into positive mood states once you feel better.

Epilogue

Although you have read about many different people in this book, you have followed in detail the progress of Ben, Linda, Marissa, and Vic. You may be curious to know what happened to them. This Epilogue describes their lives as time went by.

BEN: *Older and better.*

Ben conquered his depression by testing his thoughts on Thought Records and by doing experiments to learn new ways of interacting with his children and grandchildren. He also found completing Activity Schedules and keeping a gratitude journal very helpful. By the end of therapy, he felt much happier. He resumed meeting with his friends, tinkering with projects in his garage, and doing a variety of activities with his wife, Sylvie. In addition, Ben and Sylvie talked about how they would each cope if the other died first. While Ben hoped Sylvie would live as long as he, he felt more certain that he could learn to enjoy his life even if she died first.

The dramatic improvement in his mood pleased and surprised Ben. He sprang up from his chair at the end of his last therapy session and gave his therapist a firm handshake: "Thank you, Doctor. You've been a terrific help, and you know I didn't believe therapy could help." Ben's therapist smiled and told Ben, "Well, you deserve the credit. You worked very hard to feel better."

Ben *had* worked hard in therapy. Almost every day he made some attempt to feel better. Some days he identified his moods and thoughts; other days he increased his activities or experimented with new behaviors. As described in Chapter 13, Ben especially increased activities that gave him a sense of pleasure or accomplishment, and those that led him to approach rather than avoid life challenges. Ben also paid attention to what he valued most (i.e., family and friends) and made sure his activities kept him connected to them. Even with this consistent effort, Ben's improvement varied from week to week. Figure E.1 shows the graph of Ben's depression scores on the *Mind Over Mood* Depression Inventory (Worksheet 13.1) for the time he was in CBT.

Usually people do not improve every single week on a depression score graph. Notice that Ben might have thought he wasn't making any progress in week 3, when his depression score actually went up several points. But over time, Ben's depression decreased,

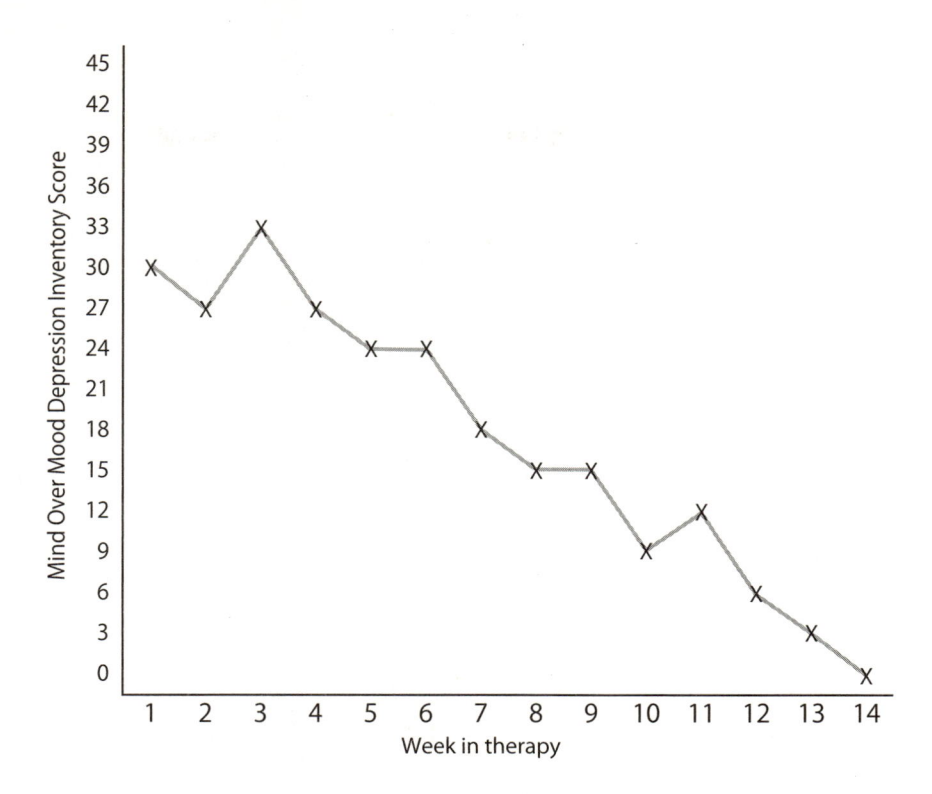

FIGURE E.1. Ben's weekly depression scores.

especially after week 6 when he learned to use Thought Records. Even though Ben's depression scores sometimes increased or stayed the same, over time he felt better.

MARISSA: *Finally my life seems worth living.*

As you see from Marissa's depression score chart (Figure E.2 on p. 294), her improvement pattern was quite different from Ben's. Marissa's depression scores went up and down quite a lot over the time she was in therapy. During particularly difficult times (e.g., when she was getting critical feedback at work, when she and her therapist were discussing her childhood abuse, when Marissa became discouraged and stopped doing Thought Records), her depression scores were higher (she was more depressed). As Marissa improved her ability to use problem solving, Thought Records, and experiments, her depression scores were lower (she was less depressed).

At times, Marissa's depression scores were as high as when she started therapy, but you can see that her scores were mostly lower in the later weeks of therapy. In the first ten weeks, Marissa's depression scores were above 30 for seven weeks. In the next ten weeks, Marissa's scores were above 30 for only four weeks. In the next ten weeks, her scores were above 30 in only one week. So, although Marissa continued to struggle with depression for months, her chart helped her see that she had fewer very depressed weeks as she practiced using Thought Records and the other skills she learned. As is often the

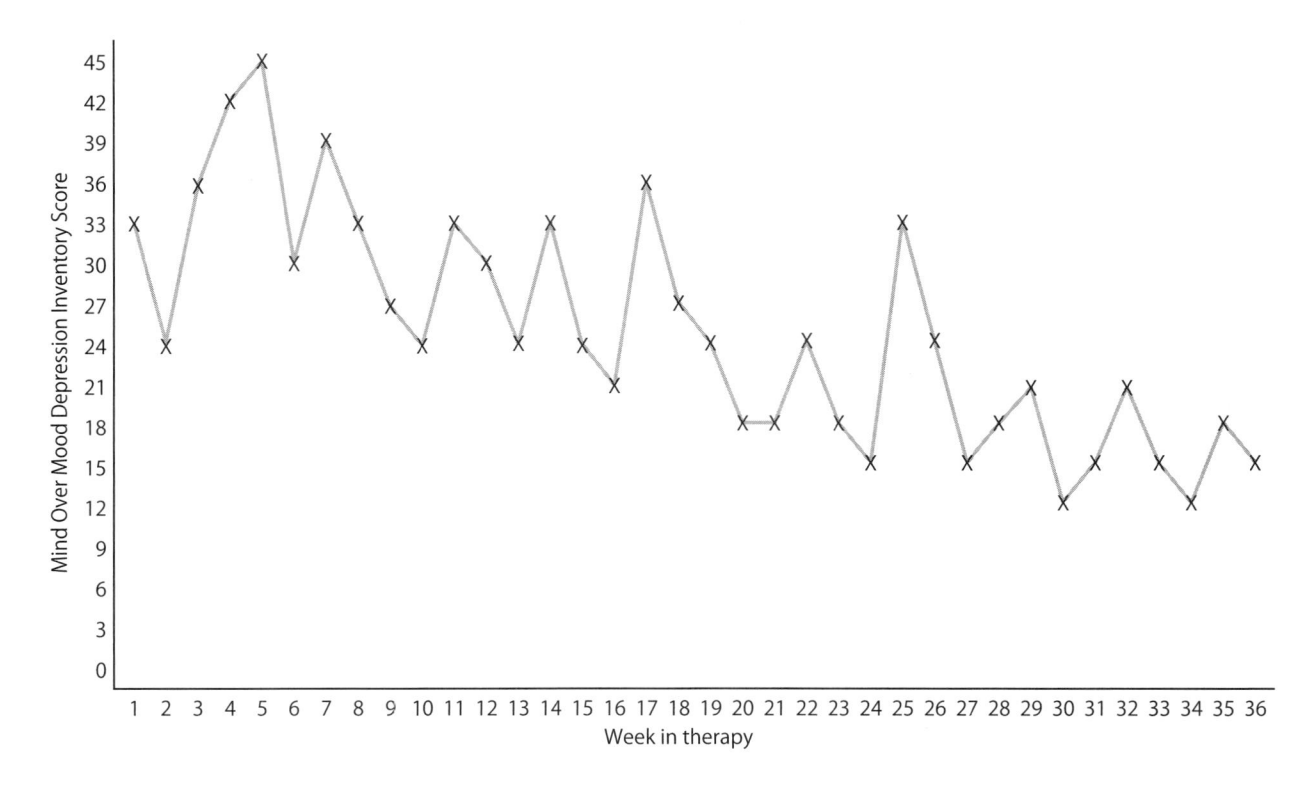

FIGURE E.2. Marissa's weekly depression scores.

case for people who learn to use *Mind Over Mood* skills, Marissa noticed that she felt depressed less often and that when she did experience worse moods, these were not as severe and did not last as long.

At her most recent follow-up, Marissa had been using the strategies described in *Mind Over Mood* for over three years. She was using the methods on her own now, although she went back to see her therapist for help with problem solving when she felt stuck. Marissa had not made any suicide attempts in the previous three years. She no longer felt guilty or ashamed about her childhood abuse history. She had done well in her job and received positive evaluations from her supervisor. Her second child had entered college, and with both children living away from home, Marissa had moved to a smaller apartment in a building where she could keep a garden. Marissa was living alone for the first time in her life. She had made some new friends and felt more hope for the future.

LINDA: *Frequent flyer.*

As you learned in Chapter 11, Linda was successful in overcoming her panic attacks and her fear of flying. Three key steps led to her success:

1. Linda identified the physical sensations (e.g., rapid heart rate) that frightened her, and her catastrophic fears (e.g., "I'm having a heart attack") about these sensations.

2. With the help of her therapist, Linda constructed alternative explanations (e.g., a rapid heart rate can be caused by anxiety, excitement, or coffee) for the sensations she experienced.

3. Linda did a number of experiments to gather information and to test whether her catastrophic beliefs or alternative explanations matched her life experiences better. These experiments were done in the therapist's office, in imagery, at home, and on airplanes.

Over time, Linda became confident that the physical sensations she experienced were fueled by anxiety, not physical danger. She learned and practiced a number of strategies for reducing her anxiety. She was flying with comfort a few months after beginning therapy.

Linda kept her job promotion and became regional supervisor for her company. She was able to use the skills she learned in *Mind Over Mood* to identify and change her thoughts and feelings in ways that helped her manage the additional pressures of her new job.

VIC: *The perfect solution – to be imperfect.*

Vic initially went into treatment wanting to feel more confident, to feel better about himself, to manage his anger, and to get help in maintaining his sobriety. As time passed, some of Vic's therapy goals changed. He remained steadfast in his commitment to sobriety. However, he began to realize that his problems with anger, depression, and anxiety were threatening his marriage.

Vic addressed each of these issues in turn. His progress was characterized by hard work, sustained effort, and steady improvement, interrupted by two episodes of binge drinking and significant deterioration in his life. After completing approximately 35 Thought Records, Vic developed a good ability to identify and test the thoughts that contributed to his moods, low self-esteem, and drinking. Anticipating difficult events and using imagery to prepare for them helped Vic control his urges to drink and minimized the frequency of his anger outbursts.

Vic also used the Core Belief Record (Worksheet 12.6) to record evidence supporting his new sense of competence (Figure E.3 on p. 296).

After his second episode of binge drinking, Vic was successfully able to control his urges to drink and maintain his sobriety. He attributed his sobriety to learning multiple strategies to manage his moods in healthier ways. One of these strategies was learning to recognize and shift the thoughts and beliefs that increased his negative moods and urges to drink.

In addition, Vic and Judy decided that couple therapy would be helpful. Couple therapy taught them how to improve their communication, express their feelings clearly, and test the accuracy of their thoughts about each other. Furthermore, therapy helped

> **New Core Belief:** *I am competent.*
>
> **Evidence or experiences that support my new belief:**
>
> 1. *My daughter and I visited a college she was considering attending. I helped her get acquainted and ask questions. She told me she appreciated my help.*
> 2. *I helped my son with a science project he was working on. I didn't do the project for him, but I helped him think it through in a way that helped him do it himself.*
> 3. *Judy expressed admiration for my continuing sobriety.*
> 4. *I sold products to four new accounts last month.*
> 5. *I was asked by the minister at my church to help organize a meeting for new church members.*
> 6. *I attended an AA meeting Tuesday night when I felt like drinking.*
> 7. *I got my monthly reports in on time.*
> 8. *I stayed calm when Judy and I were discussing our bills.*

FIGURE E.3. Vic's new Core Belief Record.

Vic and Judy repair their trust, which had been weakened by years of anger and alcoholism.

As his therapy was coming to an end, Vic realized that he would continue to face challenges on a daily basis. As part of his relapse management plan, Vic decided to write out Thought Records periodically when he was unable to test out his thoughts in his head. Rather than trying to be perfect, he worked on accepting his imperfections and continued to gather and review the data on his new Core Belief Record to help him stay aware of the ways he was competent. Vic attributed his ongoing sobriety, improved marriage, and increased sense of happiness to these strategies and methods.

CHANGE HOW YOU FEEL BY CHANGING THE WAY YOU THINK

Chapter 1 of *Mind Over Mood* described how an oyster turns an irritant into a valuable pearl. Our hope is that *Mind Over Mood* has helped you learn new skills to transform irritants and problems in your life into new coping strategies and strengths. You are now more capable of evaluating your thoughts, managing your moods, and changing your life. We hope that you have resolved the problems that led you to *Mind Over Mood,* and that in that resolution you have gained insight, understanding, skills, and methods to transform future irritants into valuable pearls.

Appendix
Duplicate Copies of Selected Worksheets

Worksheet 9.2.	Thought Record	*299*
Worksheet 10.2.	Action Plan	*311*
Worksheet 11.2.	Experiments to Test an Underlying Assumption	*313*
Worksheet 12.6.	Core Belief Record: Recording Evidence That Supports a New Core Belief	*315*
Worksheet 12.7.	Rating Confidence in My New Core Belief	*316*
Worksheet 12.8.	Rating Personal Experiences	*317*
Worksheet 12.9.	Behavioral Experiments to Strengthen New Core Beliefs	*318*
Worksheet 13.1.	*Mind Over Mood* Depression Inventory	*319*
Worksheet 13.2.	*Mind Over Mood* Depression Inventory Scores	*320*
Worksheet 13.6.	Activity Schedule	*322*
Worksheet 14.1.	*Mind Over Mood* Anxiety Inventory	*324*
Worksheet 14.2.	*Mind Over Mood* Anxiety Inventory Scores	*325*
Worksheet 14.4.	Making a Fear Ladder	*326*
Worksheet 14.5.	My Fear Ladder	*327*
Worksheet 15.1.	Measuring and Tracking My Moods	*328*
Worksheet 15.2.	Mood Scores Chart	*329*
Worksheet 15.4.	Writing a Forgiveness Letter	*330*
Worksheet 15.9.	Forgiving Myself	*331*
Worksheet 16.2.	My Plan to Reduce Relapse Risk	*332*

WORKSHEET 9.2. **Thought Record**

THOUGHT RECORD

1. Situation	2. Moods	3. Automatic Thoughts (Images)	4. Evidence That Supports the Hot Thought	5. Evidence That Does Not Support the Hot Thought	6. Alternative/Balanced Thoughts	7. Rate Moods Now
Who were you with? What were you doing? When was it? Where were you?	Describe each mood in one word. Rate intensity of mood (0–100%). Circle or mark the mood you want to examine.	Answer one or both of the questions below, and then some or all of the questions (on p. 54) specific to the mood you circled or marked: What was going through my mind just before I started to feel this way? What images or memories do I have in this situation?	Circle hot thought in previous column for which you are looking for evidence. Write factual evidence to support this conclusion. (Try to write facts, not interpretations, as you practiced in Worksheet 8.1 on p. 72.)	Ask yourself the questions in the Helpful Hints (p. 75) to help discover evidence that does not support your hot thought.	Ask yourself the questions in the Helpful Hints in Chapter 9 (p. 100) to generate alternative or balanced thoughts. Write an alternative or balanced thought. Rate how much you believe each alternative or balanced thought (0–100%).	Copy the moods from column 2. Rerate the intensity of each mood (0–100%), as well as any new moods.

Copyright 1983 by Christine A. Padesky. Reprinted in *Mind Over Mood, Second Edition*. Copyright 2016 by Dennis Greenberger and Christine A. Padesky. Purchasers of this book can photocopy and/or download additional copies of this worksheet (see the box at the end of the table of contents). All other rights reserved.

299

WORKSHEET 9.2. **Thought Record**

THOUGHT RECORD

1. Situation	2. Moods	3. Automatic Thoughts (Images)	4. Evidence That Supports the Hot Thought	5. Evidence That Does Not Support the Hot Thought	6. Alternative/Balanced Thoughts	7. Rate Moods Now
Who were you with? What were you doing? When was it? Where were you?	Describe each mood in one word. Rate intensity of mood (0–100%). Circle or mark the mood you want to examine.	Answer one or both of the questions below, and then some or all of the questions (on p. 54) specific to the mood you circled or marked: What was going through my mind just before I started to feel this way? What images or memories do I have in this situation?	Circle hot thought in previous column for which you are looking for evidence. Write factual evidence to support this conclusion. (Try to write facts, not interpretations, as you practiced in Worksheet 8.1 on p. 72.)	Ask yourself the questions in the Helpful Hints (p. 75) to help discover evidence that does not support your hot thought.	Ask yourself the questions in the Helpful Hints in Chapter 9 (p. 100) to generate alternative or balanced thoughts. Write an alternative or balanced thought. Rate how much you believe each alternative or balanced thought (0–100%).	Copy the moods from column 2. Rerate the intensity of each mood (0–100%), as well as any new moods.

Copyright 1983 by Christine A. Padesky. Reprinted in *Mind Over Mood, Second Edition*. Copyright 2016 by Dennis Greenberger and Christine A. Padesky. Purchasers of this book can photocopy and/or download additional copies of this worksheet (see the box at the end of the table of contents). All other rights reserved.

WORKSHEET 9.2. Thought Record

THOUGHT RECORD

1. Situation	2. Moods	3. Automatic Thoughts (Images)	4. Evidence That Supports the Hot Thought	5. Evidence That Does Not Support the Hot Thought	6. Alternative/Balanced Thoughts	7. Rate Moods Now
Who were you with? What were you doing? When was it? Where were you?	Describe each mood in one word. Rate intensity of mood (0–100%). Circle or mark the mood you want to examine.	Answer one or both of the questions below, and then some or all of the questions (on p. 54) specific to the mood you circled or marked: What was going through my mind just before I started to feel this way? What images or memories do I have in this situation?	Circle hot thought in previous column for which you are looking for evidence. Write factual evidence to support this conclusion. (Try to write facts, not interpretations, as you practiced in Worksheet 8.1 on p. 72.)	Ask yourself the questions in the Helpful Hints (p. 75) to help discover evidence that does not support your hot thought.	Ask yourself the questions in the Helpful Hints in Chapter 9 (p. 100) to generate alternative or balanced thoughts. Write an alternative or balanced thought. Rate how much you believe each alternative or balanced thought (0–100%).	Copy the moods from column 2. Rerate the intensity of each mood (0–100%), as well as any new moods.

Copyright 1983 by Christine A. Padesky. Reprinted in *Mind Over Mood, Second Edition*. Copyright 2016 by Dennis Greenberger and Christine A. Padesky. Purchasers of this book can photocopy and/or download additional copies of this worksheet (see the box at the end of the table of contents). All other rights reserved.

WORKSHEET 9.2. **Thought Record**

THOUGHT RECORD

1. Situation	2. Moods	3. Automatic Thoughts (Images)	4. Evidence That Supports the Hot Thought	5. Evidence That Does Not Support the Hot Thought	6. Alternative/Balanced Thoughts	7. Rate Moods Now
Who were you with? What were you doing? When was it? Where were you?	Describe each mood in one word. Rate intensity of mood (0–100%). Circle or mark the mood you want to examine.	Answer one or both of the questions below, and then some or all of the questions (on p. 54) specific to the mood you circled or marked: What was going through my mind just before I started to feel this way? What images or memories do I have in this situation?	Circle hot thought in previous column for which you are looking for evidence. Write factual evidence to support this conclusion. (Try to write facts, not interpretations, as you practiced in Worksheet 8.1 on p. 72.)	Ask yourself the questions in the Helpful Hints (p. 75) to help discover evidence that does not support your hot thought.	Ask yourself the questions in the Helpful Hints in Chapter 9 (p. 100) to generate alternative or balanced thoughts. Write an alternative or balanced thought. Rate how much you believe each alternative or balanced thought (0–100%).	Copy the moods from column 2. Rerate the intensity of each mood (0–100%), as well as any new moods.

Copyright 1983 by Christine A. Padesky. Reprinted in *Mind Over Mood, Second Edition*. Copyright 2016 by Dennis Greenberger and Christine A. Padesky. Purchasers of this book can photocopy and/or download additional copies of this worksheet (see the box at the end of the table of contents). All other rights reserved.

WORKSHEET 9.2. **Thought Record**

THOUGHT RECORD

1. Situation	2. Moods	3. Automatic Thoughts (Images)	4. Evidence That Supports the Hot Thought	5. Evidence That Does Not Support the Hot Thought	6. Alternative/Balanced Thoughts	7. Rate Moods Now
Who were you with? What were you doing? When was it? Where were you?	Describe each mood in one word. Rate intensity of mood (0–100%). Circle or mark the mood you want to examine.	Answer one or both of the questions below, and then some or all of the questions (on p. 54) specific to the mood you circled or marked: What was going through my mind just before I started to feel this way? What images or memories do I have in this situation?	Circle hot thought in previous column for which you are looking for evidence. Write factual evidence to support this conclusion. (Try to write facts, not interpretations, as you practiced in Worksheet 8.1 on p. 72.)	Ask yourself the questions in the Helpful Hints (p. 75) to help discover evidence that does not support your hot thought.	Ask yourself the questions in the Helpful Hints in Chapter 9 (p. 100) to generate alternative or balanced thoughts. Write an alternative or balanced thought. Rate how much you believe each alternative or balanced thought (0–100%).	Copy the moods from column 2. Rerate the intensity of each mood (0–100%), as well as any new moods.

Copyright 1983 by Christine A. Padesky. Reprinted in *Mind Over Mood, Second Edition*. Copyright 2016 by Dennis Greenberger and Christine A. Padesky. Purchasers of this book can photocopy and/or download additional copies of this worksheet (see the box at the end of the table of contents). All other rights reserved.

WORKSHEET 9.2. **Thought Record**

THOUGHT RECORD

1. Situation	2. Moods	3. Automatic Thoughts (Images)	4. Evidence That Supports the Hot Thought	5. Evidence That Does Not Support the Hot Thought	6. Alternative/Balanced Thoughts	7. Rate Moods Now
Who were you with? What were you doing? When was it? Where were you?	Describe each mood in one word. Rate intensity of mood (0–100%). Circle or mark the mood you want to examine.	Answer one or both of the questions below, and then some or all of the questions (on p. 54) specific to the mood you circled or marked: What was going through my mind just before I started to feel this way? What images or memories do I have in this situation?	Circle hot thought in previous column for which you are looking for evidence. Write factual evidence to support this conclusion. (Try to write facts, not interpretations, as you practiced in Worksheet 8.1 on p. 72.)	Ask yourself the questions in the Helpful Hints (p. 75) to help discover evidence that does not support your hot thought.	Ask yourself the questions in the Helpful Hints in Chapter 9 (p. 100) to generate alternative or balanced thoughts. Write an alternative or balanced thought. Rate how much you believe each alternative or balanced thought (0–100%).	Copy the moods from column 2. Rerate the intensity of each mood (0–100%), as well as any new moods.

Copyright 1983 by Christine A. Padesky. Reprinted in *Mind Over Mood, Second Edition*. Copyright 2016 by Dennis Greenberger and Christine A. Padesky. Purchasers of this book can photocopy and/or download additional copies of this worksheet (see the box at the end of the table of contents). All other rights reserved.

WORKSHEET 9.2. Thought Record

THOUGHT RECORD

1. Situation	2. Moods	3. Automatic Thoughts (Images)	4. Evidence That Supports the Hot Thought	5. Evidence That Does Not Support the Hot Thought	6. Alternative/Balanced Thoughts	7. Rate Moods Now
Who were you with? What were you doing? When was it? Where were you?	Describe each mood in one word. Rate intensity of mood (0–100%). Circle or mark the mood you want to examine.	Answer one or both of the questions below, and then some or all of the questions (on p. 54) specific to the mood you circled or marked: What was going through my mind just before I started to feel this way? What images or memories do I have in this situation?	Circle hot thought in previous column for which you are looking for evidence. Write factual evidence to support this conclusion. (Try to write facts, not interpretations, as you practiced in Worksheet 8.1 on p. 72.)	Ask yourself the questions in the Helpful Hints (p. 75) to help discover evidence that does not support your hot thought.	Ask yourself the questions in the Helpful Hints in Chapter 9 (p. 100) to generate alternative or balanced thoughts. Write an alternative or balanced thought. Rate how much you believe each alternative or balanced thought (0–100%).	Copy the moods from column 2. Rerate the intensity of each mood (0–100%), as well as any new moods.

Copyright 1983 by Christine A. Padesky. Reprinted in *Mind Over Mood, Second Edition*. Copyright 2016 by Dennis Greenberger and Christine A. Padesky. Purchasers of this book can photocopy and/or download additional copies of this worksheet (see the box at the end of the table of contents). All other rights reserved.

WORKSHEET 9.2. **Thought Record**

THOUGHT RECORD

1. Situation	2. Moods	3. Automatic Thoughts (Images)	4. Evidence That Supports the Hot Thought	5. Evidence That Does Not Support the Hot Thought	6. Alternative/Balanced Thoughts	7. Rate Moods Now
Who were you with? What were you doing? When was it? Where were you?	Describe each mood in one word. Rate intensity of mood (0–100%). Circle or mark the mood you want to examine.	Answer one or both of the questions below, and then some or all of the questions (on p. 54) specific to the mood you circled or marked: What was going through my mind just before I started to feel this way? What images or memories do I have in this situation?	Circle hot thought in previous column for which you are looking for evidence. Write factual evidence to support this conclusion. (Try to write facts, not interpretations, as you practiced in Worksheet 8.1 on p. 72.)	Ask yourself the questions in the Helpful Hints (p. 75) to help discover evidence that does not support your hot thought.	Ask yourself the questions in the Helpful Hints in Chapter 9 (p. 100) to generate alternative or balanced thoughts. Write an alternative or balanced thought. Rate how much you believe each alternative or balanced thought (0–100%).	Copy the moods from column 2. Rerate the intensity of each mood (0–100%), as well as any new moods.

Copyright 1983 by Christine A. Padesky. Reprinted in *Mind Over Mood, Second Edition*. Copyright 2016 by Dennis Greenberger and Christine A. Padesky. Purchasers of this book can photocopy and/or download additional copies of this worksheet (see the box at the end of the table of contents). All other rights reserved.

WORKSHEET 9.2. Thought Record

THOUGHT RECORD

1. Situation	2. Moods	3. Automatic Thoughts (Images)	4. Evidence That Supports the Hot Thought	5. Evidence That Does Not Support the Hot Thought	6. Alternative/Balanced Thoughts	7. Rate Moods Now
Who were you with? What were you doing? When was it? Where were you?	Describe each mood in one word. Rate intensity of mood (0–100%). Circle or mark the mood you want to examine.	Answer one or both of the questions below, and then some or all of the questions (on p. 54) specific to the mood you circled or marked: What was going through my mind just before I started to feel this way? What images or memories do I have in this situation?	Circle hot thought in previous column for which you are looking for evidence. Write factual evidence to support this conclusion. (Try to write facts, not interpretations, as you practiced in Worksheet 8.1 on p. 72.)	Ask yourself the questions in the Helpful Hints (p. 75) to help discover evidence that does not support your hot thought.	Ask yourself the questions in the Helpful Hints in Chapter 9 (p. 100) to generate alternative or balanced thoughts. Write an alternative or balanced thought. Rate how much you believe each alternative or balanced thought (0–100%).	Copy the moods from column 2. Rerate the intensity of each mood (0–100%), as well as any new moods.

Copyright 1983 by Christine A. Padesky. Reprinted in *Mind Over Mood, Second Edition*. Copyright 2016 by Dennis Greenberger and Christine A. Padesky. Purchasers of this book can photocopy and/or download additional copies of this worksheet (see the box at the end of the table of contents). All other rights reserved.

WORKSHEET 9.2. **Thought Record**

THOUGHT RECORD

1. Situation	2. Moods	3. Automatic Thoughts (Images)	4. Evidence That Supports the Hot Thought	5. Evidence That Does Not Support the Hot Thought	6. Alternative/Balanced Thoughts	7. Rate Moods Now
Who were you with? What were you doing? When was it? Where were you?	Describe each mood in one word. Rate intensity of mood (0–100%). Circle or mark the mood you want to examine.	Answer one or both of the questions below, and then some or all of the questions (on p. 54) specific to the mood you circled or marked: What was going through my mind just before I started to feel this way? What images or memories do I have in this situation?	Circle hot thought in previous column for which you are looking for evidence. Write factual evidence to support this conclusion. (Try to write facts, not interpretations, as you practiced in Worksheet 8.1 on p. 72.)	Ask yourself the questions in the Helpful Hints (p. 75) to help discover evidence that does not support your hot thought.	Ask yourself the questions in the Helpful Hints in Chapter 9 (p. 100) to generate alternative or balanced thoughts. Write an alternative or balanced thought. Rate how much you believe each alternative or balanced thought (0–100%).	Copy the moods from column 2. Rerate the intensity of each mood (0–100%), as well as any new moods.

Copyright 1983 by Christine A. Padesky. Reprinted in *Mind Over Mood, Second Edition*. Copyright 2016 by Dennis Greenberger and Christine A. Padesky. Purchasers of this book can photocopy and/or download additional copies of this worksheet (see the box at the end of the table of contents). All other rights reserved.

WORKSHEET 9.2. **Thought Record**

THOUGHT RECORD

1. Situation	2. Moods	3. Automatic Thoughts (Images)	4. Evidence That Supports the Hot Thought	5. Evidence That Does Not Support the Hot Thought	6. Alternative/Balanced Thoughts	7. Rate Moods Now
Who were you with? What were you doing? When was it? Where were you?	Describe each mood in one word. Rate intensity of mood (0–100%). Circle or mark the mood you want to examine.	Answer one or both of the questions below, and then some or all of the questions (on p. 54) specific to the mood you circled or marked: What was going through my mind just before I started to feel this way? What images or memories do I have in this situation?	Circle hot thought in previous column for which you are looking for evidence. Write factual evidence to support this conclusion. (Try to write facts, not interpretations, as you practiced in Worksheet 8.1 on p. 72.)	Ask yourself the questions in the Helpful Hints (p. 75) to help discover evidence that does not support your hot thought.	Ask yourself the questions in the Helpful Hints in Chapter 9 (p. 100) to generate alternative or balanced thoughts. Write an alternative or balanced thought. Rate how much you believe each alternative or balanced thought (0–100%).	Copy the moods from column 2. Rerate the intensity of each mood (0–100%), as well as any new moods.

Copyright 1983 by Christine A. Padesky. Reprinted in *Mind Over Mood, Second Edition*. Copyright 2016 by Dennis Greenberger and Christine A. Padesky. Purchasers of this book can photocopy and/or download additional copies of this worksheet (see the box at the end of the table of contents). All other rights reserved.

WORKSHEET 9.2. Thought Record

THOUGHT RECORD

1. Situation	2. Moods	3. Automatic Thoughts (Images)	4. Evidence That Supports the Hot Thought	5. Evidence That Does Not Support the Hot Thought	6. Alternative/Balanced Thoughts	7. Rate Moods Now
Who were you with? What were you doing? When was it? Where were you?	Describe each mood in one word. Rate intensity of mood (0–100%). Circle or mark the mood you want to examine.	Answer one or both of the questions below, and then some or all of the questions (on p. 54) specific to the mood you circled or marked: What was going through my mind just before I started to feel this way? What images or memories do I have in this situation?	Circle hot thought in previous column for which you are looking for evidence. Write factual evidence to support this conclusion. (Try to write facts, not interpretations, as you practiced in Worksheet 8.1 on p. 72.)	Ask yourself the questions in the Helpful Hints (p. 75) to help discover evidence that does not support your hot thought.	Ask yourself the questions in the Helpful Hints in Chapter 9 (p. 100) to generate alternative or balanced thoughts. Write an alternative or balanced thought. Rate how much you believe each alternative or balanced thought (0–100%).	Copy the moods from column 2. Rerate the intensity of each mood (0–100%), as well as any new moods.

Copyright 1983 by Christine A. Padesky. Reprinted in *Mind Over Mood, Second Edition*. Copyright 2016 by Dennis Greenberger and Christine A. Padesky. Purchasers of this book can photocopy and/or download additional copies of this worksheet (see the box at the end of the table of contents). All other rights reserved.

> **EXERCISE: Making an Action Plan**
>
> Identify a problem in your life that you would like to change, and write your goal on the top line on Worksheet 10.2. Complete the Action Plan, making it as specific as possible. Set a time to begin, identify problems that could interfere with completing your plan, develop strategies for coping with the problems if they should arise, and keep written track of the progress you make. Complete additional Action Plans for other problem areas of your life that you would like to change.

WORKSHEET 10.2. Action Plan

Goal: _____

Actions to take	Time to begin	Possible problems	Strategies to overcome problems	Progress

From *Mind Over Mood, Second Edition*. Copyright 2016 by Dennis Greenberger and Christine A. Padesky. Purchasers of this book can photocopy and/or download additional copies of this worksheet (see the box at the end of the table of contents).

> **EXERCISE: Making an Action Plan**
>
> Identify a problem in your life that you would like to change, and write your goal on the top line on Worksheet 10.2. Complete the Action Plan, making it as specific as possible. Set a time to begin, identify problems that could interfere with completing your plan, develop strategies for coping with the problems if they should arise, and keep written track of the progress you make. Complete additional Action Plans for other problem areas of your life that you would like to change.

WORKSHEET 10.2. Action Plan

Goal: _____

Actions to take	Time to begin	Possible problems	Strategies to overcome problems	Progress

From *Mind Over Mood, Second Edition*. Copyright 2016 by Dennis Greenberger and Christine A. Padesky. Purchasers of this book can photocopy and/or download additional copies of this worksheet (see the box at the end of the table of contents).

WORKSHEET 11.2. Experiments to Test an Underlying Assumption

ASSUMPTION TESTED					
Experiment	Predictions	Possible problems	Strategies to overcome these problems	Outcome of experiment	What have I learned from this experiment about this assumption?
				What happened (compared to your predictions)? Do the outcomes match what you predicted? Did anything unexpected happen? If things didn't turn out as you wanted, how well did you handle it?	
ALTERNATIVE ASSUMPTION THAT FITS WITH THE OUTCOME(S) OF MY EXPERIMENT(S)					

From *Mind Over Mood, Second Edition*. Copyright 2016 by Dennis Greenberger and Christine A. Padesky. Purchasers of this book can photocopy and/or download additional copies of this worksheet (see the box at the end of the table of contents).

WORKSHEET 11.2. Experiments to Test an Underlying Assumption

ASSUMPTION TESTED					
Experiment	**Predictions**	**Possible problems**	**Strategies to overcome these problems**	**Outcome of experiment**	**What have I learned from this experiment about this assumption?**
				What happened (compared to your predictions)? Do the outcomes match what you predicted? Did anything unexpected happen? If things didn't turn out as you wanted, how well did you handle it?	
ALTERNATIVE ASSUMPTION THAT FITS WITH THE OUTCOME(S) OF MY EXPERIMENT(S)					

From *Mind Over Mood, Second Edition*. Copyright 2016 by Dennis Greenberger and Christine A. Padesky. Purchasers of this book can photocopy and/or download additional copies of this worksheet (see the box at the end of the table of contents).

WORKSHEET 12.6. Core Belief Record: Recording Evidence That Supports a New Core Belief

New Core Belief: _____

Evidence or experiences that support my new belief:

1. _____
2. _____
3. _____
4. _____
5. _____
6. _____
7. _____
8. _____
9. _____
10. _____
11. _____
12. _____
13. _____
14. _____
15. _____
16. _____
17. _____
18. _____
19. _____
20. _____
21. _____
22. _____
23. _____
24. _____
25. _____

From *Mind Over Mood, Second Edition*. Copyright 2016 by Dennis Greenberger and Christine A. Padesky. Purchasers of this book can photocopy and/or download additional copies of this worksheet (see the box at the end of the table of contents).

EXERCISE: Rating Confidence in New Core Beliefs over Time

On the first line of Worksheet 12.7, write the new core belief you identified and have been strengthening on Worksheet 12.6. Then enter the date and rate the new core belief by placing an × on the scale above the number that best matches how much you think this new belief fits with your current experiences. If you don't believe the new core belief at all, mark your × above 0 on the scale. If you have total confidence in your new core belief, put your × above 100 on the scale. To measure your progress in strengthening your new core belief, rerate the new core belief every few weeks.

WORKSHEET 12.7. Rating Confidence in My New Core Belief

New core belief: _____

Ratings of confidence in my belief

Date:

0%　　　　　25%　　　　　50%　　　　　75%　　　　　100%

Date:

0%　　　　　25%　　　　　50%　　　　　75%　　　　　100%

Date:

0%　　　　　25%　　　　　50%　　　　　75%　　　　　100%

Date:

0%　　　　　25%　　　　　50%　　　　　75%　　　　　100%

Date:

0%　　　　　25%　　　　　50%　　　　　75%　　　　　100%

Date:

0%　　　　　25%　　　　　50%　　　　　75%　　　　　100%

Date:

0%　　　　　25%　　　　　50%　　　　　75%　　　　　100%

From *Mind Over Mood, Second Edition*. Copyright 2016 by Dennis Greenberger and Christine A. Padesky. Purchasers of this book can photocopy and/or download additional copies of this worksheet (see the box at the end of the table of contents).

> **EXERCISE: Rating Behaviors on a Scale instead of in All-or-Nothing Terms**
>
> On Worksheet 12.8, identify some of your own behaviors related to your new core belief. For example, if you are trying to develop a new core belief that you are lovable, you might rate your social behavior or things you do that you think would make you lovable. If you are trying to develop a new core belief that "I am a worthwhile person," you could focus on behaviors that you think demonstrate your worth. Choose behaviors that you tend to evaluate in all-or-nothing terms. For each scale, describe the situation and write what behavior you are rating. Notice how it feels to rate your behavior on a scale instead of evaluating yourself in all-or-nothing terms. After you have rated several behaviors on these scales, summarize what you have learned at the bottom of Worksheet 12.8.

WORKSHEET 12.8. Rating Behaviors on a Scale

Situation: _____   Behavior I am rating: _____
0%   25%   50%   75%   100%
|——————————|——————————|——————————|——————————|

Situation: _____   Behavior I am rating: _____
0%   25%   50%   75%   100%
|——————————|——————————|——————————|——————————|

Situation: _____   Behavior I am rating: _____
0%   25%   50%   75%   100%
|——————————|——————————|——————————|——————————|

Situation: _____   Behavior I am rating: _____
0%   25%   50%   75%   100%
|——————————|——————————|——————————|——————————|

Situation: _____   Behavior I am rating: _____
0%   25%   50%   75%   100%
|——————————|——————————|——————————|——————————|

Situation: _____   Behavior I am rating: _____
0%   25%   50%   75%   100%
|——————————|——————————|——————————|——————————|

Summary: _____
_____
_____
_____

From *Mind Over Mood, Second Edition*. Copyright 2016 by Dennis Greenberger and Christine A. Padesky. Purchasers of this book can photocopy and/or download additional copies of this worksheet (see the box at the end of the table of contents).

WORKSHEET 12.9. Behavioral Experiments to Strengthen New Core Beliefs

Write down the core belief(s) you want to strengthen: _____

List two or three new behaviors that fit with your new core belief. These might be behaviors you would do if you had confidence in your new core belief. They might be behaviors that you feel reluctant to do and yet they would strengthen your new core belief if you did them: _____
_____

Make predictions about what will happen, based on your old and new core beliefs.

My old core belief prediction:
_____
_____

My new core belief prediction:
_____
_____

Results of my experiments with strangers (write down what you did, who you did it with, and what happened):

Results of my experiments with people I know (write down what you did, who you did it with, and what happened):

What I learned (do the results support my new core beliefs even partially?):

Future experiments I want to do:

From *Mind Over Mood, Second Edition.* Copyright 2016 by Dennis Greenberger and Christine A. Padesky. Purchasers of this book can photocopy and/or download additional copies of this worksheet (see the box at the end of the table of contents).

WORKSHEET 13.1. *Mind Over Mood* Depression Inventory

Circle or mark one number for each item that best describes how much you have experienced each symptom over the last week.

	Not at all	Sometimes	Frequently	Most of the time
1. Sad or depressed mood	0	1	2	3
2. Feelings of guilt	0	1	2	3
3. Irritable mood	0	1	2	3
4. Less interest or pleasure in usual activities	0	1	2	3
5. Withdrawing from or avoiding people	0	1	2	3
6. Finding it harder than usual to do things	0	1	2	3
7. Seeing myself as worthless	0	1	2	3
8. Trouble concentrating	0	1	2	3
9. Difficulty making decisions	0	1	2	3
10. Suicidal thoughts	0	1	2	3
11. Recurrent thoughts of death	0	1	2	3
12. Spending time thinking about a suicide plan	0	1	2	3
13. Low self-esteem	0	1	2	3
14. Seeing the future as hopeless	0	1	2	3
15. Self-critical thoughts	0	1	2	3
16. Tiredness or loss of energy	0	1	2	3
17. Significant weight loss or decrease in appetite (do not include weight loss from a diet plan)	0	1	2	3
18. Change in sleep pattern – difficulty sleeping or sleeping more or less than usual	0	1	2	3
19. Decreased sexual desire	0	1	2	3
			Score (sum of item scores)	

From *Mind Over Mood, Second Edition*. Copyright 2016 by Dennis Greenberger and Christine A. Padesky. Purchasers of this book can photocopy and/or download additional copies of this worksheet (see the box at the end of the table of contents).

WORKSHEET 13.2. *Mind Over Mood* Depression Inventory Scores

Score														
57														
54														
51														
48														
45														
42														
39														
36														
33														
30														
27														
24														
21														
18														
15														
12														
9														
6														
3														
0														
Date														

From *Mind Over Mood, Second Edition*. Copyright 2016 by Dennis Greenberger and Christine A. Padesky. Purchasers of this book can photocopy and/or download additional copies of this worksheet (see the box at the end of the table of contents).

EXERCISE: Activity Scheduling

Before filling out Worksheet 13.6 on the next page, write down at least several activities you want to plan for each day. You might find it helpful to review Worksheet 13.5 on page 208, especially your answers to questions 3, 6, and 8. It is helpful to think of several activities in each of the following categories and spread them out throughout the week.

Pleasurable activities: _____

_____

_____

_____

_____

Activities that accomplish something: _____

_____

_____

_____

_____

What I can do to begin to approach things I have been avoiding: _____

_____

_____

_____

_____

Activities that fit with my values: _____

_____

_____

_____

_____

Some activities could fit in a variety of categories. For example, walking or exercising may be pleasurable for one person, may be an accomplishment for someone else, and may fit with a value of doing healthy activities for yet another person. If you have been avoiding exercise for some time, it may even be overcoming avoidance. Put activities in whatever category makes sense to you. The important thing is to do activities in each of the four areas throughout the week.

WORKSHEET 13.6. Activity Schedule

Referring to the "Activity Scheduling" exercise (p. 213), use this worksheet to schedule some activities. Write down the times and days of the week you plan to do these activities. If something more enjoyable or more important comes along, you can do that activity instead during that time period. If you do something different during any time period, put a line through what you had planned and write down what you actually did. For each time period in which you planned an activity, write down: (1) Activity. (2) Mood ratings (0–100).

(Mood I am rating: _____)

Time	Monday	Tuesday	Wednesday	Thursday	Friday	Saturday	Sunday
6–7 A.M.							
7–8 A.M.							
8–9 A.M.							
9–10 A.M.							
10–11 A.M.							
11 A.M.–12 noon							
12 noon–1 P.M.							
1–2 P.M.							

2–3 P.M.							
3–4 P.M.							
4–5 P.M.							
5–6 P.M.							
6–7 P.M.							
7–8 P.M.							
8–9 P.M.							
9–10 P.M.							
10–11 P.M.							
11 P.M.–12 midnight							
12 midnight–1 A.M.							

WORKSHEET 14.1. *Mind Over Mood* Anxiety Inventory

Circle or mark one number for each item that best describes how much you have experienced each symptom over the past week.

	Not at all	Sometimes	Frequently	Most of the time
1. Feeling nervous	0	1	2	3
2. Worrying	0	1	2	3
3. Trembling, twitching, feeling shaky	0	1	2	3
4. Muscle tension, muscle aches, muscle soreness	0	1	2	3
5. Restlessness	0	1	2	3
6. Tiring easily	0	1	2	3
7. Shortness of breath	0	1	2	3
8. Rapid heartbeat	0	1	2	3
9. Sweating not due to the heat	0	1	2	3
10. Dry mouth	0	1	2	3
11. Dizziness or light-headedness	0	1	2	3
12. Nausea, diarrhea, or stomach problems	0	1	2	3
13. Increase in urge to urinate	0	1	2	3
14. Flushes (hot flashes) or chills	0	1	2	3
15. Trouble swallowing or "lump in throat"	0	1	2	3
16. Feeling keyed up or on edge	0	1	2	3
17. Being quick to startle	0	1	2	3
18. Difficulty concentrating	0	1	2	3
19. Trouble falling or staying asleep	0	1	2	3
20. Irritability	0	1	2	3
21. Avoiding places where I might be anxious	0	1	2	3
22. Thoughts of danger	0	1	2	3
23. Seeing myself as unable to cope	0	1	2	3
24. Thoughts that something terrible will happen	0	1	2	3
	Score (sum of item scores)			

From *Mind Over Mood, Second Edition.* Copyright 2016 by Dennis Greenberger and Christine A. Padesky. Purchasers of this book can photocopy and/or download additional copies of this worksheet (see the box at the end of the table of contents).

WORKSHEET 14.2. *Mind Over Mood* Anxiety Inventory Scores

Score														
72														
69														
66														
63														
60														
57														
54														
51														
48														
45														
42														
39														
36														
33														
30														
27														
24														
21														
18														
15														
12														
9														
6														
3														
0														
Date														

From *Mind Over Mood, Second Edition*. Copyright 2016 by Dennis Greenberger and Christine A. Padesky. Purchasers of this book can photocopy and/or download additional copies of this worksheet (see the box at the end of the table of contents).

> **EXERCISE: Making My Fear Ladder**
>
> Make your Fear Ladder by filling out Worksheets 14.4 and 14.5. Worksheet 14.4 helps you brainstorm and rate situations you avoid because of anxiety. Once this is done, put on Worksheet 14.5 the item you rated with the highest anxiety on the top step, and the item you rated with the lowest anxiety on the bottom step. Fill in the other steps from high to low based on your anxiety ratings. If you rated some items equally, put them in the order that makes most sense to you, so that your Fear Ladder steps move from your least feared at the bottom to your most feared situations at the top of the ladder. It's OK if some of your steps are blank.

WORKSHEET 14.4. Making a Fear Ladder

1. First, brainstorm a list of situations, events, or people that you avoid because of your anxiety. Write them in the left-hand column below, in any order.

2. After you complete your list, rate how anxious you feel when you imagine each of the things listed in the first column. Rate these from 0 to 100, where 0 is no anxiety and 100 is the most anxious you have ever felt. Write these ratings next to each item in the right-hand column.

What I avoid	Rate anxiety (0–100)

From *Mind Over Mood, Second Edition*. Copyright 2016 by Dennis Greenberger and Christine A. Padesky. Purchasers of this book can photocopy and/or download additional copies of this worksheet (see the box at the end of the table of contents).

WORKSHEET 14.5. My Fear Ladder

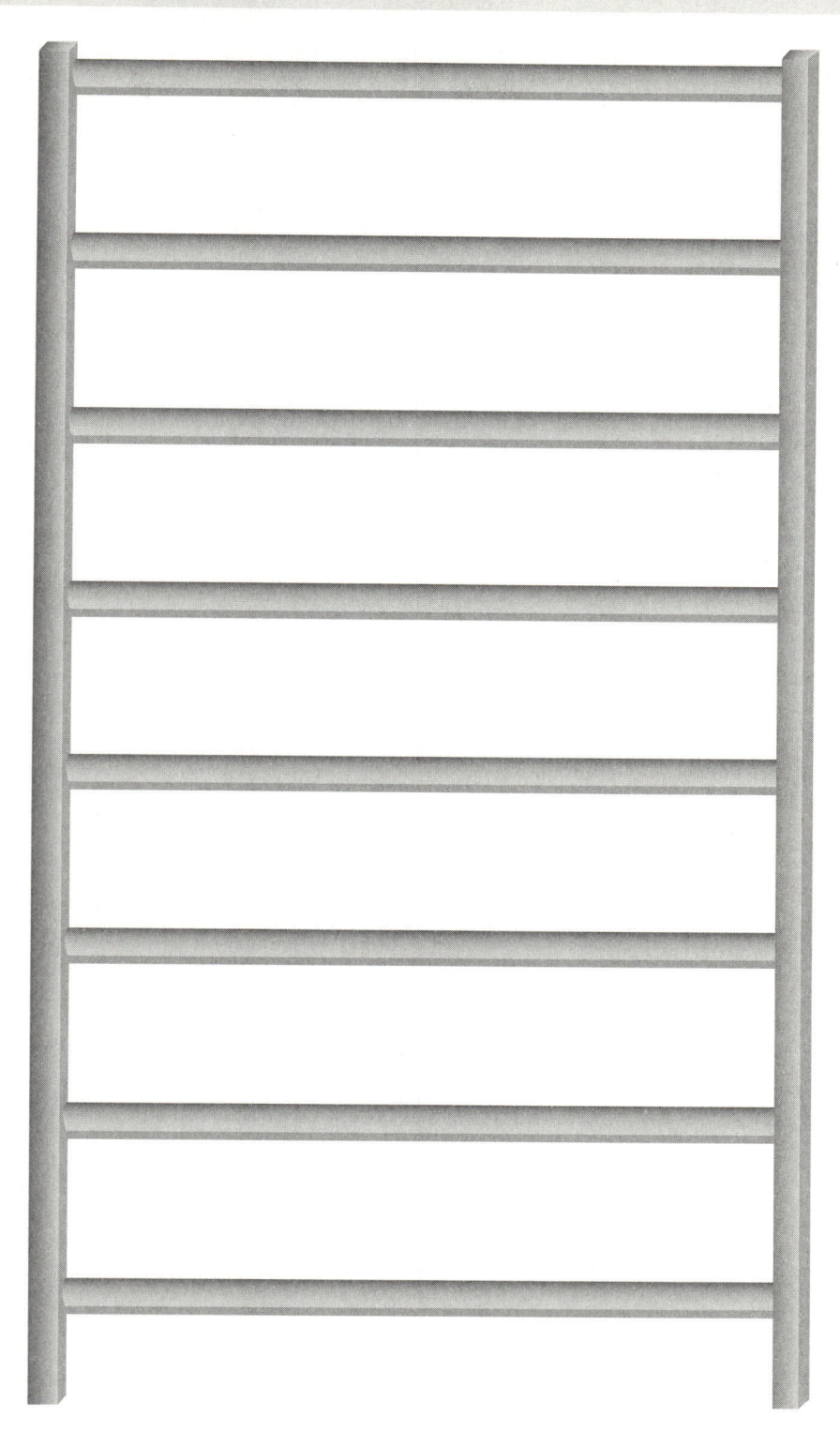

From *Mind Over Mood, Second Edition*. Copyright 2016 by Dennis Greenberger and Christine A. Padesky. Purchasers of this book can photocopy and/or download additional copies of this worksheet (see the box at the end of the table of contents).

WORKSHEET 15.1. Measuring and Tracking My Moods

Use this worksheet to measure and track the frequency, strength, and duration of any mood you want to improve. This worksheet can also be used to measure and track positive emotions, including happiness.

Mood I am rating: _____

FREQUENCY

Circle or mark the number below that most accurately describes how often you experienced this mood this week:

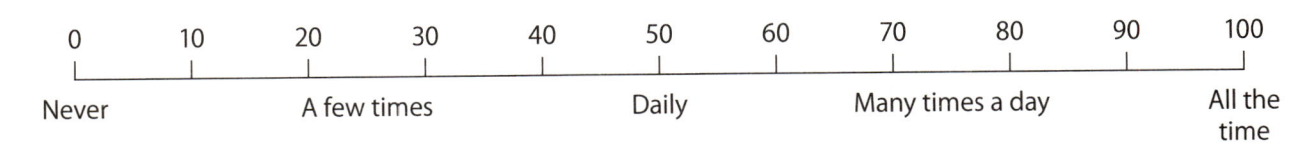

```
0     10    20    30    40    50    60    70    80    90    100
|—————|—————|—————|—————|—————|—————|—————|—————|—————|—————|
Never           A few times         Daily         Many times a day        All the
                                                                           time
```

STRENGTH

Circle or mark below how strongly you felt this mood this week. Rate the time when your mood was the strongest, even if most of the time you did not experience it this strongly. A score of 0 would mean that you did not feel the mood this week. A score of 100 would show that it was the strongest you have ever felt this mood in your life. Strongly felt moods will score higher than 70. If you felt the mood at a medium level of strength, give it a rating between 30 and 70. Rate a mild mood between 1 and 30.

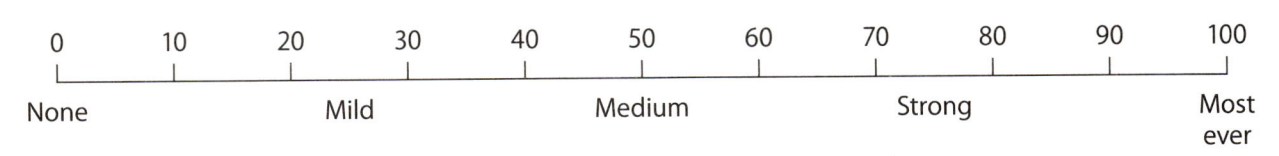

```
0     10    20    30    40    50    60    70    80    90    100
|—————|—————|—————|—————|—————|—————|—————|—————|—————|—————|
None            Mild              Medium            Strong           Most
                                                                     ever
```

DURATION

Circle or mark the number below that matches how long your mood lasted. Again, make this rating for the time during the week when you felt this mood most strongly (think about the rating you gave this mood on the Strength scale above). If you did not experience the mood this week, circle 0.

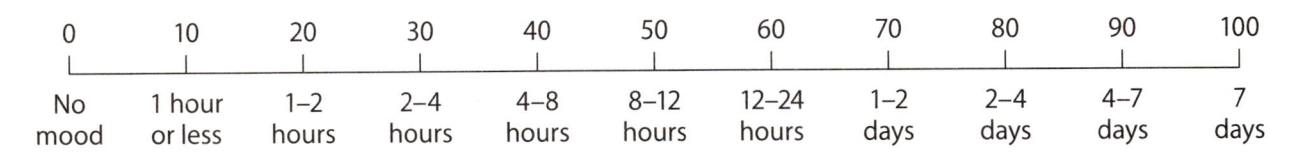

```
0      10      20     30      40     50     60      70     80     90     100
|——————|——————|——————|——————|——————|——————|——————|——————|——————|——————|
No    1 hour   1–2    2–4     4–8    8–12   12–24   1–2    2–4    4–7     7
mood  or less  hours  hours   hours  hours  hours   days   days   days   days
```

From *Mind Over Mood, Second Edition*. Copyright 2016 by Dennis Greenberger and Christine A. Padesky. Purchasers of this book can photocopy and/or download additional copies of this worksheet (see the box at the end of the table of contents).

EXERCISE: Mood Scores

Use Worksheet 15.2 to record your scores on the frequency, strength, and duration of the mood(s) you are rating on Worksheet 15.1. You can label them F (frequency), S (strength), and D (duration) on Worksheet 15.2, or you can use different colors for each. By tracking all three types of mood ratings on the same chart, you will be able to see your progress as you learn *Mind Over Mood* skills. Use a different copy of Worksheet 15.2 for each mood you are rating. For example, you might be rating both shame and happiness, and you want to track each on a different Worksheet 15.2.

WORKSHEET 15.2. Mood Scores Chart

Mood I am rating:

100														
90														
80														
70														
60														
50														
40														
30														
20														
10														
0														
Date														

From *Mind Over Mood, Second Edition*. Copyright 2016 by Dennis Greenberger and Christine A. Padesky. Purchasers of this book can photocopy and/or download additional copies of this worksheet (see the box at the end of the table of contents).

WORKSHEET 15.4. Writing a Forgiveness Letter

1. This is what you did to me:

2. This is the impact it has had in my life:

3. This is how it continues to affect me:

4. This is how I imagine my life will be better if I'm able to forgive you:

5. (Forgiveness often begins with a compassionate understanding of persons who have hurt you. Write about any life experiences the other person or persons had that might have contributed to the ways they hurt or mistreated you.) This is how I can understand what you have done:

6. (Everyone hurts someone else sometimes. When you hurt someone else, how would you want that person to think about you?) This is how I would want to be viewed if I hurt someone:

7. (Forgiveness does not mean that you approve of, forget, or deny what was done and the pain you have experienced. Instead, forgiveness means finding a way to let go of your anger and understand the events from a different perspective.) This is how I can forgive what you have done:

8. These are the qualities I have that will allow me to move forward:

From *Mind Over Mood, Second Edition*. Copyright 2016 by Dennis Greenberger and Christine A. Padesky. Purchasers of this book can photocopy and/or download additional copies of this worksheet (see the box at the end of the table of contents).

> **EXERCISE: Forgiving Myself**
>
> Some people have great difficulty forgiving themselves; they may have harsh and critical internal voices. If you are able to forgive others for their faults, but you have a hard time forgiving yourself, you can benefit from practicing self-forgiveness. This involves learning to view yourself with the same kindness or compassion with which you view others. Worksheet 15.9 on the next page can guide you through this process.

WORKSHEET 15.9. Forgiving Myself

1. This is what I need to forgive myself for:

2. This is the impact that what I did has had on me and others in my life:

3. This is how it continues to affect me and others:

4. This is how I imagine my life will be better if I'm able to forgive myself:

5. Forgiveness often begins with understanding. What life experiences have I had that might have contributed to what I did?

6. How would I think about someone else who did this?

7. What positive aspects of myself and my life do I tend to ignore when I'm feeling guilt or shame?

8. Forgiveness does not mean that you condone, forget, or deny what was done and the pain you have experienced. Instead, forgiveness means finding a way to let go of your guilt and shame, and understand your actions from a different perspective. Write with a kind, compassionate voice about how I can forgive myself for what I have done:

9. These are the qualities that I have that will allow me to move forward:

From *Mind Over Mood, Second Edition*. Copyright 2016 by Dennis Greenberger and Christine A. Padesky. Purchasers of this book can photocopy and/or download additional copies of this worksheet (see the box at the end of the table of contents).

WORKSHEET 16.2. My Plan to Reduce Relapse Risk

1. My high-risk situations:

_____
_____
_____
_____
_____
_____
_____
_____

2. My early warning signs:

_____
_____
_____
_____
_____
_____
_____
_____

Rate my moods on a regular basis (monthly, for example). My warning score is _____

3. My plan of action (review Worksheet 16.1 on pp. 282–285 for ideas):

_____
_____
_____
_____
_____
_____
_____
_____

From *Mind Over Mood, Second Edition*. Copyright 2016 by Dennis Greenberger and Christine A. Padesky. Purchasers of this book can photocopy and/or download additional copies of this worksheet (see the box at the end of the table of contents).

Index

Acceptance
   anxiety and, 241–242, 245–246
   core beliefs and, 164, 283
   no change in mood after completing a Thought Record and, 106, 107
   overview, 126–130, 131, 152, 154, 290
   paths to, 129, 131
Action Plan
   no change in mood after completing a Thought Record and, 106
   overview, 119–125, 130, 131, 290
   relapse prevention and, 287–288
Activity planning, 210–216, 216–217, 218. *See also* Behavioral activation
Activity schedule, 210–215, 218, 324–326
Alcohol use, 1, 3, 4. *See also* Vic (case example)
Alternative assumptions, 150. *See also* Underlying assumptions
Alternative/balanced thoughts. *See also* Strengthening new thoughts; Thought Record; Thoughts
   Action Plan and, 119–125
   gathering new evidence and, 95–100
   no change in mood after completing a Thought Record, 106–112
   overview, 95, 99–113, 116–118, 131
   support for hot thoughts and, 112–113
Anger. *See also* Moods; Vic (case example)
   assertive responses and, 261–263
   automatic thoughts and, 56, 257–258
   forgiveness and, 263–264
   management strategies, 258–264
   multiple moods and, 31
   overview, 1, 4, 252, 255–267, 279
   testing angry thoughts, 257–260
   warning signs of, 260–261
Anxiety. *See also* Linda (case example); Moods; Vic (case example)
   acceptance of, 127–128
   behaviors, 225–228
   Fear Ladder and, 235–241
   goal setting and, 34
   medication use and, 248–249
   multiple moods and, 31
   overcoming, 233–249
   overview, 1, 4, 219–225, 249–251
   symptoms of, 220–223
   thoughts and, 24, 55–56, 61–63, 229–234, 247–248
   underlying assumptions and, 134
Assertion, 261–263
Assumptions, underlying. *See* Underlying assumptions
Automatic thoughts. *See also* Core beliefs; Evidence for or against a thought; Thought Record; Thoughts; Underlying assumptions
   behavior and, 18–19
   downward arrow technique and, 156–163
   hot thoughts, 61–67
   identifying, 52–60, 64–67
   overview, 50–52, 68, 153, 187
   Thought Record, 39–46
Avoidance
   anxiety and, 225–226, 251
   changing the way you think and, 24
   Fear Ladder and, 240–241
   overcoming, 234–235

333

B

Balanced thoughts. *See* Alternative/balanced thoughts
Bannister, Roger, 18
Beck, Aaron T., 194, ix–xi
Behavior. *See also* Thought–behavior connection
  anger and, 255
  anxiety and, 224–228, 251
  depression and, 193
  mood identification and, 27
  thought–behavior connection, 18–20
  underlying assumptions and, 134
Behavioral activation, 198–199, 201–217, 290
Behavioral experiments. *See also* Underlying assumptions
  do the opposite and see what happens experiment, 144–148
  does "then . . ." always follow "if . . ."? experiment, 142–145, 148
  overview, 134–137, 148, 150–151, 290
  planning, 137–138
  strengthening new core beliefs with, 172–174
Behaviors in the five-part model, 6–11, 13–15. *See also* Five-part model to understand life experiences
Beliefs. *See* Core beliefs; Thoughts; Underlying assumptions
Ben (case example)
  alternative/balanced thoughts, 101–103
  behavioral activation, 201–203, 208–211
  depression and, 188, 201–203, 211
  evidence for or against a thought, 74–77
  mood identification and, 27, 28
  overview, 5–6, 292–293
  rating the intensity of moods, 29
  relapse management and, 286, 287
  strengthening new thoughts and, 118
  Thought Record first three columns, 46
  thought–behavior connection, 19–20
  understanding Ben's problems, 6–8
Binges, 3
Breathing strategies, 243

C

Case examples. *See* Ben (case example); Linda (case example); Marissa (case example); Vic (case example)

Cognitive-behavioral therapy (CBT) overview, 1–2, 4
  anxiety and, 249
  depression and, 199, 218
  resources for, 291
Communication, 261–264
Confidence, 1, 117–118, 169
Coping
  anxiety and, 227–228, 248, 251
  relapse prevention and, 289
  thoughts and, 229
Core beliefs. *See also* Automatic thoughts; Downward arrow technique; Underlying assumptions
  acts of kindness and, 184–186
  behavioral experiments and, 172–174
  gratitude and, 175–183
  identifying, 156–165
  no change in mood after completing a Thought Record and, 106
  overview, 152–155, 158, 164, 186, 187
  strengthening new core beliefs, 165–174
  testing, 163
Couple therapy, 267

D

Depression. *See also* Ben (case example); Marissa (case example); Moods; Vic (case example)
  activity scheduling, 210–217
  automatic thoughts and, 55
  medication use and, 199–200
  multiple moods and, 31
  overview, 1, 4, 188–194, 218
  thoughts and, 194–198
  treatment for, 198–217
Downward arrow technique, 156–163. *See also* Core beliefs
Drug use, 1, 3, 4

E

Eating issues, 3–4
Emotions. *See* Moods
Enjoyable activities, 210–215, 212, 216–217, 218. *See also* Activity planning; Behavioral activation
Environment, 24. *See also* Thought–environment connection
Environmental/life changes/situations in the five-part model, 6–11, 13–15. *See also* Five-part model to understand life experiences

Evidence for or against a thought. *See also* Gathering new evidence; Thought Record; Thoughts
  core beliefs and, 163, 165–167
  interpretations and, 98
  no change in mood after completing a Thought Record, 106–112
  overview, 69–86, 94
  support for hot thoughts and, 112–113
Examples. *See* Ben (case example); Linda (case example); Marissa (case example); Vic (case example)
Experiments, behavioral. *See* Behavioral experiments
Exposure, 234–235, 251

F

Facts, 72–74
Family therapy, 267
Fear Ladder, 235–241, 251
Feelings. *See* Moods
Fight, flight, and freeze responses, 223–224. *See also* Anxiety
Five-part model, 6–11, 13–15
Forgiveness, 263–264, 277–278
Future, thinking about, 195–196

G

Gathering new evidence. *See also* Evidence for or against a thought
  core beliefs and, 163
  overview, 95–100, 131
  strengthening new thoughts and, 118–119
Generalized anxiety disorders, 234. *See also* Anxiety
Goal setting, 33–38
Gratitude, 175–183, 187
Gratitude journal, 176, 187, 287
Guilt. *See also* Moods
  automatic thoughts and, 56
  multiple moods and, 31
  overview, 1, 252, 267–278, 279

H

Happiness. *See also* Moods
  gratitude and, 175
  multiple moods and, 31
  overview, 3, 280–285, 289–291

Health worries, 234. *See also* Anxiety
Hierarchy, 235–241, 251
Hopelessness, 194. *See also* Thoughts
Hot thoughts. *See also* Automatic thoughts
  alternative/balanced thoughts, 101–105, 110–111
  automatic thoughts and, 68
  evidence for or against a thought and, 86, 112–113
  gathering new evidence and, 99–100
  identifying, 61–67
  interpretations and, 98
  no change in mood after completing a Thought Record, 106–112
  support for, 112–113

I

"I" statements, 262, 264
Identification of automatic thoughts. *See* Automatic thoughts
Identification of moods. *See* Moods
Imagery, 244–245, 260
Images, 18, 24, 40, 44, 52, 54–55, 62, 68, 223, 229–231, 234, 247–248, 251, 256, 260–261, 266, 279, 282–284, 290, 295. *See also* Automatic thoughts
Improvement, noticing, 37–38
Intensity of moods, 29–31, 43–44. *See also* Moods; Moods, rating strength
Interpretations, 72–74, 95–100

J

Jealousy, 1

K

Kindness, acts of, 184–187

L

Life situations
  acceptance and, 126–131
  anxiety and, 223
  changing the way you think and, 24
  depression and, 195
  relapse prevention and, 286
Linda (case example)
  alternative/balanced thoughts, 107–111

Linda (continued)
    anxiety and, 231
    evidence for or against a thought, 82–85
    overview, 7–8, 219, 294–295
    positive thinking disadvantages and, 23
    relapse management and, 286
    Thought Record first three columns, 46
    thought–physical reactions connection, 20–21
    underlying assumptions and behavioral experiments and, 134–137
    understanding Linda's problems, 9–10

M

Maintaining gains, 280–285, 289–291. *See also* Relapse management
Marissa (case example)
    Action Plan and, 119–122
    alternative/balanced thoughts, 104–106
    automatic thoughts, 50–51
    core beliefs, 155, 163, 164, 167
    depression, 188–189, 194
    downward arrow technique and, 156–158
    evidence for or against a thought, 77–81
    guilt or shame and, 252, 272–273
    overview, 9–10, 293–294
    relapse management and, 286
    Thought Record first three columns, 39–45
    thought–environment connection, 21
    thought–mood connection, 17–18
    understanding Marissa's problems, 10–11
Medication use
    anxiety and, 248–249, 251
    depression and, 199–200
Mindfulness, 241–242, 245–246, 251, 284, 290
Moods. *See also* Anger; Anxiety; Depression; Guilt; Happiness; Moods in the five-part model; Shame; Thought Record; Thought–mood connection
    acceptance and, 126–131
    anger profile and, 255
    anxiety profile and, 224, 251
    depression profile and, 193
    identifying, 25–29
    list of moods, 25
    multiple moods, 31–32
    rating the intensity or strength of, 29–31, 43–44, 252–254
    Thought Record, 39–46, 106–112
    thoughts and, 16–18, 55–56, 61–67, 68
Moods in the five-part model, 6–11, 13–15. *See also* Five-part model to understand life experiences; Moods
Multiple moods, 31–32. *See also* Moods
Muscle relaxation, 243–244

N

Negative automatic thoughts. *See* Automatic thoughts
Negative core beliefs. *See* Core beliefs
Negative thoughts. *See* Thoughts

O

Overeating, 3

P

Panic, 1, 21, 34, 36, 44, 55, 230, 234, 236, 251
Panic attacks, 136, 234, 236. *See also* Linda (case example)
Panic disorder, 234. *See also* Anxiety
Perception of events, 2, 229–230, 247, 257, 279. *See also* Thoughts
Perspective, 105–106, 112, 130, 164, 175, 259, 264
Phobias, 219, 234. *See also* Anxiety
Physical reactions. *See also* Thought–physical reactions connection
    anger and, 255
    anxiety and, 224, 251
    depression and, 193
    mood identification and, 26
    Thought Record, 44
Physical reactions in the five-part model, 6–11, 13–15. *See also* Five-part model to understand life experiences
Plan of action. *See* Action Plan
Pleasurable activities, 210–218
Positive moods, 3. *See also* Happiness
Positive thinking, disadvantages of, 23
Posttraumatic stress disorder, 234. *See also* Anxiety
Practicing skills, 3, 4, 280–285, 287, 289–291
Predictions, 55, 137, 142–151, 150
Problem solving, 138
Professional help, 291
Progressive muscle relaxation, 243–244
Purging, 3

Q

Questions to help
  acceptance and, 129
  evidence for or against a thought, 75, 86
  gathering new evidence and, 98–100
  identifying automatic thoughts, 54–56, 64–67. See also Automatic thoughts
  no change in mood after completing a Thought Record and, 107

R

Relapse management, 281, 285–289. See also Maintaining gains
Relationship problems. See also Vic (case example)
  anger and, 255–260, 262–265
  anxiety and, 230
  depression and, 200–201
  overview, 1, 3
  underlying assumptions and, 134
Relaxation methods, 241–246
Responsibility pie, 272–274

S

Safety behaviors, 226–228
Secretiveness, 276–277
Self-criticism, 194. See also Ben (case example); Marissa (case example); Thoughts; Vic (case example)
Self-esteem, 1, 3, 4. See also Vic (case example)
Self-forgiveness, 277–278. See also Forgiveness
Setting goals, 33–38
Shame, 1, 56, 252, 267–279. See also Marissa (case example); Moods; Vic (case example)
Situational factors. See also Thought Record
  mood identification and, 27
  overview, 39
  Thought Record, 39–46
  thoughts and, 51–54, 61–67
Social anxiety, 225–228, 234, 235–236. See also Anxiety
Strengthening new thoughts, 117–125. See also Alternative/balanced thoughts; Thoughts
Stress management, 1, 4, 24

T

Thankfulness. See Gratitude
Thought Record. See also Alternative/balanced thoughts; Automatic thoughts; Evidence for or against a thought; Moods; Situational factors
  alternative/balanced thoughts, 101–113, 116
  anger and, 259–260
  anxiety and, 231, 248
  evidence for or against a thought, 69–86
  gathering new evidence and, 95–100
  hot thoughts and, 61–68
  no change in mood and, 106–112
  overview, 39–46, 49, 112
  relapse prevention and, 287
  underlying assumptions and, 134
Thought–behavior connection, 18–20, 23. See also Behavior; Thoughts
Thought–environment connection, 21–22. See also Environment; Thoughts
Thought–mood connection, 16–18, 22. See also Moods; Thoughts
Thought–physical reactions connection, 20–21, 23. See also Physical reactions; Thoughts
Thoughts. See also Alternative/balanced thoughts; Automatic thoughts; Evidence for or against a thought; Perception of events; Strengthening new thoughts; Thought–behavior connection; Thought–mood connection; Thought–physical reactions connection; Thoughts in the five-part model
  acceptance of, 126–131
  Action Plan and, 130
  anger and, 255, 257–260
  anxiety and, 224, 229–234, 247–248, 251
  changing the way you think, 24
  depression and, 193–198
  guilt and, 267
  hot thoughts, 61–67
  overview, 2
  positive thinking disadvantages and, 23
  shame and, 267
  testing angry thoughts, 259–260
  Thought Record, 39–46
  thought–behavior connection, 18–20
  thought–environment connection, 21–22
  thought–mood connection, 16–18
  thought–physical reactions connection, 20–21
Thoughts in the five-part model, 6–11, 13–15. See also Five-part model to understand life experiences; Thoughts
Timeouts, 261. See also Anger

Trauma, 223. *See also* Marissa (case example)
Treatment interventions
　for anger, 258–267
　for anxiety, 233–249
　for depression, 198–218
　for guilt, 267–276, 277–278
Triggers, 139, 141, 219, 260

U

Underlying assumptions. *See also* Behavioral experiments; Core beliefs
　downward arrow technique and, 156–163
　identifying, 139–142, 151
　overview, 133–137, 150–152, 187

V

Vic (case example)
　Action Plan and, 121, 123–124
　anger and, 252
　automatic thoughts, 51–52
　core beliefs, 155, 163, 169–170
　depression, 188, 201
　downward arrow technique and, 157, 158
　evidence for or against a thought, 69–74
　gathering new evidence and, 95–100
　guilt or shame and, 273
　hot thoughts, 61–63
　mood identification and, 26, 28
　overview, 11–12, 295–296
　relapse management and, 286
　Thought Record first three columns, 45
　thought–environment connection, 22
　understanding Vic's problems, 13

W

Warning signs, relapse management and, 286–287
"What if . . . ?" thinking, 229–230, 251. *See also* Anxiety
Worksheets, xix–xx
　2.1. Understanding My Problems, 13–15
　3.1. Thought Connections, 22–23
　4.1. Identifying Moods, 27–29
　4.2. Identifying and Rating Moods, 29–31
　5.1. Setting Goals, 34
　5.2. Advantages and Disadvantages of Reaching and Not Reaching My Goals, 35–36
　5.3. What Will Help Me Reach My Goals? 36
　5.4 Signs of Improvement, 37–38
　6.1. Distinguishing Situations, Moods, and Thoughts, 47–48
　7.1. Connecting Thoughts and Moods, 57
　7.2. Separating Situations, Moods, and Thoughts, 58–59
　7.3. Identifying Automatic Thoughts, 59–60
　7.4 Identifying Hot Thoughts, 64–67
　8.1. Facts versus Interpretations, 72–74
　9.1. Completing Linda's Thought Record, 107–110, 108–109
　9.2. Complete Thought Record, 114–115, 298–309
　10.1. Strengthening New Thoughts, 119
　10.2. Action Plan, 125, 310–312
　11.1. Identifying Underlying Assumptions, 140–142
　11.2. Experiments to Test an Underlying Assumption, 136–137, 142–149, 313–314
　12.1. Identifying Core Beliefs, 159
　12.2. Downward Arrow Technique: Identifying Core Beliefs about Self, 160
　12.3. Downward Arrow Technique: Identifying Core Beliefs about Other People, 161
　12.4. Downward Arrow Technique: Identifying Core Beliefs about the World (or My Life), 162
　12.5. Identifying a New Core Belief, 165
　12.6. Core Belief Record: Recording Evidence That Supports a New Core Belief, 165–167, 315
　12.7. Rating Confidence in My New Core Belief, 168–170, 316
　12.8. Rating Behaviors on a Scale, 171, 317
　12.9. Behavioral Experiments to Strengthen New Core Beliefs, 318–320
　12.10 Gratitude about the World and My Life, 176, 177
　12.11. Gratitude about Others, 176, 178
　12.12. Gratitude about Myself, 176, 179
　12.13. Learning from My Gratitude Journal, 176, 180
　12.14. Expressing Gratitude, 181–183
　12.15. Acts of Kindness, 185
　13.1. *Mind Over Mood* Depression Inventory, 190–193, 321
　13.2. *Mind Over Mood* Depression Inventory Scores, 192, 322–323
　13.3. Identifying Cognitive Aspects of Depression, 197–198
　13.4. Activity Record, 201–207, 218
　13.5. Learning from My Activity Record, 208–210

13.6. Activity Schedule, 210–215, 218, 324–326
14.1. *Mind Over Mood* Anxiety Inventory, 220–223, 327
14.2. *Mind Over Mood* Anxiety Inventory Scores, 222, 328
14.3. Identifying Thoughts Associated with Anxiety, 232
14.4. Making a Fear Ladder, 238, 329
14.5. My Fear Ladder, 235–241, 329
14.6. Ratings for My Relaxation Methods, 245–246
15.1. Measuring and Tracking My Moods, 253, 331
15.2. Mood Scores Chart, 254
15.3. Understanding Anger, Guilt, and Shame, 256–257, 268
15.4. Writing a Forgiveness Letter, 264–265, 333
15.5. Ratings for My Anger Management Strategies, 266
15.6. Rating the Seriousness of My Actions, 270–271
15.7. Using a Responsibility Pie for Guilt or Shame, 272–274
15.8. Making Reparations for Hurting Someone, 275–276
15.9. Forgiving Myself, 277–278, 334
16.1. *Mind Over Mood* Skills Checklist, 282–285
16.2. My Plan to Reduce Relapse Risk, 287–289, 335
key, duplicates of, 297–332
overview of, 3–4

About the Authors

Dennis Greenberger, PhD, a clinical psychologist, is the founder and Director of the Anxiety and Depression Center in Newport Beach, California. He is a past president and Founding Fellow of the Academy of Cognitive Therapy, and has practiced cognitive-behavioral therapy for more than 30 years. His website is *www.anxietyanddepressioncenter.com*.

Christine A. Padesky, PhD, a clinical psychologist, is the cofounder of the Center for Cognitive Therapy in Huntington Beach, California, the coauthor of five books, and an internationally renowned speaker. She is a recipient of the Aaron T. Beck Award for significant and enduring contributions to the field of cognitive therapy from the Academy of Cognitive Therapy and the Distinguished Contribution to Psychology Award from the California Psychological Association. Her website is *www.mindovermood.com*.